Healing Massage:
A Simple Approach

MARSHA JELONEK WALKER
RN, PhD(c), HNC, RMT

JONATHAN D. WALKER
M Ed, RMT

THOMSON

DELMAR LEARNING

Australia Canada Mexico Singapore Spain United Kingdom United States

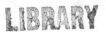
JUN 0 2 2003

THOMSON
™
DELMAR LEARNING

Healing Massage: A Simple Approach

by Marsha Jelonek Walker, PhD(c), HNC, RN
Jonathan D. Walker, MEd, RMT

Executive Director:
William Brottmiller

Executive Editor:
Cathy L. Esperti

Acquisitions Editor:
Matt Filimonov

Developmental Editor:
Maria D'Angelico

Executive Marketing Manager:
Dawn F. Gerrain

Marketing Coordinator:
Kip Summerlin

Editorial Assistant:
Patricia Osborn

Executive Production Manager:
Karen Leet

Art/Design Coordinator:
Jay Purcell

Production Coordinator:
Cathy Ciardullo

Project Editor:
Bryan Viggiani

Library of Congress
Cataloging-in-Publication Data

Walker, Marsha Jelonek.
 Healing massage : a simple approach /
Marsha Jelonek Walker, Jonathan D. Walker.
  p. cm.—(Healer series)
Includes bibliographical references and index.
 ISBN 0-7668-0692-8 (alk. paper)
 1. Touch—Therapeutic use. 2. Massage
therapy. 3. Healing. 4. Massage. I. Walker,
Jonathan D. II. Title. III. Series: Nurse as
healer series.

RZ401 .W356 2002
615.8'22—dc21

                                2002035153

NOTICE TO THE READER

INTRODUCTION TO THE HEALER SERIES

LYNN KEEGAN, PhD, RN, Series Editor
Director, Holistic Health Consultants
Port Angeles, Washington

Most healthcare professionals care for others with compassion; they begin their formal education with this ideal. Many retain this orientation after graduation, and some manage their entire careers under this guiding principle of caring. Many of us, however, tend to forget this ideal in the hectic pace of our professional and personal lives. We may become discouraged and feel a sense of burnout.

I have spoken at many conferences with thousands of caregivers. Their experience of frustration and failure is quite common. These professionals feel themselves spread as pawns across a healthcare system too large to control or understand. In part, this may be because they have forgotten their true roles as healers.

When individuals redirect their personal vision and empower themselves, an entire pattern may begin to change. And so it is now with the healthcare profession. Most of us conceptualize our roles as much more than a vocation. We are greater than our individual roles as scientists, specialists, or care deliverers. We currently search for a name to put on our new conception of the empowered caregiver. The recently introduced term *healer* aptly describes the qualities of an increasing number of clinicians, educators, administrators, and practitioners. Today most caregivers are awakening to the realization that they have the potential for healing.

It is my feeling that, when awakened and guided to develop their own healing potential, most will function as healers. Thus, the concept of caregiver as healer is born. When we realize we have the ability to evoke others' healing, as well as care for them, a shift of consciousness begins to occur. As individual awareness and changes in skill building occur, a collective understanding of this new concept emerges. This knowledge, along with a shift in attitude and new kinds of behavior, allows empowered healthcare providers to renew themselves in an expanded role. The Healer Series is born of the belief that caregivers are ready to embrace guidance that inspires them to their journeys of empowerment. Each book in the series may stand alone or be used in complementary fashion with other books. I hope and believe that information herein will strengthen you both personally and professionally, and provide you with the help and confidence to embark upon the path of a healer.

Titles in the Healer Series:

Healing Touch: A Resource for Healthcare Professionals, 2nd Edition
Healing Life's Crises: A Guide for Nurses
The Nurse's Meditative Journal
Healing Nutrition, 2nd Edition
Healing the Dying, 2nd Edition
Awareness in Healing
Creative Imagery
Profiles of Nurse Healers
Healing Addictions
Healing & the Grief Process
Healing with Complementary & Alternative Therapies
Spirituality: Living Our Connectedness
Healing Meditation
Energetic Approaches to Emotional Health
Taking Charge of the Change: A Holistic Approach to the Three Phases of Menopause

Dedication

This book is dedicated to our parents,
who taught—and still teach us—about love.

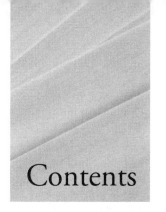

Contents

PART II   SIMPLE MASSAGE TECHNIQUES THAT WORK

PART III   MASSAGE AS A BRIDGE FOR CONNECTING

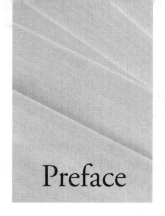

Preface

Most of us can remember a time when we had pain in our back muscles, or a headache that just wouldn't go away. Some days are so stressful that we feel emotionally exhausted by the time they are over. For times like these, few things in this world feel better, and do more for you than a slow, relaxing massage. There are also few things that are as rewarding for the person giving the massage. Using only your two hands, you see a person's face light up, and their body relax right before your eyes. Another wonderful benefit of giving a massage is that, when you massage someone else, you become relaxed right along with them.

As nurses, we play many different roles in a 24-hour day. Many of those scenarios involve people who could use a little help getting through a tough afternoon, or a tough week. Our work environment, by its very nature, puts us in contact with people who are tense and stressed. Clients are often in pain, have trouble sleeping, and may feel anxious about their future. We also care for the families of our clients. One of the greatest concerns of many of these families is wanting to *do something* to help their loved one feel better. Our colleagues at work might also welcome something to relieve tight shoulders or a stiff neck. Our lives don't end when we leave the work place. Most of us go home to our own families, who may have also had a stressful day. A friend might stop by with a nagging headache. The five-minute massage in this book is designed specifically to show you how to help people in all of these situations.

Sometimes when life gets stressful, we need something that can bring a little relaxation and peace, right away, no matter what the circumstance. A short massage can truly work wonders. A massage that takes only five minutes could be a welcomed addition, not only in the healthcare setting, but in all areas of life where we have the opportunity to give and to care. Teaching this short massage to a friend, or someone in your own family, may also help you receive that shoulder rub you need when you come home after a hard day.

INTEGRATIVE CARE

Before the 1970s, the backrub was taught in nursing schools as a standard part of evening care. Both clients and nurses benefited from that time together. As technology became an increasing part of health care, the evening backrub faded into the background. Nurses are now realizing that they, and their clients, need a balance. As a result, many nurses are exploring holistic, or integrative, health care, not only to use in the care of their clients, but for their personal lives as well. The American Holistic Nurses Association now has approximately 3,000 members, and is growing.

Integrative health care incorporates a philosophy and modalities that nurture the body, mind, emotions, and spirit of the client, his family, and the nurse. This type of health care is not only being embraced by nurses, but is being sought after and demanded by clients. In 1997, 42% of the people in the United States tried integrative modalities. Massage, relaxation techniques, and chiropractic care were the top three techniques used (Eisenberg, et al., 1998). People seem to be searching for promotion of health and well-being, as well as the healing of disease. We are witnessing a transformation in health care. Hopefully, we will see Western and integrative methods merging as equal partners, using the best of both to help people truly heal. Nurses are at the crest of this wave.

The Healer series introduces nurses to many aspects of holistic philosophy and different modalities of care that address the mind, body, and spirit. Massage is one such modality that nurses can use in almost all areas of nursing practice, as well as in their personal lives.

ORGANIZATION

This book is divided into three parts. In Part I, Massage as a Healing Tool, we begin our journey into the world of massage. Since touch is the foundation of massage, we begin with simple touch, and why it is a necessary part of our lives for healthy growth and development. Many people find massage to be a comfortable and socially appropriate way to touch and be touched. Part I goes on to explore massage, what it actually is, and how it can be used in a nurse's daily life. We then discuss ways in which massage benefits our health, as discovered both through our own direct experience and some of the current research, including studies that address massage in a variety of conditions.

Part II, Simple Massage Techniques That Work, describes the massage strokes and suggested routines. In the first chapter, we discuss some things you might do to create the most healing environment possible for your client as they receive their massage. The next chapter offers a few pointers to keep in mind as you give the massage that help the movements feel even better.

Next, you find the two technique chapters. Most people carry tension in the back, neck, shoulders, head, hands, or feet, so these are the areas we include. We describe the strokes in great detail and include as many photos and illustrations as necessary so that those who have no massage experience will find the hand movements easy to visualize, learn, and perform. In a very short time you can help relieve stress and headaches, and relax tight muscles. Perhaps most importantly, if someone is "having a bad day," you will be able to bring a smile to their face.

The first of the two technique chapters includes strokes to be applied "dry," that is, without using lotion. These techniques are very relaxing and can be performed in almost any setting, with the client fully clothed. The next chapter describes strokes that are applied with a small amount of lotion to reduce friction on the skin. Some of these strokes use a long, gliding motion for the more superficial musculature, and others allow you to reach a little deeper into the layers of muscles. Each of these chapters also includes an outline for the major steps of the routine so you can quickly refer to it while you are giving the massage. For either massage, you can do all of the strokes if you have time, or you can choose whatever areas of the body best suit your situation and the amount of time you have. We also explore how to make the best use of limited time.

Following the techniques in Part II, we elaborate briefly on this suggestion: The "practice" of massage includes much more than just "giving it" to people. Continual learning is an important part of any kind of practice, and there are no better ways to really learn massage than by receiving it and showing someone else how to give it.

If you have received much massage, you know that most are good, but some make you feel indescribably wonderful. A great massage is more than just technique. Part III, Massage As a Bridge for Connecting, explores what we believe makes some massage feel like a truly healing experience, for both the giver and the receiver. In our opinion, the key is what the giver is thinking, feeling, and intending while they are in the receiver's presence.

In the first chapter on Psychoneuroimmunology (PNI), we see how the thoughts we think and the feelings we have affect the overall health of the body, including stress levels and immune function. This is very practical information because so many nurses are experiencing the effects of increasing stress in their work setting. The second chapter discusses techniques for becoming more aware of what we are thinking, and how we can start learning to intentionally choose our thoughts and feelings, especially in stressful circumstances. It is especially important to be able to notice what we are thinking and feeling as we massage a client because our internal thinking-feeling state greatly affects the quality of the massage we give.

In the third chapter of Part III, The Energy Field, Spirituality, and Connection, we look at the energetic nature of life and how we are constantly interacting with others through this very real, dynamic field of energy. New areas of research, including distant intentionality and distant healing, suggest that we are connected to each other in ways we are just beginning to understand. Is it possible that what the nurse is thinking and feeling actually affects the client? This chapter discusses ways in which our thoughts and feelings may be able to affect the people around us, including the receiver of your massage. We briefly discuss different types of energy-based therapies, and how they can enhance the massage you give. Our discussion of energy fields and healing leads to spirituality. We explore how a connection with spirit, our own spiritual nature as well as a Higher Power, brings another dimension to massage.

Chapter 12 introduces HeartTouch, an "internal maneuver" that builds on all of the information in Part III. This easy to learn technique is designed to be practiced in many different situations whenever a heart connection might be beneficial. Chapter 13 describes how to incorporate the HeartTouch technique into the massage in Part II to give a massage *with heart* that is healing for both the giver and receiver.

In summary, we are going to use massage as a vehicle to learn how to:

1. Ease the physical tension of others, helping them feel better in body and mind

2. Intentionally choose life-affirming, healing thoughts and feelings more often

3. Connect with others, heart-to-heart

4. Further realize our connection with a benevolent Higher Power

WHY WE WROTE THIS BOOK

Over the last 25 years, we have continually experienced the healing benefits of massage, as giver and receiver. Most people today experience extreme stress, including clients and nurses in healthcare settings, and families in daily life. All of us need the relief massage can bring. As mentioned, massage is a traditional nursing intervention, but has not been focused on for many years. We thought how wonderful it would be to offer a short collection of very effective massage techniques that nurses and families could easily learn and use to help one another. Hence, this book.

From the very beginning, we want you to know that this is not intended to be a formal textbook. For us, talking about, and giving, massage is a personal interaction, so the voice of this book is intentionally casual and informal. Although we will not get to know you as we would in a face-to-face situation, perhaps we can still connect in a very real way.

We also do not intend to teach a detailed, full-body massage. There are many excellent books, and courses of instruction, if you are interested in learning a long massage. Most books on massage teach a routine designed to be given in one to one and a half hours. If you have ever practiced nursing, you know that most nurses will never have time to give a massage much longer than about five minutes. In fact, nurses really need to know some relaxing massage strokes they might do in 1–2 minutes that will help their clients. If you decide to teach a few massage techniques to the family members of a client for their use at home, they probably will not have time to give a massage that is longer than 5–10 minutes. Also, if you and a colleague decide to trade a shoulder massage at work, you might have two minutes. And when you give, or receive, a short backrub within your own family, or with a friend, a 5-minute massage may be about all you can fit into those precious moments you have together. Therefore, the massage we offer in this book includes some of our favorite strokes that are very effective in 1–10 minutes.

Another reason for a short, yet effective massage is so that it might more easily be included in the curricula of nursing schools. Nursing students could then learn how to give a massage they would realistically use in their practice, as well as providing them with another way to connect with clients in a meaningful way. If a long, full-body massage is taught, the new nurse soon finds there is never enough time for it. Massage ends up being forgotten. If massage cannot be taught within the formal curriculum, this book is written so instructors can recommend it to their students as a supplementary text so they can learn massage at home.

Even though massage therapists usually want a longer routine than this book offers, the HeartTouch technique and all of the information in Part III could enhance each massage they give and offer a greater understanding of stress and the role our thoughts and feelings play in health and well-being. Part III might be helpful for anyone who encounters others in a professional helping scenario, as well as those who appreciate massage but who just don't practice it professionally.

SPECIAL FEATURES

Since the beginning of time, people have shared stories as a way to learn new things. Since we both really enjoy stories, most of the chapters contain one or more. Many are in the original words of the storyteller to best convey their own experiences. Some of the topics we cover are difficult to completely describe in words, but easy to feel in the heart, and stories help us share feelings. For the same reason, we also include a number of photographs.

At the end of each chapter, you will find a few suggested activities that can be practiced in just a few minutes. We hope they help you begin to use the ideas in these chapters in your daily work and personal life.

In Chapter 8 you will find some specific suggestions to help you decide which massage strokes might be most effective depending on the amount of time you have to give a massage. This simple approach will essentially eliminate time as a stressor when you are helping your clients with touch.

HOW TO BEST USE THE BOOK

To get the most benefit out of this book we suggest that you start at the beginning, finding out why touch and massage are such powerful healing tools. Most of us are much more likely to take the time to incorporate a new skill into our lives when we realize how much it can help others, and ourselves.

Next, read through the two massage technique chapters, start to finish, taking time to study the photos. Most importantly, picture the hand movements of each step in your mind as you read. Next, with the book beside you, practice the strokes on a friend or family member. Encourage them to give you honest feedback about how it feels to receive it. Practice the techniques in both the "with" and "without" lotion chapters. Be sure to read Chapters 4 and 5 for special tips on creating an environment most conducive for massage and ways to enhance the massage you give. After you become comfortable with the hands-on techniques, Part III describes how to give a massage *with heart*. Decide for yourself whether these ideas are helpful to you, and if so, incorporate them as you give your massage.

Finally, give your massage to clients. Use the information in Chapter 8 to help you choose which strokes, and how many, are appropriate for your situation. When you feel familiar with the techniques, teach some of them to the families of your clients so they can use them at home. For your own benefit, teach the massage to some of your colleagues and your own family members so you can receive a massage when you need it. If you are not able to teach the massage to others, you might suggest they read the book.

Most importantly, don't worry about needing to perform any part of this massage "perfectly" before you start practicing it with someone. If you give these ideas and techniques a try, even in the beginning, you will be amazed at the appreciative responses you receive, and the amount of good you can do.

ABOUT THE AUTHORS

Massage has woven itself throughout our lives like a thread connecting the different events and stages. Both of us received backrubs as children and realized how wonderful they felt. We soon began giving them to family members, and saw that in a couple of minutes we could help somebody else feel much better.

In the Fall of 1977, as Marsha was finishing her degree in nursing, we took our first massage class. That little class, looking back on it, was a major fork in the road for us both. In a massage class, in addition to giving the massage, you also get to receive a lot of it. This allowed us to personally experience the depths of physical and mental relaxation that massage can bring. We started to see more clearly how the body, mind, and spirit are intimately connected, and that by affecting one, we affect them all. From that time forward, this point of view has been a guiding force in our work and our personal lives.

About a year after that first class, we realized we wanted to broaden our repertoire of techniques for working with the body. We studied deep tissue massage with Robert Brown at the Soma School of Massage in Oakland, California. There we became aware of the power of relaxed, focused intention as you are giving a massage. We later studied a technique similar to reflexology, called "VitaFlex," from its originator, Stanley Burroughs.

In 1978 and 1979, we studied Therapeutic Touch with Dora Kunz and Dolores Krieger. These two wonderful women taught us that almost everyone can learn how to use their hands to feel the human energy field and help bring it back into balance.

We soon began teaching massage, VitaFlex, and Therapeutic Touch to nurses and community groups in several cities around the United States as well as a few in Canada. In 1980, we became Registered Massage Therapists and began a private practice where we offered massage, Vitaflex, stress management, and energy-based therapies.

By 1992, Marsha had received her Master's Degree in Nursing, which focused on Psychoneuroimmunology (PNI). In 1994, she also helped develop a Holistic Nursing Series for the Continuing Education Department at the University of Texas School of Nursing in Austin, and taught several of the workshops in the series over the five years it was offered. She continues to enjoy her private practice and is on the faculty of the Lauterstein-Conway School of Massage in Austin. In 1997, she became a Certified Holistic Nurse and is now working on her Ph.D. in Holistic Adult Nursing.

In 1994, after practicing and teaching massage for 14 years, Jonathan received his Master's Degree in Education with a focus on Instructional Design for Learning Technologies. In addition to his continuing interest and involvement in spirituality, healing, and teaching, he has worked as a freelance writer and designer in instructional media.

So, as you can see our journey began with a simple massage. Massage continues to be an ally as we travel down this road called life, relaxing our bodies in times of stress, and reminding us of our closeness in those moments when we feel alone. When the world outside gets hectic, massage clears the mind and quiets the noise so we can better listen to the Spirit within. Through it all, that Spirit remains with us.

Our dream is to help fill healthcare facilities and homes with people touching and appreciating each other, and using a short, easy-to-learn massage to do it. We want to see massage return to nursing. When we give and receive massage, our thoughts, words, and actions all become much more caring and kind. Kindnesses have a way of spreading out, one kindness leading to another. Like pebbles in the pond, one simple massage ripples out, connecting friend to friend on this little blue planet of ours spinning around our star. Realizing how interconnected we all are brings a new meaning to life, and helps us remember that we are never alone.

We have a wonderful friend, George Goodwin, who is fond of saying, "The *main* thing, is to keep the main thing, the main thing." Being there to lend a hand when times are tough, offering kind words, a loving touch, and maybe a prayer. What else is there, really?

ACKNOWLEDGMENTS

Over the last 25 years of giving massage we have met many wonderful people. We have learned so much from each one of them, and we are deeply grateful for their presence in our lives. From our students we have learned to cherish the thirst for learning, and that sharing knowledge is really about giving away what we have come to love most. They have helped us realize that we may have something to share that others want to hear. This book exists largely because of the feedback and encouragement from our clients and students.

We thank our family and friends for their continual support, patience, and understanding throughout the writing of this book. Our photographer, Susan Gaetz, brought her expertise to help us get just the right images. And thanks to all the people who gave their time, and so kindly consented to letting us include their photos: Barbara, Diana, Doug, John, Florian, Tracy, Eli, Katie, Henry, Claire, Shannon, Lete, Venus, Winston, and Sophie. We also thank those who so gladly and openly shared their personal stories: Florian, Betty, Lou, Vicki, May, Diana, Kathy, and Marsha C. Also, we thank those whose names we did not cite in the text.

John Conway's support of our work, and especially the writing of this book, has always been greatly appreciated. The moral support of Pat, Marsha C., Debra, and Joan was invaluable. We are also grateful to all of our teachers, who taught us so much through their work, and even more by their example: Zach Elrod, Bob Brown, Stanley Burroughs, Helen Erickson, Dolores Krieger, Dora Kunz, Beth Gray, Bob Buckalew, Liu Min, and John Trimble.

We also want to acknowledge Dr. Ashley Montagu, Dr. Candace Pert, D.L. Childre, and Dr. William Glasser, who, although we have never met them personally, have influenced us, and this book, through their research and writing.

And finally, this book would probably never have come into being without the caring expertise of our editor, Jill Rembetski.

So, what is the "Main Thing," the main message of this book?

You can help people feel better with your hands—and you can touch them with your heart. As a result, you both win. And that will make this world an even better place.

We hope the massage we offer, and all of the information that accompanies it, enriches your life as much as it has our own.

Marsha and Jonathan Walker
Austin, Texas

REVIEWER ACKNOWLEDGMENTS

We would like to thank the following reviewers:

Sue C. DeLaune, MN, RNC
President, SDeLaune Consulting
Adjunct Faculty, William Cray College School
   of Nursing
New Orleans, LA

Renee Geel, MA, BA
Freelance Editor
Delmar, NY

Merla R. Hoffman, MSN, RN, CHTP/I, HNC
Nursing Educator
Colorado Springs, CO

Lynn Keegan, RN, PhD, HNC, FAAN
Editor, Healer Series & Director, Holistic
   Nursing Consultants
Port Angeles, WA

Gail S. Kozlowski, RN, MS, HNC, CHPN
Holistic Nurse Specialist
Community Hospice
Albany, NY

Melanie L. Moffat, RN, BS, LMT, CHTP
Nursing Supervisor, Memorial Behavioral
   Health Instructor,
Blue Cliff School of Therapeutic Massage
Gulfport, MS

Dana L. Moorman, LMT
Director of Education
Phoenix Therapeutic Massage College
Scottsdale, AZ

Fredonna Newton
Executive Director
Phoenix Therapeutic Massage College
Scottsdale, AZ

PART

I

Massage as a
Healing Tool

INTRODUCTION TO PART I

The purpose of Part I is to introduce you to massage and why it is a companion you will enjoy having by your side for the rest of your life. We begin by exploring touch, the underlying foundation of all massage. We then discuss what massage is, give a little history, and an introduction to the strokes you will be learning in Part II. The role of massage in nursing includes how massage is used currently in the profession, and how it benefits your practice and personal life, both as a giver and receiver. Finally, the physical, mental, and emotional benefits of massage are presented in detail, including current research findings for specific conditions and populations.

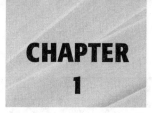

CHAPTER 1

The Healing Power of Touch

Learning to learn, learning to love and to be kind are profoundly interwoven with the sense of touch. Where touching begins, there love and humanity also begin.

—Ashley Montagu

OBJECTIVES

1. Explore what healing means to you.
2. List three ways physical touch affects the health of the body.
3. Discuss why touch can be a way to connect with others in a meaningful way.
4. Discuss the relationship between the quality of touch we receive as children and its potential effects on adult behavior.
5. Describe how touch can benefit nursing practice in neonatal, geriatric, and cardiovascular settings.

We begin our journey of life as a tiny, fragile, and most precious bundle. Held securely in loving hands, we feel ourselves loved back into that warm and comforting peace (Figure 1-1).

For the rest of our lives, simple touch has the power to calm us when we feel afraid, comfort us when we feel sad, and fill us with love. It nurtures the body and soul, and first inspires us to connect. The healing power of touch is a gift we all possess. There are only two steps: (1) extend a hand and touch another; (2) wish them well from the heart.

I began to learn this lesson when I worked as a nurse's aide in the summer between my two years of pre-nursing courses. I was on the cardiac floor at Methodist Hospital in Houston, Texas. It was 1973, and Dr. Debakey was pioneering open heart surgery. People came from all over the world to get a new

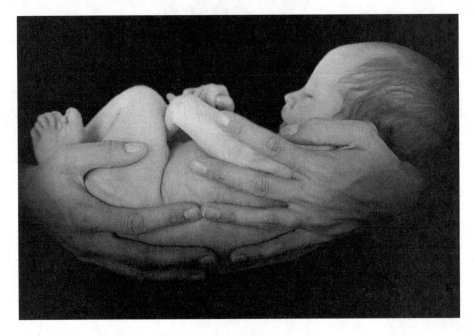

Figure 1-1

heart and a new lease on life. In my third week of working there I was assigned to Mr. C., a man from Italy. His wife would be joining him, but in the beginning, he was alone. I couldn't speak Italian, and he couldn't speak English. Whenever I passed his room, I stuck my head in, smiled, and waved. Often I would go in for a minute, sit on the bed, and hold his hand. We laughed, we cried, he squeezed my hand, and we got our messages across.

He had heart surgery, and it was successful. The day he was scheduled to go home, his wife, who spoke a little English, pulled me aside. She told me how much those few minutes had meant to her husband in the days before she arrived. We parted with tears and hugs. I knew then that nursing was the perfect profession for me.

What was it about my time with Mr. C. that was so powerful?

It had nothing to do with perfectly performed procedures or saying just the right words. Touch and time spent conveyed more than words ever could have.

—Marsha

When we think of being touched, each one of us has many memories that come to mind. We have all experienced a time in our lives when touch was not a pleasant experience. It can create fear and sadness. We realize that not all touch is positive, however, in this book, when we mention "touch," we are not referring to those kinds of situations. Later in the chapter, we will address the topic of when touch is appropriate, and when it is not. Our purpose here is to focus on the healing aspects of touch, those that help us remember, and connect with, our own wholeness.

As nurses, we continually look for ways to help our clients heal in body, mind, and spirit. When they are not feeling well, most want to be comforted. Being touched by a loving hand or a kind word helps them know they are cared about. When they feel cared for, it helps them heal. One of the great benefits of touch is that it goes two ways. When we touch another, whether with hand or heart, we are touched in return. This exchange of caring and healing is why many of us continue to be nurses.

The purpose of this chapter is to help us: (1) realize that touch often conveys what words cannot; (2) realize that touch seems to be a "universal communicator"; (3) become aware of how necessary touch is for health and happiness, throughout our lives. Since massage is touch of a specific nature, every time we give or receive a massage, we experience the many benefits of touch.

WHAT DOES IT MEAN TO HEAL?

What do we mean by healing? According to Webster's dictionary, the words "heal" and "holy" both come from the Old English word "Hal" (pronounced *hale*), which means "to make whole." Whole is defined as a complex unity, a coherent system working together as one. "Working as one" means that all aspects of the whole function in a constantly changing, harmonious way, each interdependent on the others. The aspects of our coherent system include all that we are: our physical body, our thoughts, our emotions or feelings, and our spirit, or essence. Our environment also contributes to who we are. When imbalances occur in the way these aspects work together, there is then a need for healing, or reestablishing harmony. Imbalances can occur due to what we think, feel, do, eat, the company we keep, and myriad other factors.

We often think of healing as the cure of a disease of the physical body, however healing does not always mean that the body is pain-free or disease-free. Healing can mean clarity for a mind that is worried or the calming of emotions in turmoil, even in the presence of physical illness or disability. To help bring about healing, we consider what the body needs, what the mind needs, and what the spirit needs, so they can once again work together harmoniously as a unified whole.

It is the natural state of the body to heal itself, have abundant energy, and feel no pain. Sadness, constipation, pain, anger, and low energy are wake-up calls. If we make the necessary changes when we receive these early signals, we can often prevent chronic illness. Imbalance, or disease, occurs when we deprive the body of physical, mental, emotional, or spiritual needs. If we recognize and work to remove the resistances we may have, and provide the nourishment we need, the mind and immune system are powerful allies to restore and maintain health.

What can we use to guide us as we discover what we need? Remember that "holy" also means reestablishing a sense of wholeness, or health. Holy is further defined as sacred and having a divine quality. Even if the body is broken or the mind is distraught, our true self, or essence, is always, and forever, whole and complete. Healing is about turning our attention inward and reconnecting with our inner self. When we remember our divine inner self, we remember that wholeness is our natural state. Comparing our outward daily lives to this inner state helps us realize where disharmony lies. We can then choose if, or how, we want to change to bring ourselves back into balance and health. When we remember that we are part of, or one with, a Greater Whole, this memory brings about changes in our thoughts, feelings, and physical body. In remembering this oneness, we heal.

Throughout the ages people have used loving intention to help others heal. Clergy counseled and prayed with people. Country doctors came to patients' houses and sat with them, listening to their concerns. Since the early days, a nurse's primary focus has been to nourish and care for the patient. Every time a parent holds a crying child, loving intent is helping that child to heal. Helping people heal includes being with them, listening, and caring. We do all we can to help them meet their needs, and realize their own unique goals for health. Helping people heal can also mean being with them and comforting them as they die. It is possible to die from a disease and be emotionally and spiritually healed. No one can ever be sure what healing looks like for another. By accepting clients as they are and seeing them as whole persons in body, mind, and spirit, we help them remember that unity or wholeness is who they truly are. The more they remember, the more healing is possible in their lives.

The Nurse Healer

What is a nurse healer? According to Webster's dictionary, nurses are those who support, encourage, nurture, cherish, and look after carefully to promote growth and development. Healing means to become whole. A nurse healer could be defined as one who helps others to become whole, or to heal, by cherishing, nurturing, promoting growth, and encouraging and empowering others to discover what they need to heal and to meet those needs.

Some may think that being a nurse healer means being proficient in a number of holistic, or integrative, modalities such as energy-based therapies, guided imagery, or massage. Learning techniques can be very helpful; however, modalities alone are not enough. A nurse can hold a client's hand, or have a short conversation with a client and her family, and be a nurse healer. A nurse healer is willing to really connect with the client. This does not mean just giving. It means being willing to open a two-way connection, sharing with, and receiving from, the client. This connection might be sharing experiences or just sitting in silence. A nurse healer helps the client discover what he believes he needs to feel whole by helping him realize that he has the power to make choices in his life, and that he deserves happiness. A nurse healer also empowers clients to help themselves by teaching them tools to change their lives.

Healing comes from within the client. This healing can be aided and inspired by other people, helpful information, massage, surgery, laughter, good food, and love. As nurse healers, we do not "heal" others. We support and encourage the client in his own unique healing journey.

Another important aspect of being a nurse healer is being willing to explore our inner self and discover where we need to heal. Part of this healing includes becoming aware of our thoughts and feelings and learning to intentionally choose them, even in stressful situations. These inner choices affect how clients experience us. These choices also create a presence that has an especially great impact on people who are vulnerable and not feeling well. We also ask ourselves what we need in order to live a happy, fulfilling life, and take steps to meet those needs. Having the desire to heal is doing all we can to realize our greatest potential by drawing ourselves ever closer to the heart.

A Moment for Reflection

1. Have you ever worked with a client who felt he had a healing experience even though his physical illness had not changed?
2. Recall an interaction with a client that felt healing. What about it was most memorable?
3. Focus on your inhale and exhale for a few breaths. Now consider these questions, one at a time:
   - What is one thing in my life that is not working the way I would like?
   - How would it look and feel, if instantly, the situation changed, and I had what I need?
   - What is one thing I can do to help make that happen?

What Is the Healing Power of Touch?

Imbalances in body, mind, and spirit often come from years of habitual thoughts and feelings that hold pain, hurt, and fear inside. We may feel isolated and alone, and need a helping hand to guide us back along our way. Touch helps us enter a place within ourselves where words often cannot reach. Here we feel safe and can release old, unwanted habits and fears. We often realize changes that must be made for healing to occur. Touch can help create relaxation and convey love and caring. Often when the body is relaxed and the spirit feels cared for, the mind becomes clear and the heart opens. Balance and healing occur.

The best way to experience the healing power of touch is to receive it from a caring individual. Since a book can't offer you that, we tried to decide what would be the next best way to help you have that experience. This chapter could have been all stories of people telling how touch affected them and their lives. It could have been a chapter of nothing but pictures of individuals touching in different ways, or a discussion of studies reporting the ways in which touch affects physical health and emotional development. So, we decided to include all three, hoping that by the end of the chapter you will have an experience of the healing power of touch.

IS TOUCH NECESSARY FOR HEALTH AND HAPPINESS?

Most people would agree that air, water, and food are necessary components of life. But touch? It may be nice, but is it necessary? In this section, we look at touch from several points of view, and attempt to answer this question.

Touch permeates our lives in a very subtle, yet influential way—our language. "Touch" is one of the longest entries in the Oxford English Dictionary (1989), with 14 full columns devoted to it. When we try to convey an idea, and the other person does not understand, we often say, "I tried so hard to *reach* him," as we might reach out with a hand. We use phrases like, "He *rubs* me the wrong way," or, "I've been trying to *get in touch* with you."

Touching is as old as life itself. As long as there have been two individuals, touch has brought people together for comfort and healing of the body, mind, and spirit. Something usually continues generation after generation because it contributes greatly to our survival. The oldest written document describing the use of touch for healing is said to be the *Huang Ti Nei Ching*, a book of internal medicine written about 5,000 years ago in China. In ancient Greece, touch therapies were used in healing centers, and to assist people who wanted to transition to a higher level of consciousness (Keegan, 1995). In the Bible, Matthew 8–9 speaks of Jesus bringing about instantaneous healing of leprosy, palsy, fever, blindness and mental illness by touching the person or holding his hand. Today, many different religions, as part of their ministry, have members who offer the "laying on of hands" to help the sick.

Seeing a behavior in many different species is another indication of its importance for health and well-being. Individuals throughout the plant and animal kingdoms seem to be "hard wired," or designed, for touch. Many varieties of plants thrive in the presence of caring touch (Tompkins and Bird, 1973). Insects, reptiles, birds, fish, and mammals (including humans) all seek out, and seem to enjoy, giving and receiving touch. Physical bodies are designed so that caring touch is vital for the most healthy functioning. Not only does the body need touch to be healthy, but when youngsters receive loving touch they are better able to establish and maintain cooperative, loving relationships as adults. Some species groom each other for hours, others lay on top of each other in piles or engage in very physical play.

Touch serves as a universal communicator, so that no matter what language we speak, or what species we are, we can communicate with each other. It is a heartwarming experience to see a cat and dog sleeping curled up together, or a parrot tenderly rubbing the cheek of its favorite human.

Many species have at least one especially sensitive part of their body with which they explore their world and communicate with others (see Figure 1-2). If a honey bee lands on your hand and you hold very still, you will feel its tiny tongue delicately exploring the pores of your skin. People have extremely sensitive fingers and hands at the ends of long arms. Plants send out roots and runners.

Types of touch communicate similar feelings in many species. Hard, abrupt touching usually creates feelings of caution, anger, or fear. Slow stroking conveys safety, peacefulness, and love. Although touch communicates many different feelings, it is widely used in times when comfort and caring are needed (Figure 1-3).

So, to answer the question, "Is touch necessary?", it may be. It permeates our language and our lives, has been around forever, and is used by individuals to communicate and connect, within and between many different species. Let's take a closer look at specifically how touch affects the health of animals and people.

Animal Studies Related to Touch

Animals are our teachers. From them we learn forgiveness, trust, patience, unconditional love, and unbridled play. They honor us with their presence and their touching. By noticing how animals touch, we realize how much all of us have in common. By realizing how touch affects the health and well-being of animals, we learn more about the importance of touch for our own well-being. As we mentioned previously, most animals, even hedgehogs and porcupines, seek out touch, and need it to survive and thrive.

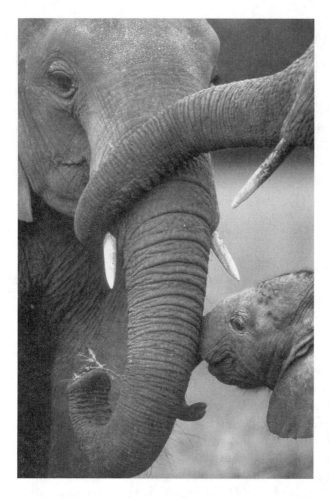

Figure 1-2 Elephants use their trunks to hold each other and share feelings. (Copyright Tom and Pat Leeson Nature Wildlife Photography. Used with permission.)

With animals, just as with humans, receiving touch as infants affects the development of normal healthy behaviors as adults (Figure 1-4).

In Harlow's classic study of monkeys, an amazing finding was that the infants chose softness (touch) over food! The infants who were deprived of soft contact began to show signs of trauma and depression with high levels of cortisol and other stress hormones. The researchers brought in an older monkey who constantly hugged and cuddled the babies. The hugging stopped the secretion of stress hormones, and the stress symptoms were reversed.

Schanberg (1994) found that it is not just generic touch, but touch that conveys nurturing to the individual, that makes the difference. There is even a gene that responds to touch that contributes to the making of protein, which contributes to

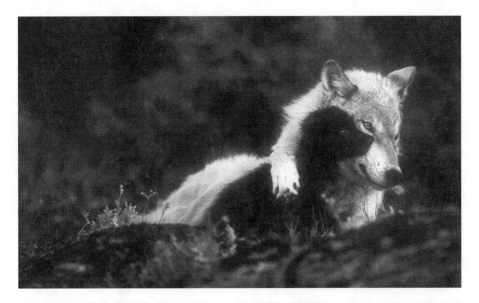

Figure 1-3 Mothers of many species put an arm around their children to comfort them in times of fear. (Copyright Carl R. Sams II/Peter Arnold, Inc. Used with permission.)

growth! The symptoms of decreased growth and behavioral development produced in baby rats (Figure 1-4) who had been removed from their mothers were very similar to characteristics seen in children with failure-to-thrive syndrome.

Schanberg's research with rats suggests that we are genetically designed so that touch affects all aspects of the healthy functioning of the body since protein is necessary for all growth and healing. His findings may offer an explanation for the results of a study conducted by Dieter, Field, and Hernandez-Reif discussed in Field (1998). They found that only one week of stroking with pressure created a 46% weight gain in premature human infants. Similarly, Meaney's study with rats, mentioned in Figure 1-4, may offer some insight into the findings of Modi and Glover (Field, 1998). Meaney's research indicated that decreased cortisol levels may affect brain development. Modi and Glover found that pre-term human babies who were stroked with pressure had lower levels of cortisol (stress hormone) and higher development in the hippocampus of the brain, which affects memory.

In summary, many branches of science believe animals to be very similar to people, both physically and behaviorally. Several of the above studies suggest that touching decreases the effects of the stress response. Today at least 90% of all ailments of the body and mind are considered to be stress-related. If receiving loving touch can help rats survive surgery better than those who were not touched, it seems that loving touch might similarly benefit people who are ill or recovering

Researcher	Subject/intervention	Results
Harlow, 1958	Infant monkeys removed from mothers	Infants chose wire mothers covered with terry cloth and no bottle over wire mothers with a bottle of milk and no terry cloth. Females did not develop normal sexual behavior and were indifferent or abusive to their babies when they became mothers.
Hammett, 1922	Two groups of rats, Group 1 received intentional petting, Group 2 did not. Then both had thyroid gland removed.	Group 1—87% survived surgery, were relaxed, had high tolerance to stress. Group 2—21% survived surgery, highly irritable, high degree of neuromuscular tension.
Meaney, Aitken, Bhatnagar, Bodnoff, Mitchell, Sarrieau, 1990	Newborn animals: Group 1—licked and touched by mother or petted by people Group 2—no touching	Group 1 more relaxed, better response to stress, better immune function, better memory as they aged, than Group 2
Reite, 1990	Pairs of infant and mother monkeys, and peers raised together, were separated for two weeks	Immune function of both members of the pairs decreased
Suomi, 1995	Infant monkeys	More touch received during first 6 months of life, the better immune functioning
Nerem, Levesque, Cornhill, 1980	Two groups of rabbits fed high-fat, high-cholesterol diet. Group 1 held and stroked affectionately, Group 2 was not	Group 1 had half the incidence of heart disease of Group 2.
Diamond, 1990	Two groups of rats, Group 1 held and talked to, Group 2 was not	Group 1 lived longer, were smarter, and had larger cortexes in the brain (problem solving, abstract thought) than Group 2
Schanberg, 1994	Two groups of baby rats, Group 1 received licking from mothers, Group 2 removed from mothers	Group 2—Decreased secretion of ODB (growth hormone), regulation of stress response, growth of most body tissue and organs, production of protein, compared to Group 1

Figure 1-4 Summary of Research Studies.

from surgery. Heart disease is one of our greatest health concerns. If caring touch can have a positive effect on heart disease in rabbits, perhaps it can affect people in a similar way. Monkeys are our closest genetic relatives. If touch enhances immune system functioning in monkeys, it is very likely to affect people in a similar way. Perhaps loving touch is a key ingredient in the prevention and healing of many unhealthy conditions in people, as well as in animals.

Touch and the Health of the Human Body

How often we receive touch affects the functioning of many areas of the body, including the movement of the intestines, muscle tone, and the metabolism and biochemistry of the entire body (McCormack, 1990). We often overlook our need for touch in our rush through the days, weeks, and years. In days past, when there were three generations in one house, families living in close proximity, and neighbors who knew each other well, there was a greater likelihood that children and adults got enough touch. Living in our modern world it is easy to live a lifestyle that includes "touch deprivation" without our even realizing it. When we are deprived of sleep, we fall asleep even if we are driving a car. We also have very clear signals when we need more food. Yet most of us have not been taught to recognize the physical and emotional signals telling us that we do not have enough touch in our lives. As infants, we cry when we need touch. As adults, our cries for touch take many different forms. When we do not get enough touch, our behaviors often include anger, resentment, subtle manipulation, or depression. The absence of touch may contribute to tension in the body, stress in the mind, and loneliness in the heart. We sometimes attempt to satisfy our need for loving touch with excessive food, sex, drugs, alcohol, exercise, or work.

If we recognize that sometimes these feelings and behaviors are signals that we need touch, we can take steps to give and receive more of it. We often don't realize how much we have missed it until we get it. Some people hug a friend, snuggle with pets, give massage, go dancing, or nurture plants. We touch heart to heart by sharing feelings, whether we touch physically or not, with cards, phone calls, and meaningful conversations. Some people play music together as it brings about the sharing of feelings of the heart.

Ashley Montagu, an anthropologist, first began researching the importance of touch on human health in 1944. In 1953, when his first paper was published, little research existed that looked at how the touch that an infant receives, or the lack thereof, affects growth and development from birth to old age. There is no brighter star than Dr. Montagu when it comes to showing how we need touch to survive and thrive. He devoted his entire career to this topic, writing more than 60 books and teaching in a variety of universities.

In books and articles published as recently as 1999, Dr. Montagu continues to be referred to by almost everyone writing about touch, and his seminal work remains perhaps the most comprehensive resource available today on the subject. His work regarding the effects of touch on the human body and inner self is so fascinating, that we have included several of his findings illustrating the need for touch as well as the value of massage. If you are interested in reading further about this topic, his book, *Touching: The Human Significance of the Skin*, is a must.

Throughout all stages of life, the health of the body improves with touch. When nurses graduate from nursing school, we are qualified to assist the healing of people in all stages of life. We choose the developmental stage, from labor and delivery to hospice, that is of special interest to us. The following discusses how touch affects these different stages.

INFANTS NEED TOUCH TO THRIVE

Anyone who has worked in prenatal care, in labor and delivery, or with newborns has seen the dramatic effects of caring touch. The earlier a function develops in the embryo, the more vital it is to the growth and development of the entire being. Touch is the first function to develop in the human embryo (Gottfried, 1990). When the embryo is less than an inch long, with no eyes or ears, stroking the lip or nose will cause it to move away from the stimulation. At nine weeks, when the palm is touched, the fingers move to grasp (Montagu, 1986). In newborns of many species, the sense of touch is the first to develop.

Humans are born with a need for touch. In the infant, lack of touch can cause physical death. In the United States during the 1800s, more than 50% of the infants less than one year old died from a disease called marasmus, or infantile atrophy. Marasmus was even seen in infants in affluent homes and in hospitals considered to be among the best. As late as 1920, the death rate for infants under a year old in various orphanages in the United States was almost 100% (Montagu, 1986).

During this time Luther Holt, a professor of pediatrics at Columbia University, was a leading child rearing expert. His book, *The Care and Feeding of Children,* was published in 1894; by 1935, it was in its 15th edition. Holt recommended not picking the baby up when he cried, feeding him by the clock, and not "spoiling" him by holding him too much. Holt's work had a great influence in orphanages, as well as in the homes of higher-income parents.

Before the beginning of World War I, Dr. Fritz Talbot visited several children's clinics in Germany. In one such hospital he noticed a woman carrying children around on her hip. The director told Dr. Talbot that when the doctors could do no more for infants, Anna could usually love them back to health. Dr. Talbot brought Anna's tender, loving care for infants back to the United States. "Mothering" (picking infants up frequently and carrying them around) was prescribed several times a day in pediatric wards. Infant mortality dropped to 10% in many institutions. By 1938, the lack of holding and cuddling babies was believed to have been a major contributing factor to infantile atrophy.

People who were born around 1925 are in their 70s now. If their parents followed the advice of the child rearing "experts" of the day, they may not have received much touching. By now, millions of children and grandchildren have been influenced by this advice regarding the holding and touching of infants and small children. We have a friend whose child was born in 1980. She was still being advised not to hold her newborn when he cried because it would spoil him. Could these early practices regarding lack of touch with infants be causing the increased incidence of some of the physical diseases and emotional problems we see today in adults?

THE SKIN

The skin is our largest sensory organ, and the way in which we perceive touch. It is no coincidence that our bodies have no shell, fur, or scales. Instead, every inch of us is covered with this soft, sensitive receptor capable of perceiving even the most subtle touch. We are designed with extremely sensitive hands so that we are able to give touch as well. The information we gather through our skin greatly affects growth, learning, and the functioning of the entire body.

When we receive inadequate touching as an infant, the skin's ability to perceive touch as an adult is not as fully developed. This may partially explain why some people do not really enjoy massage, and why a breeze on the face, the softness of a puppy, or a caring touch often goes unappreciated or unnoticed.

The skin and nervous system both emerge out of the same layer of cells in the embryo. The central nervous system turns inward, while the skin remains on the outside. Throughout a person's life, the skin remains in intimate contact with the central nervous system, which includes the brain, giving it constant input about the outside world. A piece of skin the size of a quarter contains 3 feet of blood vessels, 12 feet of nerves, 25 nerve endings, 100 sweat glands, and about 3 million cells (Grossbart, 1993). Just as the skin sends information to the brain, the brain affects the skin. What we are feeling causes the skin to flush with embarrassment or turn white with fear. Our thoughts and feelings greatly influence the health of the skin; acne, psoriasis, herpes, and rashes often result from emotional upsets.

THE BRAIN

The area of the brain devoted to touch is extremely large. This may explain why touch has such myriad effects on the development of both the body and behavior, from birth to death.

Diana Moore has been practicing massage since she was 21, and has always worked with infants. Several years ago she heard of The Northwest Medical Teams International (NWMTI), which provides medical relief to people in needy countries. She heard of the orphanages in Romania where approximately 100,000 infants lived. They were rarely held and were left to grow up alone. Moore established the International Loving Touch Foundation, and teamed up with NWMTI to provide infant massage in orphanages in Romania. Nurses and massage therapists were among those who went. The only physical contact the babies got was when their diapers were changed three times a day. Moore educated the workers in infant massage, reflexology, and movement therapy. When asked how the babies responded, Moore said, "Their eyes sparkle, even if it's just for a moment. You know you've touched them in some way, and that you're providing love that they might not otherwise get." Many of the babies were normal at birth, but due to lack of contact and stimulation, were labeled mentally retarded as they began to grow (Jensen, 1998).

When we do not receive enough touch as babies, the brain does not develop normally, nor do the nerve connections between our brain and skin. The information gathered by the skin from all over the body is not as available to help the brain perform all of its functions. Consider the implications. An early childhood that has decreased amounts of touching affects the brain's ability to receive, process, and interpret information that comes to it from the senses. Information coming from the sense of touch is especially affected because the nerve connections between the brain and skin do not develop in an optimal way. We use this information from the senses to construct and understand what we experience each day as our reality. With decreased functioning of the brain and nerves from the skin, our ability to create solutions to problems, intentionally choose new points of view, and even what the brain allows us to notice in our environment, may be diminished.

On the other hand, an environment that includes a generous amount of touching during infancy helps create a brain more equipped to perceive a wide variety of input from the world, making our life experiences that much more rich and enjoyable. These people may be able to adapt more easily and find creative, unique solutions to dilemmas. So, the amount and quality of the touch in our lives may affect which stimuli our brain allows us to perceive from all of the available information in the world around us. Those whose lives are filled with touch may, literally, see and hear a different world than those who are touch-deprived. Luckily, the brain continues to develop until we are about 25, and continues to be flexible throughout our lives. By increasing the quantity and quality of touch we experience as adults, childhood touch inadequacies may be able to be overcome. We have the opportunity to change the way we experience our world.

The cortex and the brainstem are two areas of the brain that are greatly affected by the touch we give and receive. The functions of the cortex include personality, creativity, perception of sight and sound, language, and abstract thought. The area of the cortex devoted to the hand is 20% of the area devoted to the entire body. This suggests the importance of the hand in the gathering and processing of information that affects all of the activities of the cortex. Touch influences what we pay attention to, and the emotions we attach to incoming information from the five senses. Have you noticed that if you are talking to someone, and another person touches you, your attention is immediately drawn to the touch?

The brainstem plays a significant role in the placebo effect, which is the ability of the body to make changes in our health according to what we believe. The brainstem is also involved in perception of pain. Have you noticed how a mother's touch can magically make a child's pain disappear?

THE IMMUNE SYSTEM

No matter what area of nursing you work in, the health of the client's immune system is always a major concern. Through chemical messengers, the skin is also in constant communication with the thymus gland, one of the immune system's major control centers (Grossbart, 1993). In this way, what we perceive with our skin may directly affect immune function. There are many accounts suggesting that individuals who have greater amounts of touching have a decreased response to stress (Field, 1995; Montagu, 1986; Barnard and Brazelton, 1990; Field, 1998). From the study of psychoneuroimmunology (Chapter 9), we know that our bodies secrete large amounts of cortisol during periods of prolonged stress. Sustained cortisol secretion decreases many aspects of immune system functioning. As we have seen, touch decreases cortisol levels. It is reasonable to conclude that touch enhances immune system functioning because it helps us to handle stress more effectively.

THE HEART

No matter what client population you focus on, a simple tool that can stabilize heart function is very valuable. In "kangaroo care," a caregiver, usually the parent, holds an infant next to his or her bare skin, usually chest to chest. This approach is extremely effective with premature infants. Kangaroo care stabilizes the heart rate, respiration, and temperature of infants who are having problems so they can safely go home much sooner than is customary for premature infants. In one particular situation, a baby born prematurely at 32 weeks and given kangaroo care was discharged from the hospital 36 hours after birth (Anderson, 1995). In addition to kangaroo care being very cost effective, these babies have beautiful, relaxed expressions on their faces.

Researchers studied men and women in a hospital intensive care unit who had a significant number of irregular heartbeats. Sustained irregular heartbeats can be harmful to the functioning of the heart. When a client was touched by a nurse or doctor to take the pulse, the irregular beats subsided and sometimes disappeared. Even brief, simple touch benefited heart function (Lynch, 1998).

A study at the Institute of Heartmath suggests that when we hold and stroke animals, especially if there is a mutually caring relationship, heart rate variability improves in both the person and the animal. Improved heart rate variability can help normalize blood pressure and decrease the chances of sudden death from heart attack (Childre, 1996). It seems likely that if we hold and stroke people we care about, we would both benefit in similar ways.

RELAXATION OF TENSION

Tight muscles begin to relax when the hands are simply rested on an area of tension. Shoulders that are tense often drop down an inch or more. Warm palms, placed gently on almost any abdomen, help the intestines relax. For someone who is having trouble breathing, hands placed comfortably on the chest area help that person relax so that the breath comes more easily and deeply. Touch also encourages the release of emotional tension. When the body relaxes, it often releases feelings that we may have held onto for a long time.

Reflection

1. If you take a client's blood pressure and it is high, have you ever touched her arm or shoulder and talked to her a few minutes, and then taken the blood pressure again? If not, give it a try.
2. Why does an infant often stop crying, and go to sleep, when you pick him up and hold him?

Touch and the Development of the Inner Self

The inner self is a dynamic interaction of thoughts, feelings, and essence or spirit. It is who we are on the inside, and it determines to a large extent what our behaviors are as we interact with the world around us. As nurses, we find ourselves not only ministering to the bodies of our clients, but to their inner selves as well. Mental health nurses focus primarily on this inner self. When clients talk to us about their joys and fears of living and dying, we connect with who they are on the inside.

Touch seems to be a necessary ingredient for the healthy development of the inner self, especially with children. When the need for touch is frustrated or unsatisfied, abnormal behavior is much more likely to occur. Infants grow and develop socially through the exchange of touch with others. Whether we work directly with infants and children or in the role of teaching parents, understanding the relationship between touch and self-esteem makes a significant difference in the life of a child.

INFANTS AND YOUNG CHILDREN

The first communicative relationship an infant forms is with its mother, through skin contact. Infants and young children can tell what the person holding them feels about them by the way that person holds them (Figure 1-5).

Subtle, often unconscious, external body movements such as holding them close and secure, convey these inner feelings. Babies and young children also receive cues as to whether the outside world should be trusted or feared directly from contact with the caretaker's body through their muscle-joint behavior. If the caretaker's musculature is soft, relaxed, and slow-moving, infants learn that this is how to interact with the world. On the other hand, when the caretaker's body movements are rigid and jerky, and the muscles are chronically tense, they learn quite a different approach to interacting with the very same world (Montagu, 1986).

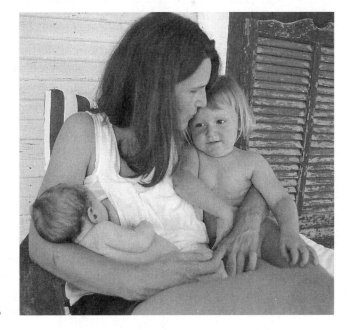

Figure 1-5

We first learn to speak by being spoken to and imitating what we have heard. As adults, we find ourselves using many of the same words, rhythms, and tones of voice that we learned as children. In much the same way, we learn to touch from how we are touched as infants, and will give touch in very similar ways as adults. Being held, hugged, and cuddled as babies determines to a large extent how comfortable we are with these behaviors as adults. Touch in childhood is the foundation for intimacy in later life, whether it is sexual intimacy or being emotionally close with friends and family.

While studying cultures worldwide, Montagu found that infants who received loving touch grew into loving, peaceful adults, as seen in the Kaingang of Brazil, the Tasaday of the Philippines, the Ganda and !Kung Bushmen in Africa, the Arapesh of New Guinea, and the indigenous people of Bali, who all had similar child rearing practices. Infants were in constant physical contact with their parents, and young children received continual stroking from adults. These children grew up to be adults who were extremely sensitive, gentle, and loving. Adults sat together, legs flung over each other, caressing each other. Loyalty to each other had its roots in the close tactile contact. Competition and aggression were rare. Violent conflict only arose between men who had never shared this close touching.

Generous touch as an infant was also found to affect the way an adult viewed many areas of life. The Netsilik in the Canadian Arctic and the Aivilik in the northwest boundary of Hudson Bay carried their babies on their backs under their parkas, directly touching their skin. The infant's needs were met before frustration developed. Adults viewed events as dynamic, changing processes, rather than as separate, rigid events. They were able to deal with very stressful situations with thoughtful composure, and were able to perceive situations from many angles, enabling them to find unique solutions to problems. Children also grew up being extremely altruistic, having an unselfish regard for the welfare of others.

When our needs are always met as infants, we learn to trust that we are secure and that the world is a safe place (Erickson, Tomlin, and Swain, 1988). We have less need to force ourselves, events, or other people around us into safe and predictable patterns.

In cultures where there was little caring touch, the picture was very different. In the 1930s, the anthropologist, Margaret Mead, found that in the Mundugumor of New Guinea, before a child was born, there was much discussion about whether the baby would be allowed to live. From birth, infants were carried in a basket that they could not see out of, with no contact with the mother's body. In the home, they were hung up in the basket and, if they cried, an adult scratched on the outside of the basket. If infants continued crying, they were nursed, but there was no fondling. As soon as they finished nursing, they were returned to the basket. There was no affection or reassurance. These children became adults who tended to be aggressive and hostile, and seemed to live in a state of constant discontent (Mead, 1935). Some of the characteristics of these child rearing practices sound alarmingly like aspects of Western culture today.

One study of 49 cultures explored the relationship between the amount of touching in the culture and the amount of aggressive behavior. In 48 of the cultures there was a highly significant relationship between the two: the greater the level of touching, the lower the level of adult aggression (Prescott and Wallace, 1976).

In the world today, violence is one of our greatest concerns. This includes violence between countries, between couples, on television, and in computer/video games. We are especially concerned about the increasing violence we see in our children. Even though every culture is different, we are all human. Touch seems to have the power to create loving children and caring, non-violent communities. We all have different challenges that come our way in life, and we must constantly choose our priorities. If caring touch can help children grow into loving, confident adults, what is a greater priority? The quality and quantity of touch we give and receive in our lives is often a habit rather than a conscious choice. We get into the habit of doing other things. Touch costs nothing. If people of all ages and ethnic backgrounds can learn to incorporate computers into so many aspects of daily life, maybe we can also learn to incorporate a greater amount of touching with our children and with each other. From observing other cultures, the effects on both the individual and society seem to be so beneficial when we do, and harmful when we don't.

TOUCH AND SELF-ESTEEM

Touch helps infants to develop an awareness of their body. Body awareness is the source of self-esteem. Body awareness begins when the skin is touched at birth, or before, and continues throughout childhood. Awareness of the body then becomes the basis of the connection between self and others. Almost every child gets showered with approval when they first reach up to touch a parent's face. Many hugs accompany the taking of their first steps. When body awareness leads to good feelings about ourselves, we develop high self-esteem (Jones, 1994; Montagu, 1986; Weiss, 1990). As we grow, body connectedness continues to include the giving and receiving of touch. When we receive caring touch from others, and when our touch is received by others, we feel deserving, accepted, and good enough. In one study investigating the relationship between self-esteem and touch in 80 male and female students, the higher a person's self-esteem, the more intimately they communicated through touch (Silverman, Pressman, and Bartel, 1973).

When we receive caring touch as children, we develop a sense of inner security, which also leads to high self-esteem. Inner security leads to feeling that the world is a safe place. When a person has not been securely and lovingly held in infancy, a fear of not being fully in control of the body can develop. This fear can be immobilizing, causing a person to retreat physically or emotionally from a situation (Montagu, 1986). This lack of feeling in control of the body can manifest in adulthood as a need to be in control of every aspect of life in order to feel safe. Sometimes words cannot calm our fears. The only thing that brings a feeling of safety and comfort is caring touch. Each day nurses encounter many circumstances in the healthcare setting when a client feels afraid. In these situations, a simple touch from the nurse often lets the client know he is not alone, and renews his courage to face what lies ahead.

OVERCOMING THE EFFECTS OF ABUSIVE TOUCHING SITUATIONS

Touch in childhood seems to influence to a great degree the health of the mind and body. What if we did not receive the kind or amount of touch as children that we would have liked? Research suggests that introducing more touching into our daily lives as adults can change patterns learned from childhood experiences. Touch deprivation is one kind of abuse. In one study, adult monkeys raised in isolation from birth, with no touching, were completely withdrawn and interested only in touching themselves. They were placed in cages with 3-month-old monkeys who touched constantly by hugging and clinging. The older monkeys who had been isolated began to return the touch and also began showing relatively normal social and emotional development. They were finally able to become loving mothers (Suomi, 1995). Perhaps for humans, as well as for monkeys, giving and receiving touch in ways that are comfortable can begin to change what we give to, and expect from, our world.

Touch involving violence or inappropriate sexual contact is another form of abuse. This one paragraph does not pretend to simplify the monumental task that is involved in recovering from abusive and traumatizing experiences. It only intends to suggest that recovery may be possible, and that comforting touch may be an aid. Ways for nurses to address the subject of touch with clients for whom it may be uncomfortable are offered in a later section.

TOUCH AND THE WISDOM YEARS

Aging is growing in wisdom. In many cultures, as people age, they are increasingly respected and valued as the keepers of knowledge, as the Elders. As the physical body declines, the growth of wisdom, of life experience, and of the ability to tell great stories abounds. These Elders, and their stories, teach and enliven us all.

As we age, the senses of seeing, hearing, tasting, and smelling often become dull. The sense of touch, however, usually remains very sensitive as long as we live. As it becomes more difficult to move about as we once did, the opportunities to touch and be touched by others decrease. Elders frequently feel trapped, isolated, and vulnerable. Many find that pets give the unconditional love that is so needed. Their eager affection can be a welcome source of contact and comfort.

There have been many studies investigating how important touch is for us all as we age. Most of these studies look at people in nursing homes and find that touch increases feelings of being cared for and valued. Residents are also less aggressive and confused (Hollinger and Buschmann, 1993; Fanslow, 1990). For those of us who have Elders in our lives as clients, friends, or family members, remembering to share a few minutes of touch can bring many needed and rewarding moments of connection, for both parties. Although it may be frail, much is said by a hand that holds so firmly, not wanting to let go. And when people don't get to move around much, the body especially loves receiving a massage.

Nana and Mandy

My grandmother was born in 1892, and touch had never been much a part of her life, especially with animals. As Nana's vision and hearing decreased, she would reach out when we came close and tightly hold our hand, as we sat with her. When Nana was 95, her hearing and eyesight were almost gone. She lived with my mother, who always had a dog around. Mandy was a 10-pound lap dog whom Nana never touched, as far as we knew. One day Nana didn't know my mother had come home from work. Mandy was sitting in Nana's lap, and they seemed to be having a lively conversation as Nana's hands never left Mandy's little head.

—Marsha

One study discovered that giving touch can be even more beneficial than receiving it. A group of Elders took a series of tests measuring depression, self-esteem, and immune function (cortisol). For one month the Elders received massage from massage therapists. The Elders were then trained to give massage to infants, and for the next month they gave massage to a group of infants. At the end of each month, they were retested. All scores improved after giving and receiving the massage, but the scores were even greater after the month of giving the massage than they were after the month of receiving it (Field, Hernandez-Reif, Quintino, et al., 1997).

We have seen that touch affects our physical, mental, and emotional development and well-being. Small children touch everything around them as they grow. When they play, they crawl all over each other, as well as their pets, toys, and parents. Many cultures, however, discourage adults from touching their friends, parents, children, and other adults. Here may be where the lack of touching begins.

As we enter our 30s, with busy work schedules, the demands of raising children, or possibly living alone, our opportunities for touch often decline. In our 40s and 50s, as children grow up and move away, parents die, and intimate relationships often change, somehow touching slips into the background, almost unnoticed. This gradual loss of touching may contribute to feelings of stress, loneliness, and dissatisfaction with life. As we move into our 70s and 80s, as friends and spouses die, we may go for weeks without being touched by, or touching, another living being. Some clients have told us that a massage is the only sustained, intentional touching they receive.

Could it be that as we decrease our touching, we initiate the aging process? What if, with less touching, the mind and body begin to decline? Perhaps receiving touch throughout our lives is the key to maintaining health and vitality of the body and mind.

IDEAS FOR PRACTICE

1. If you work in a neonatal intensive care unit, and the babies are too fragile to hold, take one or two minutes each hour to touch the foot or hand of each infant you care for. Suggest that the parents do the same when they are there.

2. If you have children as clients who are anxious or afraid, ask them if they would like a back rub, without lotion, with clothes on. Make slow circles with your palm on their back, starting from the midback and moving up toward the head, and down toward the lower back, for about two minutes.

3. If you have Elders as clients, take five minutes per client. Sit next to them and ask them about their day, their family, or how they are feeling. If you feel comfortable, touch their arm or hold their hand as they talk. You might ask them if they would like a backrub as described in #2.

Consider This One Question

If everyone in the United States were somehow able to receive a one-hour massage each month for the next year, what do you think might happen to the following statistics?

traffic accidents	suicides
health insurance claims	sick time from work
divorce	depression
violence	back pain

In light of the animal and human studies we have reviewed, it is likely that we would live in a very different world.

To Touch or Not to Touch

Healthcare providers must be mindful about touch. Some people have had painful childhood experiences involving touch, or a situation as an adult where touch did not convey caring. Some cultures and some age groups are not comfortable with touch. While touch may be welcomed immediately by some clients, it may be politely declined by others. If a client appears to be uncomfortable with the idea of physical touch, standing or sitting near them may be the best place to begin (McCorkle, 1974). As you ask them how they are, reach out to them with a loving presence. A loving presence involves giving them your full attention, accepting them as they are, making eye contact, and sending caring thoughts their way. When you feel a trusting connection has been made, a gradual offering of the most non-threatening touch, to areas such as the arm or shoulder, might open up a whole new world for them. You might offer a one-minute foot or hand massage. Touch must happen at a pace that is comfortable for the receiver.

In any situation where you wonder whether to touch, ask your heart and listen to your intuition. Caring touch, when it respects the needs of the person receiving it, engenders trust, regardless of age or habits learned in the past.

TOUCH CREATES A HEART-TO-HEART CONNECTION

We have seen how vital touch is to the health of the physical body. Being touched also contributes to the healthy development of our inner selves, enabling us to choose cooperative behaviors within our families and communities. Could touch be inherently necessary to our physical and emotional well-being because it is a pathway that leads to heart connection? This connection helps us go beyond who we are as a single individual and realize our greater potential as a spiritual being in community with a greater whole.

It is no coincidence that in the design of many animals, two appendages, or arms, extend from the area of the heart. We have a friend whose cat put her arm over our friend's neck at night when our friend was upset or especially tired. Our dog, Sophie, very gently touched our faces or arms with her hand when she especially wanted to connect with us, or was wondering if we were OK. Hens use their wings to enfold their chicks for protection. Pandas cradle their tiny infants in their massive arms. People have arms long enough to hold each other, heart to heart (Figure 1-6).

At the end of our arms we have hands, which are designed for extremely sensitive exploration and communication. The hands are not only designed to help us identify objects in our world, they are also the physical extensions of our hearts. As we learn to "listen" with our hands, they send information to our hearts

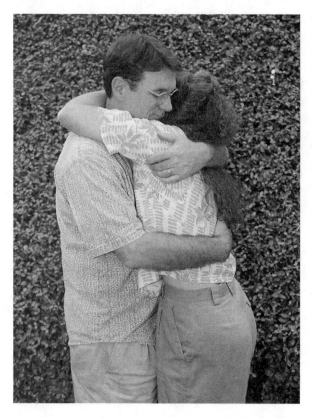

Figure 1-6

so we can better understand our world. Our hands are also transmitters, or senders, of information from our hearts to the world. Another person can feel what is in our hearts by the way our hands touch them. A handshake communicates much more than a simple hello or good-bye. Intention and character are revealed whenever two hands meet.

Nurses frequently work with clients who speak a different language than they do, or cannot speak or hear at all. We continually experience how much can be communicated through the hands (Figure 1-7).

The hand-heart connection moves in a circle. When we have heartfelt feelings for another, our hands touch them in a caring way. Their heart receives this message, and they feel loved. They then return those feelings through a look in the eyes, a kind word, or a touch of the hand. As we mentioned earlier, we touch each other in purely non-physical ways as well. We use our thoughts, feelings, and words to connect with others heart to heart, sharing the healing energy of love. This is discussed further in Part III.

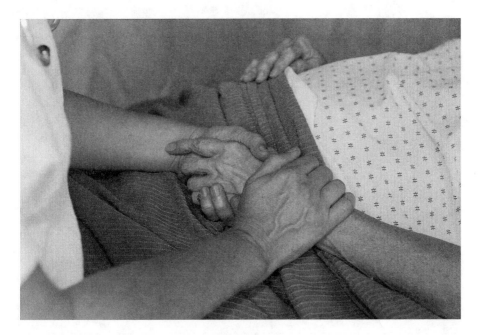

Figure 1-7

The Touch of Spirit

There is one more kind of touch that plays a vital role in the healing process. For ages, cultures worldwide have told sacred stories describing intimate relationships between a Benevolent Higher Power and rocks, plants, animals, and people. Many of these stories revolve around how we touch the Divine and the Divine touches us, for healing and guidance. Today books, television programs, and movies describe and portray conversations with God, being touched by angels, and being connected by the Force.

Many of us feel that we are more than a body, that we are a consciousness or essence, in addition to physical matter. It is with this energetic nature that we touch, heart to heart and spirit to spirit, with others, and with the Universal Life Force. Many people are curious, wanting to know more about this connection, this spiritual touching. If you have worked around people who are dying, or whose life is in great jeopardy, you have probably seen, heard, or felt unusual events that suggest the presence of Spirit. As we talk with people about this subject, more and more say they have felt the touch of God or the Holy Spirit. We believe Spirit dwells in the heart, or perhaps that we dwell in the heart of the Divine. Touch moves us to the heart. It is here that we feel Love and the Presence

Hand-Heart Connection

One summer, I experienced a hand-heart connection. In Austin, Texas, the circus comes to town in the summer. It is extremely hot, so the trains carrying all of the animals pull into town about sunrise. A small group of us are there, waiting for the train. The caretakers open the doors of the cars to give the animals fresh air while they wait for transport trucks to the circus area. I walk over to the elephant car just to be near them. I love elephants. They coo and make beautiful sounds as they talk with each other. I am standing a foot or so from the car, and suddenly, a trunk comes winding out of the opening, sniffing the breeze, and perhaps me. I reach up to touch it. As I do, it curls around my arm and begins to pull. I grasp it with my hand. When it encounters resistance, it pulls harder. I quickly realize that it can jerk my arm out of its socket as easily as it pulls trees out of the ground in its native land. Fear rushes through me. The elephant immediately releases my arm. The sensitive moist nostrils at the end of its trunk explore the palm of my hand. A massive head appears. For a brief and unforgettable moment, our eyes meet. Such kindness, such gentleness, such wisdom. A moment I will never forget.

—Marsha

The Last Breath

Betty, a nurse for 45 years, told us this story.

This is something I experienced about six years ago. My first witness of death. I don't know that I ever shared my feelings about what I experienced, but it is still with me. And it's real. I feel that it was profoundly real. My mother was 98 years old in a nursing home. She became very ill 24 hours before she passed away. She stayed with me, communicating with me until about an hour before she died. Her eyes were closed. She was very still. I knew that she was going to die, and yet I can't say I was ready. I guess you never want that to happen, you are in denial. I was watching and I was talking with her, trying to comfort her. When I would call her name, she would answer. Hmmmmmm. So I knew that she knew I was there. It seemed like not very often that she would take a breath. I realized that she was getting near the end. I didn't want to believe it. All of a sudden I was watching her, and then I realized it. She was reaching her peace. I picked her up in my arms, and she took her last breath. When she did, the Holy Spirit came and took her spirit. It was so real. And I had her. So I felt like it went through me—I was kind of with her. That I will always remember and I'm very grateful that I got to experience it.

of a Higher Power. Through this Love, we know our connection with all things. Gentle touch helps us remember our divine essence, and this remembering helps healing happen.

In the classes we teach on massage and in the massages we give, we take time to let our hands simply rest on the body. Often in the stillness, the greatest healing happens. In this stillness we become aware of the hand-heart connection. As we pay more attention to it, we notice that when two hearts open, the touch of Spirit is often present. We call this circle of connection, HeartTouch. Part III discusses HeartTouch, spiritual connection, and massage.

TOUCH IN NURSING

"Interestingly enough, the one branch of the healing community which has recognized the importance of touch is the nursing profession. . . . Being so much closer to the patient than the doctor, nurses have been in a far better position to appreciate the importance of touching in the care of the patient, in understanding that the care of the patient begins with caring for the patient. Caring is not optional, it is something that is natural and obligatory, to be caring, for which loving is another word, is to be involved, intimate."

—Ashley Montagu, *touching*

In the early days of nursing, the nurse's hands were one of the few tools she had for helping people feel better. With them she prepared meals, cleaned rooms, washed linens, made beds, cleaned wounds, and held hands. Nurses gave baths, fed people, and held them as they walked, cried, gave birth, and died. In the 1920s and as late as the 1960s (before the "technological age" and managed care), touch in the form of massage was taught in nursing schools as an essential part of evening care.

A nurse can use touch in many ways to benefit clients, including touching the arm, holding a hand, putting an arm around the shoulders, or giving a hug or a short massage. Nurses often use their intuition to know how to use touch to convey caring in different circumstances.

Research in nursing began to get under way in the 1960s, and as early as 1967 nurses were studying the effects of touch on their clients. Aguilera (1967) found that the use of touch increased verbal interactions between nurses and clients, that clients felt more positively toward the nurses who touched them, and that the nurse's touch had a calming and comforting effect on the client. McCorkle (1974) pointed out that touch communicates to people that they are valued, and because of that, it is important to touch clients in ways that convey caring, and not just in the act of doing a procedure. She suggested that touch may be the most important way to communicate to a critically ill person that he or she is valued as a human being, yet clients in critical care are seldom touched in non-technical ways. McCorkle worked with clients undergoing bone marrow transplants and suggested a gradual process in working with those who have to undergo many painful procedures. She suggests standing away from the client during initial interactions, the next time moving closer, and finally trying non-procedural touch, such as hand holding. She has observed improved self-concept, less depression, and shorter hospital stay.

Routasalo (1999) provides an excellent review of the research in the area of physical touch in nursing. For the past 30 years, nurses have been studying the touch given by nurses to all age groups and types of clients. Quantitative methods, qualitative methods, and combinations of both have been used to learn about touch. Nursing studies of touch seem to focus on three main aspects: (1) the observed effects of touch on the client; (2) the kinds of touch and how they are used; and (3) how the client experiences the touch of the nurse (as expressed by the client). Different types of touch have been classified by many different researchers, with the most common distinction being between instrumental touch and touch intended to be therapeutic. These two types of touch have been called, respectively, physical and therapeutic, instrumental and expressive, instrumental and empathetic, and procedural and expressive. Nurses rarely touch elderly clients using expressive touch and, in general, nurses touch clients using instrumental touch much more often than touch intended to be therapeutic. Some nurses never touch clients except in ways that are necessary to perform tasks. In touch intended to be therapeutic, some types intend to communicate caring or relaxation, while others have a healing intent, as in the laying on of hands or contact Therapeutic Touch. Some studies have contradictory results. For example, some studies say that critically ill clients are touched most, and some say they are touched least.

The nurse's touching style is learned and influenced by the nursing school she attended, her cultural background, and feedback from clients (Estabrooks and Morse, 1992). The way a client receives touch depends on their background and how much they need support. Clients usually feel that touch by the nurse is a positive experience, and it has a major influence on their attitude about, and their behavior toward, the nurse. If the nurse touches the client, the nurse tends to spend more time with the client, the client feels more calm and comforted, and he touches the nurse more often as well. A minority of the studies find that clients do not enjoy touching. Estabrooks and Morse (1992) are developing a theory of touching that emphasizes the touching process and acquiring a certain style of touching.

Nurses have many opportunities each day to touch others who are very vulnerable and in great need of love, support, and healing. The amount of time a nurse and a client spend together grows ever shorter. Because of this, we need to know how to make each moment spent touching the client, in any way, into a moment of connection. This type of interaction is vital not only for the client, but for the nurse to find greater meaning and fulfillment in her work. When we use any time we touch a client as an opportunity to intentionally convey feelings of acceptance and caring, the benefits flow both ways. It is this heartfelt connection that we all seek.

ON TOUCH AND MASSAGE

One of the most important reasons to learn massage is that it increases the opportunity to give and receive more touch. When we massage, we give and receive all of the value of touch, plus many benefits unique to massage. Sometimes nothing feels better than the slow, rhythmic squeezing of an area that is hurting. Massage softens muscle tension, personalities, and hearts. Massage is moving touch. For many of us, massage is a comfortable way to touch because we may feel a little uneasy when we touch someone with our hands held still for even a short amount of time. It is more comfortable to touch another, and to be touched, for longer periods of time if the hands are moving in a purposeful way, as in massage. With the hands moving, we often feel more free to send feelings of appreciation and love to the client.

Wouldn't you like to be able to do something with your hands that could help a client feel better almost immediately? Even when it lasts only a minute or two, massage fosters healing for the client, and gives the nurse a sense of truly helping in a personal, caring way. Imagine how wonderful it would feel if you and a colleague could sit down in the break room and exchange a shoulder massage

The heart uses a hand
to softly and gently
touch the heart of another
in ways
words
can never hope to understand.

—Marsha Walker

(with both parties consenting of course) when either of you needed one. A short massage is a gift that you can offer in those moments when a caring connection is what everybody needs.

SUMMARY

We return to the question, "Is touch necessary?" From the time we are born until the day we die, touch heals us and helps us connect heart to heart. We believe the answer is, yes, and every day.

We now introduce you to one of the best ways we've found to give and receive touch—massage.

PUTTING THESE IDEAS INTO PRACTICE

1. Focus your attention on the palm of your hand. Take a few breaths, allowing your exhale to travel down to your hand. Can you notice an increased awareness in your palm? Do you feel your palm begin to get a little warmer and perhaps pulsate or tingle?

2. Every day for one week, when you are not at work, touch one thing for five continuous minutes. It might be a rock, tree, pet, plant, or person. See if you notice a difference using one hand alone, or two hands, side by side. On some days, try step 1 as you are touching. Each day practice this focused touching on something new.

3. For one day, each time you touch a client, notice what thoughts are passing through your mind while you are touching him or her.

CHAPTER 2

Massage and Its Role in Nursing

A nurse who is unable to make her patient comfortable lacks one of the principal qualifications of a good nurse. Comfort is both mental and physical; one cannot be divorced from the other. Of all the measures which can be used to secure the comfort of the patient, massage ranks among the first.

—Sister Mary Agnita Claire Day, RN, MSN
Basic Science in Nursing Arts, 1947

OBJECTIVES

1. Describe the four types of techniques that contribute to the massage you will learn in this book.

2. Describe the three main strokes of Swedish Massage.

3. Discuss the role of intention in the relationship between the giver and receiver.

4. Describe two situations in your daily life where you might give and/or receive a massage.

5. Define nursing burnout and discuss two ways massage helps to prevent it.

6. Discuss three reasons why giving a massage benefits the nurse.

In this chapter we begin our exploration of massage, a very special way to touch. Massage may be one of the most important friends you add to your life. Why? We all have stress in our lives. When you receive a massage, you give your body and mind a fresh start. Tight muscles soften, and mental tension disappears. We all have people in our lives who could use a moment of relaxation and a change of perspective. Giving them a massage can offer them that needed break. With our clients, families, friends, and pets we have many opportunities to help and to care. When you take those opportunities to give a short massage, you will receive many smiles and contented groans (and a few licks and purrs).

First, let's look at what massage is and briefly review its history. We will then discuss a few different styles of massage, and how to combine some of them into the massage you will learn in Part II. Finally, we explore the role of massage in the life of a nurse.

WHAT IS MASSAGE?

The best way to answer this question is to receive one. Massage is one of those experiences in life that is hard to describe in words. Most people would agree that you should try it at least once during this journey we call life. Receiving even a short massage by someone who is relaxed and wants to help you feel better will give you a good, first hand experience.

When I was 21 years old, and traveling from Key West, Florida, to Washington, DC, I decided on the spur of the moment to spend the evening in Richmond, Virginia. That afternoon, I had my first massage from a professional masseur at the local YMCA. He was an older fellow who really knew his business, had done it for a while, and seemed to really enjoy his work. Lying there on that massage table it occurred to me what a good and valuable thing massage really was. Of course, I didn't have any idea at the time exactly why massage was good for my health, but I knew it felt great. Afterward, I slept like a baby for about twelve hours. I was impressed.

—Jonathan

Massage Is Many Things to Many People

"I feel like myself again." Pauline, restaurant owner

"I'm in much better shape than I was 18 years ago, before I started getting massage. I know I wouldn't be walking, or dressing myself, or getting out of bed without it. Well, I probably wouldn't be here." Elizabeth, at 90 years old

"That's exactly what I needed. It was kind of an out of body experience." Joan, mother of three young children

"Massage is my heaven on Earth." Kathy, human resources program director

"I have no words." Marsha C., Director of Communication

According to Webster's dictionary, massage is formally defined as: the systematic manipulation of the body's soft tissues for preventive or remedial purposes by rubbing, stroking, tapping, and/or kneading with the hands. Some people get massage for this reason, that is, to rub the pain and tight spots out of their muscles. Massage also means to stroke and to coax, as in stroking gently, coaxing the body and mind to relax and let go. In this vein, for some people massage is an opportunity to find an inner place of peace, allowing the brain to move from the active state of daily life to a state of stillness, contemplation, and creativity. For some, as the muscles relax, anxious thoughts and feelings are resolved and released through conversation. For others, massage is like a vacation. It is a chance to remember who they really are, allowing all the irritation, falsely placed priorities, and hurry, to evaporate. During a massage, some go within and reconnect with Spirit. Massage can be any, or all, of these things.

Many methods for reducing stress require the receiver to perform some activity, as in biofeedback training, physical exercise, or visualization. To enjoy the benefits of massage, all a person has to "do" is lie there and be willing to receive. This makes massage an excellent way to relax and unwind for people of varying occupations, ages, and states of health.

The receiver is not the only one who benefits during a massage. Giving a massage is an opportunity to focus the mind on thoughts that are kind and helpful which, in turn, relaxes the body and touches the heart of the giver. The giving of massage is a way to show that you care. In this kind of giving, you also receive.

HISTORY OF MASSAGE

Massage, or rubbing on a sore spot, is instinctual. When dogs and cats are in pain, or have a wound that is healing, it is almost impossible to keep them from licking the area. When children have a stomach ache, or fall and hurt their knee, it is instinctive for a parent to rub or touch the painful area. When we hit our head on the corner of a cabinet door we automatically begin rubbing it. This instinct to "touch the hurt" is built into the body, and so there has probably been massage in some form for as long as we have had injuries and sore muscles.

Massage in Ancient Times

As long ago as 2760 B.C. a medical text in China known as the *Nei Ching* contained descriptions of massage (DeDomenico and Wood, 1997). Massage treatments were used in India and were included in the book, "Ayur-Veda" (Art of Life), a work setting out an entire philosophy of health and healing said to have been written around 1800 B.C. In ancient Greece, Hippocrates (460–377 B.C.) suggested that massage should be one of the primary skills of any physician. The Roman physician, Celsus (25 B.C.–25 A.D.), compiled a series of books entitled *De Medicina* which spanned the medical knowledge of his time. Seven of those eight books focused on therapeutics and prevention, and included outlining the use of the hands to rub the body for therapeutic benefit.

The sciences suffered during the Dark Ages (475 A.D.–1000 A.D.) because few books were published and much of the written history available was either lost or destroyed. The medical traditions of Greece and Rome all but fell from view. Massage came to be viewed as more a part of folk medicine than as having any place of significance in the established medical practices of the day.

Massage in Modern Times

Credit for the development of Swedish Massage (the basis of the massage in this book) is generally given to Pehr Henrik Ling (1776–1839) of Sweden. Though he did not originate the practice in its entirety, he experimented with many of the known massage techniques of his time. Ling taught his new composite system to physicians from England, Germany, Austria, and Russia. This led to the adoption of a more scientific view and approach toward massage, thus helping it to take root in the medical practices of those countries.

In Holland, Dr. Johann Metzger (1839–1909) was the first to use the French terms, effleurage and petrissage (terms used almost universally in Swedish massage) for gliding and kneading strokes, respectively. He also established massage for the treatment of disease as a scientific subject for physicians. Metzger and Ling are both credited for having planted the seeds of modern massage therapy.

In 1858, two physicians, Charles and George Taylor introduced Ling's "Swedish Movement Cure" into the United States by incorporating it into their medical practice in New York. From about 1850 to 1920, the actual practice of massage evolved from a semi-skilled trade into a legitimate field of medical healthcare.

During World War I (1914–1918) and World War II (1939–1945), massage was used in the hospitals of the armed forces. After World War II, massage began to take a secondary role in medical practice in the United States. Massage in nursing is discussed at the end of the chapter.

During the 1950s, two outstanding leaders in the field of massage education, Frances Tappan and Gertrude Beard, wrote massage texts that are still in publication today. Though there are many massage textbooks that provide a current perspective on massage as a healing art, Tappan's *Healing Massage Techniques* and Wood and Becker's *Beard's Massage* are highly recommended for anyone wanting to learn more about full body massage.

In the early 1970s the Holistic Health movement began. As the healthcare community began to focus more on technological advances, the public began to explore ways of promoting their own health that addressed not only the body, but the mind, emotions, and spirit. In addition to treating disease, prevention of illness and promotion of health gained much attention. People began to seek out body therapies such as massage and acupuncture, and energy therapies such as Therapeutic Touch. They explored modalities such as meditation, yoga, imagery, and the use of herbs and nutrition.

The Holistic Health movement continues to thrive, with its name changing to alternative, then complementary, and now integrative. In Germany, Japan, China, and the former Soviet countries, massage therapists work with doctors as part of the healthcare team. In one Shanghai hospital the massage department covers two floors, with nurses giving massage (Collinge, 1996). In 1997, 42% of the American public used at least one form of integrative therapy (Eisenberg, et al., 1998). The research budget of the Center for Complementary and Alternative Medicine at the National Institute of Health has grown from $2 million in 1992 to $50 million in 1999 (Schroeder and Likkel, 1999).

With this increased interest in holistic healing, massage has seen a renaissance in the United States. Under the direction of Tiffany Field, Ph.D., the Touch Research Institute at the University of Miami School of Medicine conducts controlled studies to examine the effects of massage in healthcare (See Appendix A for internet address). In a survey of the American public, the top three integrative therapies used were massage, relaxation techniques, and herbal medicine (Eisenberg et al., 1998). When we first began practicing massage in 1977 there were only a few massage schools in the United States, now most states have at least one, if not several. Many massage schools graduate around 200–300 students each year, most of them becoming licensed as Registered Massage Therapists (RMT). In addition to massage schools, many nursing schools are once again including massage in their undergraduate curricula as well as providing continuing education programs in massage.

As we strive to create the ideal healthcare delivery system of the future, considering a combination of traditions from both the East and the West may provide the most effective approach. Some of these methods will probably include massage, acupuncture, herbs, meditation, energy therapy, and prayer, along with prescription drugs and surgery when necessary. It is becoming clear that our focus must shift toward prevention of illness and promotion of health, rather than waiting until we are ill and trying to fix the problem. We are learning that a large factor in the promotion of health is how we interact with the stressors in our lives. Massage is an excellent way to replace stress with relaxation, in body and mind. With more people learning and giving massage, more people are able to receive it.

As more of us give and receive massage, the world becomes a healthier and happier place to live.

TYPES OF MASSAGE

As you are learning massage and beginning to offer it to others, keep in mind that when many people think of massage they envision a person on television pounding away at someone on a massage table. If a prospective receiver has never had a massage, you might need to inform them that the majority of massage strokes are slow and soothing. The slow, rhythmic stroking, kneading, and rubbing of the body's skin and muscle tissue, when done properly and with caring intent, can be one of the most comforting and relaxing experiences life has to offer. There are few experiences in the typical clinical setting that are as relaxing as a good massage.

Throughout history, massage has undergone much change. What began as rubbing a sore spot has evolved into many unique and beneficial styles of massage and bodywork. The goal of most types of bodywork is to help release tension and restore a relaxed, balanced state. Different techniques approach this goal in different ways.

Although there are many types of bodywork, we now offer a brief introduction to four styles that are in some ways, a foundation of the massage you will learn in Part II.

The Esalen-style Massage

The Esalen-style massage was originated and popularized during the 1960s at the Esalen Institute located in Big Sur, California. Situated along the rocky Pacific coast, Esalen is famous for its breathtaking, panoramic view of the ocean, spectacular sunsets, natural hot springs, towering redwood trees—and its massage. Molly Day Shackman was one of the developers of the Esalen massage, which was a combination of Swedish massage technique and Charlotte Selver's Sensory Awareness Training.

The technique consists primarily of long, slow, gliding strokes. In addition to applying the strokes, practitioners might allow their hands to simply rest on the receiver's body. The purpose being to relax the receiver's body and to help her experience herself as an integration of body, mind, feelings, and spirit. This focus on the quality of touch fosters a nurturing sense of security, which in turn encourages the awakening of our own personal awareness.

The Esalen approach was developed using communication between the person giving the massage and the person receiving it. As you will find, this two way communication is vital as you begin practicing massage, and it will remain a key ingredient to help you continually improve the massage you give.

We can benefit by keeping this image of the Esalen-style massage in mind as we learn and give massage. Whenever there is a question of how firm the pressure of your touch should be, remember that a light touch and long strokes can induce relaxation quite well, and that they bring with them a sense of safety and comfort. People who are fragile in any way, including infants, some Elders, and anyone who is debilitated, cannot tolerate deep massage. Long, slow strokes create the desired relaxation and sense of being cared for which is the most important thing.

Myotherapy

In 1980, Bonnie Prudden introduced her unique form of hands-on bodywork called myotherapy, which focuses on small, discrete areas of tension. The goal of myotherapy is to erase these "trigger points," which are "highly irritable spot(s) in a muscle which contribute to pain." They often feel like small pebbles or areas of greater hardness in the tissue. The receiver may not have been aware of them before you touched them. These trigger points "are laid down in muscles throughout our lives" in virtually any area of the body by such things as strains, accidents, disease, and the ways the body is used at work. Even the trauma of birth can lay down trigger points on the body's muscular system. These points lie dormant until the right physical and/or emotional climate causes them to "fire," throwing the muscle, and often the area around it, into spasm (Prudden, 1980).

Trigger points can be located using a "seeking" technique. The fingers and thumb are used to explore a large area, searching for these small, tight spots. When a trigger point is located a steady pressure is applied to it. This method is very effective in helping to release, or "erase," the tense area, as well as the surrounding musculature that is connected with it.

Sometimes trigger points are sensitive to touch. In our experience, if massaging any area causes the client to wince in pain or tighten up, the amount of pressure being applied is counterproductive. It should be lessened or stopped. The purpose of your massage is to encourage the body to release and let go. It may take more than one session for a trigger point to completely relax.

Reflexology

Reflexology is the application of pressure with the thumb or finger to specific areas on the foot or hand. These areas correspond to, and create change in, other areas of the body. For example, the bone in the arch of the foot that extends from the heel to the ball of the foot corresponds to the spine. Pressing on this area of the foot beneficially affects the area of the spine. There are points on the feet and hands corresponding to almost all areas of the body. Reflexology is relaxing, reduces pain, and speeds healing.

Pressing on the feet to stimulate healing has been around a long time. Wall paintings in an Egyptian tomb, called the Physician's Tomb, dating around 2,330 B.C., show a practitioner using the thumb to apply pressure to the feet. In 1900, William Fitzgerald, M.D., began applying pressure to areas on the hands for anesthesia and to decrease pain that his patients were having. Eunice Ingham worked in the office of Joe Riley, M.D., who used these techniques in his practice. Ms. Ingham began using this approach on Dr. Riley's patients and expanded the practice to include specific points on the feet, making detailed maps of foot/body correspondences. She is considered to be the originator of the system she called reflexology.

In 1938, after 18 years of mapping the feet and hands and coordinating points with the clients' experiences, Ms. Ingham wrote *Stories the Feet Can Tell* and *Stories the Feet Have Told.* Her books can still be purchased unedited, with her writing style taking you back to the 1930s. She describes physicians adding reflexology to their "herbal powders" as another healing tool. Her books are full of love for her craft and for the people she helped. We highly recommend her books for a unique perspective on healing and greater detail about reflexology (Ingham, 1984). Dwight Byers, her nephew, continues her work and teaches at the Institute of Reflexology in Florida (Byers, 1983).

Knowing reflexology is very helpful when you cannot massage the area that is painful, or in need of healing, such as with burns, broken bones, or problems with internal organs. You can instead work on the spot on the hand or foot that corresponds to the problem area. If you would like to try this technique, but don't want to try to remember which point corresponds to what area, just work on the entire foot and you will affect the entire body. Although we will not describe reflexology specifically in this book, we do encourage a very thorough foot massage. There is something very special about holding and ministering to someone's feet. It is a gesture of humble service.

Swedish Massage

As mentioned earlier, what became widely known as Swedish-style massage has evolved out of the work of Pehr Henrik Ling and Johann Metzger in the early nineteenth century. Swedish massage is the foundation of many of the massages you receive. Most practitioners learn it first and then add other techniques to it, or branch out from it into other forms of bodywork. Generally, Swedish massage is a thorough working of the skin and muscles. It is intended to increase the circulation of the blood and lymph, and relieve soreness due to tight or over-worked muscles. It usually leaves the receiver feeling very relaxed and refreshed in body and mind.

It is helpful for anyone learning massage to become familiar with the basic strokes that characterize Swedish massage: Effleurage, Petrissage, Friction, and Tapotement. *Effleurage* is a gliding motion with the palms of the hands moving smoothly over some portion of the client's body while applying a light to moderate pressure. If you have only a short amount of time, repeating only the effleurage stroke several times has a very soothing, almost hypnotic effect on the receiver, and the giver as well. *Petrissage* is a kneading motion in which the tissue is squeezed, lifted, and released. A *friction* stroke moves one layer of muscles against another. This is a more specific type of stroke than the other two, focusing on very small areas, one at a time. It can be applied with greater pressure to relax deeper layers of muscle. Friction is often performed using the pads of the thumbs to make small circular movements, or to press and slide across the tissue for short distances. It can also be used to work on "trigger points". Because friction can be a deeper stroke, it is important to get feedback from the receiver as to their comfort level.

These three strokes are discussed in great detail, with photos, in Part II. *Tapotement* is a pounding motion that will not be included in the massage in this book.

THE MASSAGE YOU WILL LEARN IN THIS BOOK

We have discussed Swedish massage, Esalen massage, myotherapy, and reflexology because we have found that certain techniques from each of these methods create an excellent combination that is both relaxing and very effective at releasing muscle tension. Swedish massage, with its characteristic strokes, is the foundation of our massage. You will see the gentle, nurturing, gliding strokes of the Esalen style, and the more specific techniques draw on principles from myotherapy and reflexology. This introduction to a myotherapy and reflexology will enrich your practice of the rotating thumb friction stroke and a thorough foot massage, respectively.

The massage begins with general strokes (effleurage), allowing the body to get used to being touched. The next strokes are somewhat deeper (petrissage), encouraging the body to gradually let go. Once the muscles are more relaxed, the most specific stroke (friction) addresses deeper tension. The massage ends with general strokes once again, for a feeling of completion and comfort.

You can adapt the massage to your time frame and the condition of the receiver by choosing which areas of the body to work on and for how long. Never pass up a chance for massage because you think you don't have time. You will be surprised what a difference one minute of massage makes. We all can usually find one minute to help someone feel better. Even if you have a short amount of time, GO SLOWLY. You will see this reminder many times in the pages that follow. You are not trying to fit in as many strokes as you can into a short amount of time. If you do only one stroke, slowly, the receiver relaxes. That is your goal.

Each moment of our lives is truly a miracle. We tend to forget this sometimes. Massage is a gift that helps the giver and receiver slow down and remember.

THE RELATIONSHIP BETWEEN THE GIVER AND THE RECEIVER

Many people think that if they learn a large number of bodywork techniques, they will be able to give a great massage. We have found that technique is only a small part of a massage that feels truly healing. That is why we have included more in this book than technique alone. One of the most important considerations in massage is the relationship between the giver and receiver. A relationship is essentially the quality of the way two individuals relate or interact, whether they have known each other for a long time, or whether the two minutes during a shoulder massage is the extent of their relationship. This topic is covered in greater detail in Part III, Massage as a Bridge for Connection, however, in any discussion of what massage is, this relationship must at least be mentioned.

The giver is anyone offering to help another, in this case by offering to give a massage, or touch that is caring. The giver might be a nurse, mother, nursing assistant, father, physician, pet, friend, or child. The receiver is anyone who accepts your offer to help them feel better. They may be a client in a healthcare setting, a family member, or friend. The receiver could be your dog who gently nudges you with a paw and plops down beside you, a kitten who slips into your lap, or even your favorite house plant.

Some of the best massages we have ever received were from friends who had no formal instruction in massage, but who really wanted to help us feel better. Effective massage techniques are certainly important, however, it is the intention to help and care that is the key (Figure 2-1).

Intention

The use of intention may be a characteristic we are born with because infants as young as 18 months seem to understand and re-enact the intentions of others (Meltzoff, 1995). According to Webster's dictionary, an intention is the momen-

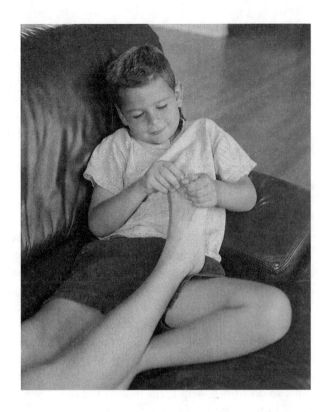

Figure 2-1

tum caused by our focused attention and willpower. Having an intention is a focusing device.

According to the dictionary, an intention is the momentum caused by our focused attention and willpower. Having an intention is a focusing device. It focuses the power of our attention and our will to create what we want in a situation. We can have the intention to really be with, listen to, and help another person. Having that intention focuses our attention on our interaction with them. The inner decision to choose how we think and feel, or what we intend to take place in a situation, manifests outwardly in many ways. Consciously intending to help affects our choice of words, tone of voice, the look in our eyes, and our body language. The receiver's reactions to us are affected by what we intend.

Nurses turn people in bed when they cannot do this for themselves, help clients hold a glass of water, and help them walk to the bathroom. In our families, we direct our children to the car, help an aging parent into their chair, touch a pet as we leave the house, or hug a spouse when they walk in the door. All too often as we do this touching we are thinking about other things, activities we need to do, or a stressful event in life.

What we consciously intend also affects the way we touch. When a nurse consciously intends to convey caring, even the shortest and most routine experiences of touch can make all the difference to a client. A simple touch while offering a sip of water can become a moment remembered years later by both nurse and client. When we have the intention to appreciate an elderly parent, the heart can hear what their words are trying to say. There is that extra five minutes to really listen to that favorite old story once again. One day that story may be very precious. We often give a friend a pat on the back or a hug hello. Intention to care causes a hand to rest just a little longer on the shoulder, and a hug becomes a prolonged moment of sharing.

INTENTION IN MASSAGE

When we are first beginning to give massage, we tend to focus mostly on technique. As we become more comfortable with technique, we can turn our attention to how to help the receiver feel cared for. Each time your hand touches the receiver during the massage you can use that physical sensation as a cue to remember your intention to help. In many cases, the intention that you, as the giver, bring to each massage makes the difference.

It can be helpful to think about what you intend for a massage beforehand. For example, when we begin each massage we intend that the receiver experience whatever degree of healing is perfect for them at that time, and that we will know what to do to best help them heal. If the receiver asks you, "Is there anything I should do during my massage?", suggest that they focus their attention on your hands, and with each movement, feel their muscles becoming warm and soft. In this way, you help them create an intention to relax and let go.

As we discuss in detail in Part III, the thoughts and feelings you have while massaging someone are very likely the most important factor in determining the way they experience the massage you give.

MASSAGE IN NURSING—PAST, PRESENT, FUTURE

As nurses, we hold people when they are most fragile. We assist them when they are most vulnerable, comforting them, and easing their pain. In all of these ways, we help them feel loved. It is this feeling of being loved and cared about that is one of the greatest healers of the body, mind, and spirit. In the beginning of the nursing profession, our hearts and hands were our most powerful healing tools. We have passed through a time when we believed technology was the answer in healthcare. Nurses and other healthcare providers are now realizing that having the greatest technology is not enough. We are coming full circle, with touch and sharing of the heart becoming equal partners with hi-tech approaches to healing. Nursing is one of the few professions bestowed with the ability, opportunity, and honor to touch others each day to help them heal. Many of us came into nursing because we wanted to do something directly to help those who are suffering. Massage gives us a tool that leaves the body relaxed, and the spirit comforted.

The intent of this section is to introduce the idea that a short, effective massage is as much a part of nursing as helping a person with a bed bath, giving medications, or charting. We also look at how massage benefits the nurse, whether she is giving it or receiving it.

One of the Earliest Nursing Interventions

Since the early days, massage has been a nursing intervention that uses the hands to help clients sleep, reduce their pain, and convey feelings of the heart. Some of the earliest nursing texts discuss massage, or the "backrub," as a valuable technique for nurses, physical therapists, and physicians. If you want to get in touch with the roots of our profession, find some of these wonderful old nursing textbooks. Their simple, yet beautiful, black and white photos, as well as the smell and faded color of their pages, will transport you back in time, and make you very proud to be a nurse (Figure 2-2).

As early as 1926, in *Text-Book of Nursing Technique*, nurses were taught to perform massage "to relieve pain, to comfort and refresh the patient, to stimulate circulation, and to lessen the danger of pressure sores" (Kelley, 1936, 3rd ed.).

Harmer and Henderson, in *The Principles and Practice of Nursing*, acknowledged that "Massage is one of the best means of stimulating the repair (of fractures), and of preventing atrophy of muscles and stiffness of joints and tendons." (p. 957). They suggested massage should be applied regularly, every day, as soon as the union of the bone was secure and there was no further danger of displacement (Harmer and Henderson, 1939, 4th ed.). In the fifth edition in 1955, massage had been expanded from a mere mention in the 1939 edition to a full chapter of its own, entitled "Massage, Therapeutic Exercise and Pressure."

In *Basic Science in Nursing Arts*, Day (1947) discusses nursing interventions saying that, "Massage ranks among the first, not only in the general care of the skin, as exemplified by the traditional back rub, but also in simple remedial massage routines which the nurse is called upon to administer." (p. 278). Day goes on to discuss the reflexive, mechanical, and physiologic effects of massage, and its benefits for the nervous system, skin, muscles, blood, and lymph. She includes detailed information on technique and a list of 22 contraindications.

Temple (1967) wrote that massage is a part of evening care that "helps the patient sleep and removes tension. Massage establishes rapport between the nurse

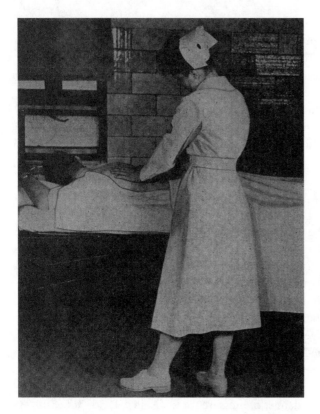

Figure 2-2 Since the early days, massage has been a nursing intervention that uses hands to help clients sleep, reduce their pain, and convey feelings of the heart. (From Day, Basic Science in Nursing Arts, copyright 1947, Mosby Publishing. Used with permission.)

and patient that would take days if words alone were used." Many nurses think that a massage takes longer than giving pain medication. Temple discovered that it took her as much time to give a pain medication as it did to give a massage when she included the time for checking to see when the last dose was given and the other preliminaries for giving a medication. She emphasized that giving a massage brought satisfaction and relaxation to the nurse as well as the patient.

Up until the early 1960s, nurses learned massage in great detail in nursing school. According to Sheryl Monfore, a labor and delivery nurse in Minnesota, "Ward Order" was attended to in the morning and evening. It required a nurse to first straighten linens and clean the patient's room—including emptying the garbage and dusting the furniture, mopping the floor, and getting fresh water. Then each person received a backrub. Marian Williams, a nurse in California, said that nursing care for the "Hour of Sleep Care" included smoothing wrinkles out of the sheets, getting patients a drink, and giving them a 5–10 minute massage for the back, neck, and shoulders (Mower, 1997).

In the 1960s time spent on massage training decreased. By the 1970s many schools eliminated it believing "there was not time for everything with the new technology." In 1975, when I entered nursing school, we didn't learn massage. During my first job as a nurse in a hospital, I saw the older nurses on the 3–11 shift giving back rubs. I asked if I was supposed to do that. They said, "Of course. All nurses do." I watched, and it made me relax just watching. They taught me, and I started offering it to my clients. I spent some of my most rewarding times giving massage.

We have now had 40 years of new nurses who were not taught massage in nursing school. When student nurses don't have a chance to give massage in school, they don't feel confident giving it to clients. When they don't receive massage in school by trading with other students, they don't get the chance to experience first hand how relaxing it is, and so don't give it priority as an intervention in their practice.

Massage was not intentionally eliminated from nursing because it didn't work or because nurses and clients didn't like it. With the emergence of new technology, nurses had to learn so many other new skills that it was just forgotten. There seemed to be less and less time to spend with clients. More sleeping pills and pain pills were given. Nurses started feeling a lack of meaning and fulfillment in their work. No one thought that perhaps the disappearance of massage could be a factor.

Massage in Nursing Today

Are you feeling more stressed than you want to? Are you feeling that your work, or your personal life, is not as meaningful as you would like it to be? If so, you might want to consider adding something new to the mix of your usual day. You may be thinking, "I can't add one more thing." Austin has a very large greenbelt with a creek, hills, and walking trails. I always enjoyed going there because you are surrounded by trees and feel like you are far from a city, but I rarely made the time to go. Well, a year ago we adopted Jasper, a very loving Golden Retriever mix. Now all of a sudden, somehow, I have an hour each morning to walk the greenbelt. What changed? My life is certainly as busy as it ever was. It's a combination of two things, the joy of watching Jasper run and jump with glee, and the fulfillment I receive walking in the woods.

So it is with massage. Although our days are very full, we could all probably use a little more joy in our lives. If you give a massage just once, the rewards both you and the receiver experience will make you take the time.

In my house-call massage practice, I have the opportunity to see people's refrigerator art. Refrigerators have become display cases where we use wonderfully varied magnets to hold photos and pieces of information that mean the most to us. We put things there we want to see many times a day. I often find jewels of wisdom. Here is one I especially like: "If you continue to do what you've always done, you get the results you've always gotten."

What a concept! Simple, yet it was new to me. Of course. How could I expect the world to change in ways I wanted it to when I insisted on doing exactly what I had always done? It just doesn't work that way.

Massage is an excellent choice to get the ball rolling in a different direction. Giving a massage has a domino effect that will initiate changes you can't imagine. One to ten minutes is all you need.

WHERE CAN WE USE MASSAGE?

Nurses care for people in such a wide variety of settings. At work, not only do we use interventions that assist the healing of the body, mind, and spirit, but we teach health promotion to clients and their families. When we go home, we care for our own families and friends. The massage in this book is designed for you to use in all of the roles you play each day, whenever people need a little relief from the stresses of life.

Our primary role as nurses is caring for clients in the healthcare setting in which we work. Chapter 3 discusses the many benefits of massage we have observed working with clients in the practice setting. It also discusses research studying the benefits of massage on specific populations and in different states of illness and wellness. Studies by nurses in nursing situations are highlighted. The bottom line is that massage relaxes the body and mind, stopping the stress response so the bodymind can heal.

Erickson, Tomlin, and Swain (1988) found that when people are impoverished, or have few resources for dealing with the stresses of their life, it is difficult to heal. Developing a trusting relationship with the nurse is a vital first step in building new resources. A trusting relationship helps the client feel that someone cares, and that there is hope and a reason to believe that healing can happen. Trust is built when a person is not discounted, but made to feel that he is important and accepted. Erickson, Tomlin, and Swain found that trust is developed in the simplest way through purposeful touch. When we touch clients in a caring way, particularly when we take the time to give them a massage, they know we value them.

How would it look to actually do massage at work? The first step in bringing about something new is seeing if we can imagine what it might look like.

Hospital

Someone called in sick again today so you are more short staffed than usual. You had an unexpected admission, and someone fell in the bathroom and may have a broken hip. A call light has been on for awhile, and you go in to answer it. A 50-year-old woman with severe burns says she is very uncomfortable and having trouble sleeping. It is not time for more pain medication. What could you do? A slow, two minute massage to each foot works wonders.

Home Health

If you do private duty nursing where you work with only one person, there are many opportunities to give a massage. Bob Hope said the reason he was so healthy for so long was that he got a massage every day. You may be one of the few nurses who has time to give a longer massage, incorporating all of the techniques in Part II.

Most nurses who do home healthcare visit the homes of many clients each day, spending only a short time with each one. Imagine this: You walk into a client's home and ask how he has been feeling. "My back has been killing me. I don't know what happened. I bent over to pick up the paper and it went out." What can you do? Before you leave, ask him if he would like a five minute back rub. Using your professional judgment, ask him to lie on his side or stomach on his bed or couch. He could also sit in a chair and lean his head on the table. Applying lotion to the tight area, massage the back, choosing a few of the strokes in Chapter 7. Five minutes of back massage goes a long way. You could also take a few minutes and teach the massage to a family member so they could give it when needed.

Nurse Practitioners

You walk into the room where a client is waiting to see you, and she is rubbing her forehead. "I'm having headaches. The other day when I woke up, my hands were numb. I'm having trouble falling asleep at night." Ask her to sit in a chair with her back facing you (clothes on) and lean her head on a pillow on the table. Using your thumbs, focus your massage on the area between the spine and shoulder blades as well as the upper trapezius on top of the shoulders. (See Chapter 6.) In addition to the neck, be sure to rub under the occipital ridge under the skull which is excellent for headaches.

Even though many nurse practitioners must stick to rigid schedules, you are the primary care provider. As part of your office visits you could choose to include a three minute massage for certain clients. You will build instant rapport, and your client may be more comfortable talking to you about her health problems because she is relaxed. Some of the complaints she came to see you about may disappear as a result of even a short massage.

Clinics, Doctor's Office

Often nurses in clinics or doctor's offices have more flexibility to be creative than they might in the hospital setting. Have you ever waited a little too long at a doctor's office? What if a nurse was in the waiting room giving short shoulder massages? There could also be a special room for massage where clients with muscle tension, headaches, and stress-related problems could receive a short massage while they wait, or a slightly longer massage by appointment at another time. Imagine how that would change the day for the clients, the nurses, and the doctor? As you look into the waiting room, even on a busy day, everyone has a smile of their face. They don't seem to mind waiting at all. You know it is because they have each spent five minutes receiving a massage from you. Another possibility would be to take the client back to the exam room and do the initial assessment and vital signs. You offer a short neck and shoulder massage to each client. Just for fun, you could recheck the vital signs to see if there was a difference.

Occupational Health

Today, many corporations have health promotion programs because they have been found to be cost effective. Stress in the workplace these days is more mental than physical, and it is unrelenting. With impossible deadlines and potential layoffs, people often come to the nurse with stress-related symptoms. For people who work long hours at computers, massage for the neck, shoulders, arms, and hands is a welcome relief.

School Nurse

Linda, who is five years old, comes in crying and grabs your hand, "I need a bandaid for my knee. I can't go back to class." Since you can't see any injury you know Linda needs more than a bandaid. You ask, "Linda would you like to lay down and rest on this couch while I rub your back?" She nods and crawls onto the couch. After a few slow circles with your palms on her back (clothes on), she stops crying and takes a deep breath. She begins to tell you about the girl who wouldn't play with her. After a few kind words, a few more palm circles, and a bandaid, Linda is ready to go back to class.

For the child or teenager who strains a muscle, has a headache, or needs comfort and encouragement, massage is an ideal way for the nurse to make contact. Often young children with aches and pains only need to be touched. Most children respond quickly to massage. Teenagers have become a little more guarded. Massage to the shoulders and neck often relaxes not only the muscles, but makes it easier to talk about pent up feelings.

Teaching Massage to Clients and their Families

You have a client who came in to the hospital for a bowel resection and expected to be going home in a week. Her bowel perforated in surgery, but no one detected it. By the time it was discovered, she had lost a lot of blood, and her body had become septic. Days in the hospital turned into weeks. Her husband had spent every night in the room. His wife had become very frail. One night you come into the room to check on her, and find him pacing. You ask, "Can I help you?" He replies, "I just don't know what to do. I feel so helpless. She seems so sad and weak." You know just the thing. "Would you like to learn some simple massage strokes that you can give your wife?" For the first time in days, a smile appears on the man's face. "Thank you so much. That would be wonderful." You take 15 minutes to teach him two minutes of massage for each area, feet, hands, back, and head. After you wash your hands, you look back. He is tenderly rubbing her feet as she smiles.

One of your roles might be to teach the family members of your clients a brief massage so they can help their loved one in the hospital, or after they go home. Often families feel helpless and really want to do something. If they learn some massage, even if it is only for the feet and hands, they can help a family member feel better. Massage can also be an "excuse" for touching, which many so desperately want to do. Some people may be taking care of a loved one for a long time at home, which becomes very stressful. Jivanjee (1994) found that family caregivers of people with Alzheimer's disease were able to enhance their own well-being by using active coping strategies, such as giving massage. When several family members learn a short massage, they can trade with each other. Massage is often a comfortable way for people to give and receive the relaxation and nurturing they need.

Nurses who work in long term care facilities or retirement homes might consider offering a class to teach clients or residents a simple massage they can give each other or a family member. Feeling that we are still helpful to others can be one of the greatest joys of life as we age.

Colleagues at Work

You walk back to the nurse's station, and a colleague is trying to squeeze her shoulder while talking on the phone. After she hangs up you ask, "Is your shoulder hurting?" She says, "It's been killing me all day. I must have slept on it wrong, now it just won't go away." You ask, "Do you have two minutes?" You go into the break room and she sits down. You slowly squeeze the shoulders, first right, then left, starting near the neck and moving out toward the shoulder joint. She begins to moan, "That feels so good." All it takes is two minutes.

Sometimes the only way nurses can make it through a tough shift is by giving each other a hand, whether that is in helping a client to the bathroom or giving each other a two minute shoulder massage. How many times would you have given anything to have someone squeeze that tight neck or shoulders? Wouldn't it feel great if a colleague knew just where to press on your back to relieve the pain?

Personal Life

A nurse is a multidimensional being. Working in a healthcare facility is only one of many roles. Nurses have personal lives, with friends and families. Massage helps others in life in addition to clients who need a change, either of a physical discomfort or a point of view. What happens at home affects all aspects of our professional lives.

Imagine that you finally have supper finished, the kids are in bed, and you and your spouse flop down on the couch for a few minutes before you go to bed. Because of your schedules, you haven't seen each other much in the last few days. You both look at each other, and say in unison, "I'm exhausted." An idea pops into your head. You go get the kitchen timer. "How about trading a five minute foot massage, and no talking about our day." Your spouse says, "Sounds great to me." You get some lotion, set the timer for five minutes, and slowly start rubbing. The groans tell you you're doing a good job. Now it's your turn. Five whole minutes of having your feet rubbed. You feel like you're in heaven. Not only are you both more relaxed, but 10 minutes of foot massage can often create more closeness than 10 minutes talking about the details of the day.

We all get so busy that sometimes we can go for days without taking the time to touch each other in a caring, supportive way. Families, couples, and friends are often looking for ways to strengthen their relationships and convey love. Massage helps us communicate our appreciation and love for each other in ways where words fall short. You can teach your family and friends a five minute massage so

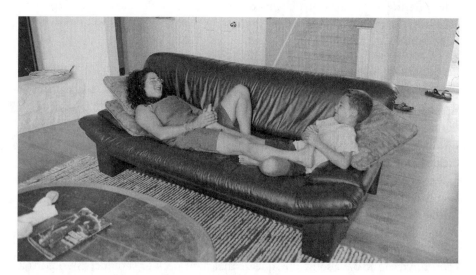

Figure 2-3

you can all give and receive it when you are in need. These days even children have complaints that come from tension and stress. Most children love massage. Children of all ages give magical massages without ever learning a technique. The love you can feel from the hands of your child will touch your heart (Figure 2-3).

MASSAGE BENEFITS THE NURSE

Usually when we think of massage in nursing, we think of it as an intervention the nurse can give to clients, colleagues, or family members to help them feel better. This alone is a good reason to learn massage. However, the other side of the coin is that we need to learn about massage because it can benefit us. With stress so high in nursing today, many experience burnout, one reason many nurses leave the profession. This section discusses the phenomenon of burnout in some detail, suggesting why giving and receiving massage may help to prevent it. For more details about stress, and how thoughts and feelings affect the stress response, immune function, and other aspects of health, see Chapter 9.

Nursing Stress and Burnout

The stress a nurse experiences in the workplace is profound. Many of us are also under more stress in our personal lives than ever before because of the fast, continuous pace. Nurses are faced every day, all day, with many of the factors determined to be the most stressful; including constant change, feeling like they have little control over their situation, and not feeling enough support. Feeling a lack of control over their practice often results in chronic anger and hostility, or even aggression (Antai-Otong, 2001). Hostility is defined as cynical mistrust, frequent angry outbursts, and/or aggression. Hostility is a predictor of coronary heart disease (Davis, Matthews, and McGrath, 2000).

One of the most influential models explaining stress in the workplace, the Job Strain Model (Karasek, 1979), suggests that staff whose jobs have high demands and low control are at greater risk for poor psychological well-being and cardiovascular disease. Landsbergis (1988) studied occupational stress among healthcare workers and found that job strain (job dissatisfaction, depression, psychosomatic symptoms) and burnout were significantly higher in jobs that combine high workload demands with low decision making authority.

In another study of job strain in health professionals (84% female), Quine (1998) found that staff in high strain jobs (high demands and low control) had the highest levels of job-induced stress. However, those who perceived a high level of social support had lower levels of job-induced stress, anxiety, depression, sickness, absence, and propensity to leave nursing. The most important sources of support were family and friends first, and then colleagues at work. Epel, McEwen, and Ickovics (1998) studied a group of women exposed to repeated stressors. Those who viewed the situation as a challenge instead of a threat did not secrete cortisol for as long as those who viewed the situation as a threat.

In some people, chronic stress, or the perception of events as stressful for long periods of time, can lead to *burnout*, a depletion of emotional resources. Burnout is typically defined as a syndrome of three factors: emotional exhaustion, depersonalization, and a reduced sense of personal accomplishment. Emotional exhaustion is when you feel emotionally over-extended and drained by contact with other people. Depersonalization is when you have a callous response toward people who are the recipients of your care. Reduced personal accomplishment is when you feel less competent in working with people (Leiter and Maslach, 1988). Burnout usually occurs among individuals who work in critical or conflicting situations and/or have an intense commitment to human beings as part of their work. Many consider emotional exhaustion to be the most influential part of burnout, and suggest that it leads to depersonalization, which is used as a coping device. Finally, feelings of reduced personal accomplishment occur (Payne, 2001).

A telling sign of burnout is that people do not realize it is happening, and deny that they are feeling burned out. Nurses are particularly susceptible to burnout because the job is emotionally demanding and stressful, and they are repeatedly confronted with people's needs, problems, and suffering (Bakker, 2000).

When someone is "burned out," physical, mental, and emotional symptoms manifest. Physical symptoms include headaches, digestive and sleeping problems, and colds of long duration. Irritability, fatigue, frustration, and a feeling of burden at the slightest strain are mental/emotional symptoms. People become cynical, meaning they take a cold, distant attitude toward work and people at work. Gradually these symptoms increase until they control feelings and actions. The personality changes. We become less open to change and new ideas, often leading to a negative view of ourselves, our work, colleagues, and clients (Leiter and Maslach, 1988).

After much research in the area of burnout, Maslach and Leiter (1997) suggest that most work situations today expect the employee to do more than they possibly can for less money than they need, and deserve. People feel overworked, not in control of job or self, and not valued as a person or appreciated for the effort given. This leads not only to the physical and mental symptoms mentioned above, but it begins to affect a person's spirit. People begin to feel ineffective, and so inadequate. They lose confidence in themselves and everything seems overwhelming. People have exhaustion that is as bad upon awakening as when they went to bed, and they are unable to unwind. I have heard many nurses sadly say they are feeling this way about work, clients, and themselves. Nurses who have been working for decades are thinking of quitting.

Many studies have attempted to discover some of the causes of burnout. Research looking at nurses in hospital settings found that burnout is more likely to occur when the nurse experiences: (1) decreased direct client contact (Kennedy and Grey, 1997); (2) poor quality of work content and low support from colleagues (Janssen, de Jonge, and Bakker, 1999); (3) decreased opportunities to care for a client's well-being and lack of effective communication with clients (Omdahl and O'Donnell, 1999); and (4) perceived imbalance of giving and receiving (Bakker, 2000).

Not all nurses respond to stress by becoming burned out. This suggests that effective coping skills may reduce the chances of burnout (Payne, 2001). As the studies above suggest, the way a nurse interprets or appraises an event plays a large role in how much stress she feels. Strategies to help the nurse appraise potentially stressful situations in positive ways decrease stress and burnout (Antai-Otong, 2001; Payne, 2001). See Chapter 10 for suggestions on how to change what you think and feel in stressful situations. Self-renewal activities help us view stressful situations in a different way. These activities are the core of stress management, and include physical, mental, social and spiritual activities. Physically renewing activities promote a sense of emotional as well as physical well-being, and increase energy. Spiritually renewing activities provide a sense of purpose and meaning in life (Antai Otong, 2001). Both the giving and receiving of massage are self-renewal activities that affect physical, emotional, social, and spiritual well-being. In addition, there is hardly any other profession more suited for promoting the benefits of massage and touch for stress and burnout.

Giving Massage is Good for the Nurse

Giving, in general, seems to benefit our health. Ornish (1998) suggests that people are hardwired to help each other. Research suggests that giving to others reduces mortality (House, Landis, and Umberson, 1988), elicits the relaxation response (Ott and Mulloney, 1998), and enhances immune function (Quinn and Strelkauskas, 1993).

Research suggests that giving massage can be even more beneficial than receiving it (Field, Hernandez-Reif, Quintino, et al., 1997). Depression, self esteem, and immune function (cortisol) were measured in a group of elderly people after receiving massage for a month, and then again after they gave massage to others for another month. All scores improved after giving and receiving the massage, but the scores were even greater after the month of giving the massage than they were after the month of receiving it.

Now let's recall the above discussion of possible causes of burnout in nursing and look at how giving massage may help to prevent it. Recall that Kennedy and Grey (1997) found that the more direct contact there was with clients, the less stress and burnout the nurse experienced. There were no differences in levels of distress, burnout, or coping strategies between work settings, indicating that it was neither the type of client nor the work setting that made the difference. One reason direct patient contact was the most satisfying part of their work was because it had immediate reward. Giving a massage is an excellent way to increase direct contact with clients.

Janssen, de Jonge, and Bakker (1999) found that high quality of work content increased intrinsic motivation (the degree to which a person wants to do a good job for internal satisfaction). Quality of work content means that the job is challenging and worthwhile, and provides a variety of tasks to perform, performance feedback, task significance, and opportunities to be creative. The greater the quality of work content the less people considered leaving the job. When you give a massage, you will have no doubt that it is worthwhile because you get immediate positive feedback. It also creates variety in your options for intervention. Higher levels of emotional exhaustion (burnout) were reported with low social support from colleagues. A short shoulder massage is a great way to support a colleague. Unrealized career expectations created higher levels of burnout and greater intention to leave nursing. For many nurses, one of the greatest career expectations is to be able to directly help people feel better. Each time you give even a one-minute massage, it is clear that you have helped your client. So giving massage may increase the quality of work content so that career expectations are better met. There may then be a greater desire to stay in nursing.

Omdahl and O'Donnell (1999) found that when nurses experienced emotional contagion (sharing the client's emotions) they were more likely to get burned out. When they felt empathic concern (being concerned for, or caring about, the client), and communicative effectiveness, fewer experienced burnout. They suggested that increasing the nurse's ability to care for the client's well-being (empathic concern) and engage in effective communication about sensitive topics (communicative effectiveness), should reduce the extent to which nurses experience the burnout symptom of depersonalizing patients, and should also enhance the sense of personal accomplishment that nurses feel. Massage is a way to increase the nurse's ability to care for the client's well-being (empathic concern) and can create a greater feeling of openness to encourage communication about sensitive issues (communicative effectiveness).

Recall that when nurses are burned out they feel ineffective, inadequate, and helpless to affect change in their environment (reduced personal accomplishment). After the nurse gives a massage, the receiver will almost always assure the nurse that she is indeed very effective at helping him, which will increase her sense of confidence and help her feel valued. Recall that one of the greatest stressors leading to burnout is the nurse's feeling that she has little control or choice in her practice. Having massage as a tool she can use in myriad situations helps the nurse feel like she has more control, realizing that at any time, she can choose to affect a great change in her environment. By giving clients a massage, she can change the way they respond to her, which changes the way she views her work experience.

Finally, a very important, but little discussed point: nurses need to receive from clients. Interpersonal exchanges trigger burnout when there is not an equal giving and receiving (Schaufeli, Van Dierendonck, and Van Gorp, 1996), and can lead to autonomic nervous system arousal, including the stress response (Siegrist et al., 1990; Siegrist, 1996). Recall Bakker's study (2000) about effort-reward imbalance. When nurses felt that they gave (effort) more than they received (reward), they were more likely to experience stress and burnout. There is a general sentiment that nurses are the givers and should not expect to receive from clients. However, giving and receiving is a circle. One can't be sustained for long unless the other is also present. Few people would ever consider doing some of

---

Burnout and Prevention

Causes of Burnout:
1. Having high job demands and feeling little control or choice over the situation
2. Decreased direct contact with clients
3. Decreased quality of work content
4. Unrealized career expectations
5. Low social support
6. Sharing client's negative emotions
7. Feeling like you give more than you receive

Ways to prevent burnout:
1. Learn ways to have more choice and to feel more in control
2. Increase direct contact with clients that is positive and rewarding
3. Increase quality of work content (which includes increased variety of skills, more feedback for performance, tasks that are significant, and ways to be creative)
4. Increase positive connection with colleagues and family
5. Increase ways to care about clients and have more effective communication
6. Feeling like there is a balance in what you receive and what you give

Massage addresses all of these concerns.

the nursing tasks involved in taking care of clients who are extremely ill. Money alone could never be enough of a reward to do what a nurse does. When a client squeezes your hand with tears in her eyes after you give her a warm face cloth, and says, "Thank you so much," it makes it all worth it. Those kinds of experiences don't usually come after an injection or inserting an IV. Perhaps as we spend less and less time with clients, we lose the opportunity to receive from them that precious gift of appreciation and gratitude. For most of us, to feel fulfilled in life, especially in a profession as stressful as nursing, there must be a circle of giving and receiving.

Massage introduces an opportunity for the nurse to help the client feel physically at ease and emotionally close to someone at a most trying time in their life. They express their appreciation with looks, words, touches, and tears. They are forever grateful. The giving and receiving circle is once again complete.

Receiving Massage Benefits the Nurse

From our discussion so far, it is probably evident that a nurse could benefit by receiving a massage. By the end of the day, and certainly the end of the week, legs hurt, feet hurt, and very often shoulders, neck, and back are painful. Neck pain often leads to headaches, irritability, and sleeping problems. You deserve something that feels absolutely wonderful, and improves your health and well-being at the same time. There is nothing we have found that is as effective at softening tight muscles and releasing emotional strain as receiving a massage. It is a self-renewal activity that reduces stress and so helps to prevent burnout.

Massage is different from many methods of relaxation because you don't have to do a thing. You can completely let go and let someone else help you relax. Many people think massage is just a luxury. If you have never received one, do yourself a huge favor and get one. The world looks very different after a massage. It is easier to entertain new points of view. A one-minute shoulder rub from a colleague in the break room changes your day. A one-hour massage by a professional or caring friend each month can change your life.

When you receive your massage, your clients also benefit. How could you describe the beauty of a rainbow to someone who has never been able to see? It is the same with massage. It cannot be described in words. Only after receiving a good massage can you truly realize how much your clients would benefit from receiving even two minutes. The experience of massage also affects how you are able to be with your clients. There is much research in the nursing literature about nursing presence and how much it affects the health and well-being of the client and the nurse (Fredriksson, 1999; Easter, 2000; Godkin, 2001). Presence is discussed in greater detail in Part III. Very simply defined, presence is "being there" for the client, including communication and task-oriented touch. Presence also includes "being with" the client, including caring, two way interaction, and connective touch. When you receive massage, you see life through different eyes, you act differently. You are better able to be present with, and for, clients.

HOW ARE NURSES CURRENTLY INVOLVED IN MASSAGE?

Nurses Using Massage in Their Practices

Nurses are the ideal healthcare professionals to reawaken the use of massage in healthcare settings. Nurses bring to massage their unique blend of the skills of assessment, the knowledge of the structure and function of the body, experience with touching the body in a therapeutic manner, and an awareness of presence. Many nurses agree that the primary focus of nursing today is caring and healing, two components of an effective massage.

Nurses are incorporating massage into their practices in many different ways. Some give excellent massages with only the few hours of training they received in nursing school, some take a continuing education workshop to learn more, and some become licensed massage therapists. As a charge nurse on an adolescent psychiatric unit, Janet Mason was part of a multidisciplinary team that developed policies for safe touch with these clients. The kids were desperate for nonsexual, nonviolent touch. Every client received a 5–10 minute back massage at bedtime. Bedtime became quieter, with fewer interventions needed for handling episodes of "acting out." The teens began asking for massage even during the day (Mason, 1999).

In 1980, the University of Akron College of Nursing in Akron, Ohio, created a Center for Nursing where advanced practice nurses work with underserved populations such as children, older adults, and the homeless. The Center provides primary care and health promotion services to the campus and local community. Since 1996, nurses have been offering massage at the clinic. They formed groups for people with specific problems, such as fibromyalgia, and talked about how massage might be helpful. Annette Mitzel-Wilkinson, an advanced practice nurse and massage therapist, discusses how a nurse can create an independent massage practice within a nursing setting, and how she balances a massage practice at the Center and a full-time teaching load at the college (Mitzel-Wilkinson, 2000).

To give you some additional ideas, Sheryl Monfore, R.N., worked four days a week in a hospital labor and delivery room in Minnesota, had a private massage practice, and ran a massage teaching and consulting business. Andy Bernay-Roman, R.N., helped start the Vital Touch Task Force at St. George's Hospital in Atlanta, Georgia to examine the role of touch in the hospital, provide general information about massage, and train healthcare providers to give various kinds of massage and touch. Jeanne Wagner, R.N., was an independent contractor to four hospitals in

Milwaukee offering massage and lifestyle education to clients. Bobbi Harris, a nurse for 30 years, has had a private massage practice for about 10 years. In 1996, she developed a type of feather-light massage called Caring Touch that she has taught to staff nurses at the Sarasota Memorial Hospital in Florida, as well as to massage therapists, home health aides, and hospice volunteers (Mower, 1997).

There are the untold numbers of nurses who quietly and lovingly massage a foot, back, or neck in the wee hours of the morning on a crowded hospital floor with only two people ever knowing it happened.

Where Nurses Can Learn Massage

We hope, of course, that you will find this book an easy and effective way to learn to give a short massage without ever leaving your home. There are, however, many other ways you can learn massage (see Chapter 8). Courses teaching full body massage and specialized types of bodywork have been developed especially for nurses. See appendix A for more information.

Continuing education classes are an excellent way for nurses to learn massage. These programs are being offered by hospitals, clinics, nursing schools, and by massage therapists in the community. Continuing education programs in massage should ideally be taught by nurses who use it in their practice. When nurses start massaging each other's shoulders, the room soon fills with laughter and groans of contentment. If you take even a short massage class, you will leave laughing and feeling great, no matter how you came in. If a massage workshop is not offered by your local CE provider, find the nearest one or request that a massage workshop be introduced.

Many nurses choose to attend a massage school and become licensed massage therapists. There are a few schools that are nationally certified, but most are regulated by a state agency. For example, the Texas Department of Health regulates the curricula for massage schools and grants licensure. Nurses often receive credit for applicable courses from nursing school and CE workshops they have taken. If you are interested in becoming a licensed massage therapist, check with the regulating body in your state, which can be found through the American Massage and Therapy Association.

Legal Considerations of Practicing Massage

The American Nurses Association has no position statement on massage in nursing. The legality of a nurse doing massage is different in each state, so check with your Board of Nurse Examiners. Since massage has always been part of nursing, as long as the nurse is functioning within her role as a nurse, massage is usually considered to be within the legal scope of practice. In most states, massage is considered an independent nursing intervention as long as the nurse feels competent, meaning that the nurse can determine which clients to give it to without an order from a physician. (See indications and contraindications in Chapter 3.) This is the case with nurses practicing many integrative therapies. The nursing profession is unique in that we can create many roles for ourselves within healthcare settings or in private practice, offering and teaching disease prevention and health promotion strategies. In most states, there are massage therapy laws that cover licensed massage therapists, so the nurse cannot call herself a massage therapist unless she has fulfilled the massage therapy requirements for that state.

Hospital-based Massage Programs

Massage is of such benefit that more and more hospitals are developing programs where inpatients, outpatients, and the community come to receive massage. The Heart Hospital in Austin, Texas, makes massage therapy available to clients. Columbia-Presbyterian Medical Center in New York has the Columbia Integrative Medicine Program headed by cardiologist, Dr. Mehmet Oz. The hosptial employs a full-time licensed massage therapist who gives free chair massage to the staff and offers massage, reflexology, acupressure, guided imagery tapes, and yoga classes for the clients. Memorial Sloan Kettering's Integrative Medicine Service offers massage for clients in the hospital and has an outpatient service.

Many nurses have initiated massage programs in the hospital setting. Michelle Bowman, R.N., (2001) is the head of one of the most successful hospital-based massage programs to date and is the Program Manager of Complementary Care at Longmont United Hospital in Colorado. They have 17 massage therapists on staff, with one nurse massage therapist. At the hospital's outreach clinic, they provide 400 massages each month. They provide massage for every mom who delivers a baby at the hospital. They also provide massage for clients at their Cancer Care center, and to hospital inpatients upon their request. Massage does not require a physician's order.

Allegheny Hospital in Pittsburgh, PA, combines integrative medicine and Western medicine to find what they feel is the best treatment for their clients. Kathleen Krebs, R.N., is the program development manager of the integrative medicine program. (See Appendix A.) She uses guided imagery and foot massage with the clients she sees in the hospital. The program includes massage, acupuncture, Oriental medicine, an Ayruvedic physician, meditation, Therapeutic Touch, and yoga. There is a physician who specializes in nutrition and wellness lifestyle, and spirituality is a large component of the program as well. Massage is offered for inpatients and outpatients by interns from the community college who are getting an associate degree in massage as part of their curriculum. Massage therapists are also available on a fee for service basis.

Hospitals are required by the Joint Commission on Accreditation and Health Care Organization to provide clients with information about non-pharmacologic pain control. Since pain relief is one of the strongest benefits of massage, a hospital-based massage program could benefit healthcare facilities as well as clients. Hospital massage programs are gradually gaining credibility with administrators. One key factor for stimulating the growth of such programs may be in providing education about the beneficial effects of massage for clients as evidenced by research studies (See Chapter 3).

Another strong point in favor of using massage in the hospital is demonstrating how it can save money in terms of shorter hospital stays and the need for fewer medications. For example, preterm infants who received 15-minute massages three times a day for 10 days while they were in the incubators averaged a 47% weight gain, had greater responsiveness, and were in the hospital 6 days less for a savings of $10,000 per infant (Field, Scafidi, and Schanberg, 1987).

For more information about massage in hospitals, contact The Hospital-Based Massage Network in Fort Collins, Colorado (see appendix A). Since 1995 the network has been "serving the integration of massage into mainstream medicine." Some of its offerings are massage research, listing of successful hospital massage programs around the country, and how to start a massage program in the hospital setting.

Professional Organizations

The interest in massage among nurses became so great that in 1987 the Georgia Association of Nurse Massage Therapists was created. Its original goal was that of creating a network which would increase the awareness of massage in nursing and to sponsor bodywork-related educational programs. The interest grew, and in 1990 the National Association of Nurse Massage Therapists (NANMT) was incorporated. The workshops in their 2001 conference focused on specific massage techniques that nurses could give to different client populations, such as infants and the elderly. One of NANMT's goals is to work with all state boards of nursing, encouraging them to recognize that holistic modalities, including massage, are part of nursing practice. They also want to educate nurses as to the value of massage in all areas of nursing practice and provide information to those who want to learn more massage than they already know. To contact NANMT, see appendix A.

In 1992, NANMT was admitted to The National Federation of Specialty Nursing Organizations. Nurse Massage Therapy is now a specialty practice within professional nursing. The American Massage and Therapy Association (AMTA) is the national organization for massage therapists and has a newsletter and yearly conferences. Each state also has a branch of the AMTA. Either organization can tell you how to find massage schools in your area if you wish to become a massage therapist. To practice massage with clients as a part of your nursing practice, you do not have to be affiliated with a professional organization. However, organized professional networks often provide rich opportunities for making contact with others who share similar interests.

Nursing in the Future, Integrative Health Care, and Massage

As mentioned earlier, the Holistic Health movement began in the 1970s with people wanting healthcare that addressed not only the body, but the mind, emotions, and the spirit. We now discuss this health paradigm shift in greater detail; first, because it is transforming the foundation of healthcare today, not only in the United States but in many areas of the world. And second, because it has dramatically affected the practice of massage. In the future, if nurses are going to continue to be integral members in the healthcare scenario, we must at least be knowledgeable of, and more likely incorporate, holistic philosophy and/or interventions into our daily nursing practice. Massage relaxes the body, mind, and spirit and so is an excellent integrative modality for nurses to use.

HOLISTIC PHILOSOPHY AND NATIONAL TRENDS TOWARD INTEGRATIVE HEALTHCARE

The holistic philosophy of healing involves considering all aspects of a person's internal and external environment that may contribute to his health and being willing to entertain a wide variety of options to help that person heal. It is looking at a person as a beautiful mosaic with each part necessary to the whole, yet the whole is greater than the sum of the parts.

The external environment includes work, home, and school. This environment contains the air we breathe, noise levels, and the water and food we take in. Sources of social support such as pets, religious affiliation, and other relationships are very important. A person's habits of daily living such as sleep, exercise, play, what his stressors are, and how he handles them are part of what creates his health.

We are multifaceted beings with all aspects of ourselves, and our lives, constantly interacting to produce varying degrees of health and illness. When assessing, planning interventions, and evaluating progress, all of these facets must be considered. A practitioner of holistic healthcare looks at all that contributes, or has contributed in the past, to making the client who she is today, and to help her discover and achieve her *unique, desired* level of wellness.

As previously mentioned, over the last 30 years holistic health has been renamed alternative, then complementary, and now integrative health. You may

---

Aspects of the Internal and External Environment

1. All concerns of the physical body, such as pain, tension, organ systems, bones, and muscles
2. The balance and movement of the energetic nature, or energy field, that permeates and surrounds the physical body
3. All aspects of the mind, such as our thoughts and what we tell ourselves
4. The feelings we have, the love in our lives, how we feel in our hearts
5. Our spiritual nature, our connection to God, a Higher Power, Nature, or our Inner Self

(Used with permission. Marsha Walker, © 1996)

---

see all of these labels used interchangeably. This reflects the attitude shift in the public and healthcare community toward the integration of mind, emotions, and spirit into the care of the physical body. It also suggests that these therapies and philosophies are being integrated more and more into Western medicine. Some people define complementary therapies as those that complement and enhance nursing and medical practice, such as massage, guided imagery, and biofeedback. Alternative therapies are often defined as those used instead of Western medicine. Although some make these distinctions, most practitioners of integrative or holistic healthcare believe that all modalities that can benefit the client should be considered, and can complement each other. Each client must be assessed individually, then the perfect combination of integrative and Western modalities is suggested for that person. It is important to keep in mind that a healthcare provider can practice an integrative healthcare modality—such as massage, herbal medicine, and guided imagery—and still not have a holistic philosophy that incorporates all aspects of the person they are caring for. The underlying philosophy is just as important as expertise with the specific modality.

To gain greater insight into the pervasiveness and reality of the current and future changes in healthcare delivery, let's look at some trends. The National Center for Complementary and Alternative Medicine at the National Institutes of Health has a steadily increasing budget for research ($50 million in 1999), and is funding research at ten Centers of Excellence around the country to evaluate the effectiveness of integrative modalities. Each center has a primary focus such as cancer or internal medicine (Giese, 2000).

In a survey on the use of integrative medicine in the United States published in JAMA in 1998, it was stated that 42% of the population used at least one integrative modality within the previous year, which was a significant increase of 9%, $p \leq .001$, since 1990. Most people used these therapies for chronic conditions such as back pain, headaches, depression, and anxiety. There was a 47% increase in total visits to integrative healthcare practitioners in the United States from 1990 to 1997, exceeding total visits to all primary care physicians. Massage therapy ranked third among the most frequently used forms of integrative healthcare, with a significant increase (4.2%) in the number of people using massage from 1990, p ≤.0001. In 1997, people paid as much out of pocket for integrative therapies as they did for primary care physician services (Eisenberg, et al., 1998).

Insurance companies are beginning to respond to public demand. Pelletier, Marie, Krasner, and Haskell (1997) performed a literature review and conducted telephone interviews of 18 insurers and a representative sample of hospitals to assess insurance coverage of integrative therapies and their availability in hospitals. A majority of the insurers offered some kind of coverage for some integrative therapies, and 12 said that market demand was their primary motivation for covering a therapy.

In 1994, the Washington State Insurance Commissioner mandated that every category of integrative healthcare provider be covered in insurance healthcare plans, including acupuncturists, massage therapists, chiropractors, and others. This response is also due to the research evidence of the cost effectiveness of these therapies. In a study of people with chronic pain, participants learned the relaxation response, yoga, communication skills, and how to avoid distressing thoughts. Over the next two years, the savings in medical care was estimated at $45,000 for all 109 participants combined. In a meta-analysis of 191 studies involving various types of surgery, holistic interventions were used, including education, breathing and relaxation, and psychosocial support. There were benefits in 80% of the studies with length of stay decreased by 1.5 days. Finally, in a meta-analysis of studies of childbirth with a doula (a supportive layperson who provides emotional support or comforting presence), Cesarean section rates, length of labor, and use of pain medication, oxytocin, and forceps decreased. Length of stay and complications for mother and baby were also reduced (Sobel, 1995).

INTEGRATIVE HEALTHCARE IN NURSING

A holistic view in nursing is not new. The nursing that Florence Nightingale taught and envisioned was holistic. She emphasized the whole person, including all aspects of their environment, their feelings, and their spiritual essence. Nursing was at the forefront of the Holistic Health Movement. The American Holistic Nurses' Association (AHNA) was founded in 1981 by Charlotte McGuire and a group of nurses "dedicated to bringing the concepts of holism to every arena of nursing practice," defining holism as a state of harmony among body, mind, emotions, and spirit within an ever-changing environment. Nurses all over the country began to remember why they became a nurse in the first place: the love of working directly with people, doing things that helped them feel better. According to the AHNA's website, (August, 2002) their mission is to "unite nurses in healing." Philosophically, the AHNA believes that "nursing is an art and a science and its primary purpose is to nurture others toward the wholeness inherent within them. Disease and distress are opportunities for increased awareness of the interconnectedness of body, mind, and spirit. AHNA is committed to unity and the healing of self, the nursing profession, and the planet." [For contact information, see appendix A.]

In December of 2000, Charlotte Eliopoulous, the president of AHNA, spoke before the White House Commission on Complementary and Alternative Medicine Policy. She emphasized the leadership role that nurses hold in the integration of complementary therapies throughout the healthcare system, and outlined therapies that nurses currently use within the scope of nursing practice. AHNA's position on the role of nurses in the practice of complementary and alternative therapies is:

> Inherent in the nursing role is the ability to touch the client's/patient's body, assess, plan, intervene, evaluate, and perform preventive, supportive, and restorative functions of the physical, emotional, mental, and spiritual domains. Therefore, it is expected that the nurse will draw upon and utilize principles and techniques of both conventional and complementary/alternative therapies, and that these would be within the scope of nursing practice.

Members of AHNA now number in the thousands. Holistic Nursing is not a mere "fringe element" within the profession. All ages, religious beliefs, and nursing specialties are represented. From nursing students and those new to the workplace to some whose time on the evening shift can be measured in decades, nurses are sensing the rise of a new vitality in the field. Many schools of nursing incorporate holistic philosophy and techniques into their curricula. The University of Texas at Galveston offers a Nursing Doctorate in Healing, and Tennessee State University in Nashville offers a Masters Degree in Holistic Nursing.

Beginning in 1995, it became possible to become a Certified Holistic Nurse (HNC). The American Holistic Nurses Certification Corporation (AHNCC) endorses BSN programs that have a curriculum based on holistic principles that prepares students to take the Holistic Nursing Certification Exam. For further information on becoming an HNC, to inquire about getting the nursing curriculum at your school endorsed, and for a list of endorsed schools, see AHNCC in appendix A.

NURSING IN THE FUTURE

Many nurses already incorporate integrative philosophy and modalities into their practices, and many more will in the future, whether they act as referral sources or as practitioners. The national sentiment of a holistic paradigm shift is spreading to nursing as a whole. For example, Giese (2000) was the first to write the new column, Complementary Healthcare Practices, in *Gastroenterology Nursing*. Massage, guided imagery, and relaxation therapy are topics that are planned for the future.

A study of 2,740 registered nurses in Ohio assessed nurses' use of integrative therapies for self and clients. The therapies most commonly used for self were prayer, diet and herbal products, imagery, meditation, and massage, in that order.

Integrative Nursing Modalities of the Future

1. Bodywork—massage, reflexology, acupressure, acupuncture
2. Relaxation techniques—meditation, progressive muscle relaxation, guided imagery, focused breathing, yoga, and the Relaxation Response
3. Energy based therapies—Therapeutic Touch, Healing Touch, Reiki, and Heart Touch
4. Aromatherapy

Nurses most commonly used diet, prayer, imagery, healing touch, and massage with clients. However, their knowledge level about the therapies and how to practice them was low. Schools of nursing and continuing education programs need to address this issue (King, Pettigrew, and Reed, 2000).

Nursing Education in the Future

Health promotion is an area of practice in which nurses must establish themselves as practitioners and role models. Toward this goal, nursing faculty must prepare new graduates for these nontraditional roles (Roberts, 1999). In many universities there are departments of Kinesiology and Health Promotion. In addition to physical education and sports, these departments are teaching physiology and mindbody health. Corporations like 3M and Motorola contact them for student interns to run their wellness programs. If nurses want to be real players in the health promotion, wellness, and integrative healthcare arena, we must make changes in undergraduate and graduate curricula, and encourage changes in nursing practice.

Forty percent of family practice physicians receive some training about integrative therapies in medical school, yet most nurses do not. As of October of 2000, a study of 73 graduate nursing students at the University of North Dakota found that fewer than 25% reported using any integrative healthcare for personal use, and 42.5% said they had no basic understanding of any integrative therapy.

Yet 82% said that it was important for healthcare professionals to understand integrative therapies commonly used by consumers (Melland and Clayburgh, 2000). If nurses want a role as providers of integrative modalities, now is the time to claim that role. "Professional nursing has a choice: we can exclusively align ourselves with Western biomedicine and miss the boat with them, or ride the crest of this new paradigm of inclusive, integrative healthcare, and thrive. Which is it going to be?" (Schroeder and Likkel, 1999).

In *Focusing Care on the Community for the 21st Century*, the Pew Commission challenged teachers of healthcare professionals to incorporate principles of community health, to promote healthy lifestyles, to put more emphasis on prevention, and to pay attention to cultural issues in program curricula. These principles are integral to most systems of integrative healthcare. In 1996, recommendations for incorporating integrative practices into medical and nursing education were issued by an interdisciplinary panel of nurses, physicians, and administrators that assembled at the National Conference on Medical and Nursing Education in Complementary Medicine. The panel recommended that medical and nursing education provide course content that includes philosophical and spiritual paradigms, scientific foundations, and research-based evidence of the effectiveness and safety of integrative practices.

Reed, Pettigrew, and King (2000) believe it is crucial to incorporate information about integrative philosophy and modalities into nursing education in the future for several reasons.

1. As was mentioned previously, about 42% of the American public used at least one integrative modality in 1997. Many of the clients nurses will work with will be using some form of integrative therapy, and nurses need to be at least knowledgeable about them and how they interact with Western medications and treatments.

2. By 2010, there will be an estimated 88% increase in the growth of integrative healthcare practitioners and only a 16% increase in physicians trained in Western medicine. Nurses are very likely to find integrative therapies as part of the healthcare delivery system within their professional careers.

3. Integrative therapies have gained recognition and governmental legitimacy, as evidenced by the creation of the Office of Alternative Medicine at the National Institutes of Health and by the budget for research into the effectiveness of integrative modalities.

4. Integrative healthcare philosophy and/or modalities have been incorporated into 75 of the 125 medical schools as of 1998 (Wetzel, Eisenberg,

and Kaptchuk, 1998). In a survey of 180 family physicians in the United States, 90% said they used some form of integrative medicine in their practices, and 73% said they did in a similar Canadian study.

Reed, Pettigrew and King (2000) recommend that categories of integrative therapies similar to those suggested by the Office of Alternative Medicine be adopted by nursing schools, such as (examples in parentheses): (1) manual healing methods (massage), (2) mindbody techniques (prayer), (3) bioelectromagnetics (magnets), (4) traditional and folk medicine (Ayurveda yoga), (5) diet and nutrition (macrobiotic diet), and (6) herbal medicine. Students must be aware that most clients using integrative therapies do not tell the healthcare provider unless asked. Nurses must therefore inquire so this information can be added to health histories, including number, kind, and frequency of use. Learning certain modalities could be part of the curricula, offered as an elective, or part of a continuing education program. Massage, reflexology, and energy-based therapies, such as Therapeutic Touch and Healing Touch, are excellent nursing interventions. Guided imagery has been very effective in many nursing situations. The beneficial effects of prayer, distant healing, and distant intentionality are new areas that will be relevant to nursing in the near future. Research into these theories and modalities could be encouraged in graduate programs.

Each nurse has her own path to walk, her own lessons to learn, in nursing and in life. You may be interested in all of the above methods, a few, or only one. Integrative principles and modalities will permeate healthcare in the future, and massage will continue to be one of the most sought after modalities. Nurses deserve to maintain and increase their role as promoters of health in this new paradigm. It is time to act.

SUMMARY

Most of us chose nursing as our career because we felt a *calling* to help others heal. A calling beckons us. It is hard to imagine doing anything other than following that call because it so enriches and fulfills us.

We know a couple who is called to grow some of the most beautiful, delicious food we have ever eaten. Each week they deliver a variety of organic vegetables to our door in a basket, hand washed, along wonderful recipes. Their food is healing. Our sister is called to groom dogs, working on "difficult" dogs without using a muzzle. Through her touch and tone of voice, they know they are safe and loved.

We believe giving massage is so rewarding because it addresses the reason many of us became nurses in the first place. We wanted to do something personally, directly, to alleviate suffering and promote peace. What may look like a simple collection of massage techniques can create a softening and opening in client and nurse alike that nurtures healing on many levels. Nurses, more than any other profession, have the opportunity to be wiht people for extended periods of time in their most vulnerable states. It is in these moments, when the mind often surrenders, that healing can happen. Embracing massage, not just as the administering of technique, but recognizing the honor of touching another, illuminates the myster of who and what we really are.

A student once asked the great Indian sage, Nem Karoli Baba, "How can I know God?" He replied, "Serve people."

In this chapter we have mentioned some of the benefits of massage. In the next chapter, we discuss the physical, mental, and emotional benefits in greater detail including findings from current research.

PUTTING THESE IDEAS INTO PRACTICE

1. Ask friends for recommendations of someone who gives massage. Make it a priority to receive at least one massage from them, even if it is only a very short one.

2. Take a few minutes and think about two situations in your personal life and two in your professional life where you believe giving a massage would make a difference.

3. Practice creating an intention. Choose a client, family member, friend, pet, or plant and set aside one to five minutes to be with them. Before you enter the room where they are, take a moment to think about what you intend the interaction to be like. It may include touching, talking, or just being together in the same room. Include in your intention how you want to feel toward them. You might think about what you want to say, and how you want to say it. Then think about how you want both of you to feel as you are ending your interaction.

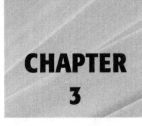

CHAPTER 3

The Physical, Mental, and Emotional Benefits of Massage: Direct Experience and Research Studies

The time that I feel most content and physically good, and able to be loving and focused is after I've had a massage.

—M.C., mother, wife, works two jobs

OBJECTIVES

1. List one physical, one mental, and one emotional benefit of massage.

2. Discuss possible causes of muscular tension and pain, and the ways in which massage can help relieve these conditions.

3. Discuss how massage can lead to increased mental clarity and creativity.

4. Describe ways in which massage contributes to feelings of greater acceptance of self and others.

5. Describe how massage is a mindbody intervention that interrupts the stress response.

6. Apply the findings of two research studies on massage to your area of practice or to a situation in your life.

As we learned in Chapter 2, people have been benefiting from massage for thousands of years. If you have ever had a massage, you know it's good for you. You feel relaxed physically, mentally, and emotionally. Considering that about 90% of all illnesses are thought to be stress related, anything that brings about relaxation is very valuable. Why does massage create relaxation, and does it have any other benefits for the body or mind? There are several ways to find these answers. One is by direct experience. When we learn by direct experience, there is no question as to what we did and what the results were. The very best way to learn about the benefits of massage, in our opinion, is to receive a massage yourself and get first-hand experience. We also learn directly by observing our life experience. You can massage others and observe the effects, listen to their spontaneous comments, and ask how they feel. A second way to find these answers is to read about or conduct research that explores the effects of massage under controlled conditions. One advantage of examining the findings of research is that you can learn about the effects of massage for certain conditions with groups of people that you may not be able to work with directly.

The first part of this chapter discusses our direct experiences of the physical, mental, and emotional benefits of massage over the last 25 years. These experiences come from what we observe and hear from clients, and how we feel both during and after receiving a massage. The second half of the chapter discusses early and current research studies on the effects of massage with specific age groups and disease conditions.

MASSAGE IS PREVENTIVE

Healthcare is focusing more and more on prevention of disease and promotion of health. The first and foremost benefit of massage, in our opinion, is that it can prevent problems from occurring. Although massage does an excellent job addressing current problems, it is always best to prevent them from ever happening. If a person gets a massage on a regular basis, even if there is no obvious pain, tension doesn't build up in the first place. Most of us have had the experience of doing something simple like bending over to pick up a piece of paper and suddenly feeling pain in the back. The body can carry much tension before the brain registers a pain signal. Muscles get tighter and tighter, and we don't even know it. Finally, one small action pushes the muscle over the edge, and we feel the pain. With a massage as infrequently as once a month, tension is prevented from building up. The body is better able to handle unexpected demands without going into spasm.

Secondly, if a person receives a massage at the first sign of discomfort, such as a slight headache or a twinge of muscle pain, it often prevents a more debilitating scenario from developing. This is especially true if there has been an accident or injury. What starts as a simple muscle strain from an accident, too many hours at the computer, or carrying a baby around for a weekend can spread to other areas. Because our muscles and nerves are so interconnected, tension between the shoulder blades, if left uncared for, can lead to breathing difficulty, a spasm in the lower back, or tension in the neck muscles. Tight muscles in the neck can lead to headaches, numbness in the hands, or tingling in the face. As we will see in the pages that follow, physical, mental, and emotional tension are all connected. If you know you are headed for a stressful time, or if a client is feeling especially anxious, a massage may prevent physical problems from arising as a result of stress.

PHYSICAL BENEFITS OF MASSAGE

Most people seek out massage because of a physical discomfort. They are pleasantly surprised when they feel relief of mental and emotional tension as well. Some of the physical effects of massage you observe, or feel with your hands, as you give a massage. Your clients are also quick to tell you about benefits they are receiving because they feel such relief. These are the physical effects of massage we most often see:

- Increased circulation of the blood and lymph
- Relief of pain and tension
- Improved sleep
- Relief of constipation

Increased Circulation of the Blood and Lymph

Massage stimulates the flow of the circulatory system, which consists of the blood vessels and the network of lymph vessels (Yates, 1989; Fritz, 1995). The evidence of increased circulation that we see is that the client's cheeks are rosy even when you don't massage the face. Their bladder often calls them to the bathroom during or immediately after the massage. We notice that the area being massaged is often redder than the surrounding tissue. When working on the neck, which is the site of many lymph nodes, clients often say they suddenly taste a bitter taste, which is caused by the movement of fluid from the nodes. Lymph nodes that are firm and enlarged often become noticeably softer after the area is massaged.

Why is increased circulation beneficial? The lymph network is part of the immune system and acts as a filter for the fluid in the body. Fluid from the blood passes into the lymph vessels and travels through the lymph nodes, which destroy abnormal cells, bacteria, pollutants, and other toxins. Since massage stimulates the movement of the fluid through the lymph vessels, it assists in this cleansing process. Immune function and overall health improves. The blood carries nutrients from the intestines and oxygen from the lungs to every cell in the body. The cells use the nutrients and oxygen for energy to do their work. The blood stream also carries off the waste products that the cells produce as they do their work, as well as toxins collected throughout the body, to the kidneys, intestines, lungs, and skin to be eliminated. With the increased supplies of oxygen and nutrients, and improved elimination of waste, cells function optimally, and people feel an overall increase in their energy level. The body and mind function more efficiently. Many of the clients a nurse works with will have some problem with the cardiovascular or immune systems, making massage a valuable tool.

When we don't move our bodies, its various functions decline. Because of the stimulation of circulation, massage is excellent for people who can't move very much due to either injury, illness, or debilitation. Massage is not a substitute for exercise, but it can keep the muscles stimulated and flexible, promote the return of venous blood to the heart, and enhance the flow of lymph. Some have voiced concern that massage, like exercise, increases circulation and energy demands and is too strenuous for people who are extremely ill or have acute cardiovascular problems. In a study of clients in an intensive care unit, when the massage was short, 1–5 minutes, and there was time to rest between activities, such as turning and suctioning, massage was considered to be beneficial, contributing to feelings of comfort and relaxation (Tyler, Winslow, Clark, and White, 1990).

Massage also increases blood flow to the specific areas being worked on. Massage to the muscles on either side of a joint can increase the removal of particulate matter in the joint area and decrease swelling. This is helpful for people with arthritis and other joint problems. After periods of extensive exercise, massage strokes applied to fatigued muscles can help shorten the amount of time needed for those muscles to recover. When the blood supply is increased to the skin, it becomes healthier and more supple. This is especially helpful for clients with dry skin. Increased blood flow to an area also helps relieve tightness and pain in that area.

Relief of Pain and Tension

An experience of pain is what brings many people to healthcare settings. Relief of tension and pain is perhaps the most popular benefit of massage. Areas in the muscles that feel like hard pebbles, or sometimes slabs of rock, literally soften and seem to melt away as you massage them. After massaging face muscles, the release of tension makes a person look like they just had 12 hours of great sleep. Worry lines soften, and the face looks years younger. There is often an almost childlike quality, with their eyes just a little bit brighter than a few minutes before. As shoulders relax, they become more even, if one was higher before you began. Headaches often disappear as neck muscles relax. Intestines relax and start to gurgle as lower back muscles release. You know a person is really relaxed when their voice is several decibels lower than normal.

Relief of Headaches

I have had headaches for 20 years. Every day I have to take 10–12 pills. I'm always dazed, and I can't get out or get anything done because I'm afraid of the pain. I am an artist and haven't been able to paint. I've tried everything. I went to a neurologist and had an MRI. I tried acupuncture. It was so bad, they were afraid that there was something wrong with my brain. There was nothing wrong. The neurologist told me he has seen 5,000 people, and only four others were as bad as me. He gave me antidepressant pills. I've tried everything really and nothing worked.

But since I had the massage, from the first time, the pain was less. The second time it was better. The third time, I took only two Advil, and I used to take something with codeine and all this heavy stuff. Every time it's getting better. I've done it only six times, and it's nearly gone.

I think it's a miracle. My husband thinks that it is a miracle.

—May H.

When people get a massage shortly after an acute situation, such as an accident or injury, massage very often greatly reduces or eliminates pain due to muscle strain. We have both found it especially helpful for "whiplash." Even chronic pain that people have had for a long time usually feels much better after only one massage. Some physical discomfort may be so long-standing that it has become hidden from conscious awareness. During a massage, people often say, "I didn't even know that area was painful until you started working on it." This is one good reason to offer a massage even if the client is not aware of any pain.

The back, shoulders, and neck are natural gathering places for muscular tension. Most people who seek out massage for the relief of discomfort have tightness, soreness, or pain in one or all of these areas. Discomfort in these areas may increase during periods of heightened physical, mental, or emotional stress, which is often experienced by clients and nurses alike.

People frequently ask, "What causes pain and tightness in my muscles?" Some people have muscle tension from an injury, lifting something that is too heavy, or from excessive or unusual exercise. We usually are aware of these causes, and they are not the remain reason people have muscle tension.

Most people have muscle tension for reasons they don't realize because there was no obvious acute situation. Most of our modern occupations require us to either stand or sit for long periods of time without stretching or changing positions. Muscles are made to move. When they move, they stay soft and pain free. If the muscles have to hold the arms, back, or any part of the body still in one position for long periods of time, they send a pain signal to wake us up. If you wonder why a muscle is hurting, first ask yourself, "What have I been doing for long periods that involves this muscle?" The spine is designed to support the head when the head is held directly over the spine. The head is very heavy, weighing 11 to 14 pounds. When the head is directly over the spine, the muscles easily help to balance the head. If we hold the head to the side or tilted forward for long periods, the muscles are not moving. They must support the head in a way they were not meant to, and become tight and sore. Activities that we don't realize cause problems include holding the phone with one shoulder while we write or long hours of computer work. A stiff neck can be caused by leaning slightly toward the light while reading in bed. Neck and shoulder tension can also be caused from carrying a shoulder purse on one shoulder all the time. When you switch your purse to the other shoulder, doesn't it fall off for awhile? The new shoulder has to learn to be tight to hold your purse on. This constant tension contributes to headaches, neck aches, and shoulder pain. If our posture is such that the chin juts out and the shoulders slump forward, the muscles of the upper back and neck have to do

Relief of Neck Pain

Back in 1994, I started experiencing pain that was shooting down my left arm and into two of my fingers. It just kept getting more and more uncomfortable, and there would be numbness. I got really concerned, so I went to my doctor and he referred me to a neurosurgeon. I got an x-ray and MRI. He told me that I had a compressed disc and it looked like it was degenerating.

He proceeded to tell me that he recommended surgery. I said, "What kind of surgery are you talking about?" He said, "Well, I would be making an incision in the front of your neck and going through to get the disc that I need to take out, and then I would take a piece of your hip bone and fuse it in between the other two disks." I was going through a divorce at the time and was very stressed. I had started a new job, and I was just devastated, especially when he said I would probably be off work for three months. I said, "Well, let me just stop you right here." I felt that if I went through with the surgery, I would die on his table. I started getting massage once a week. I think it was only after four weeks that both the shooting pain and the numbness were gone. Every time after a massage, I always felt relief, comfort, and peace. It's been seven years, and I never had the surgery. I have gotten a massage every month as a preventive measure because I feel so much better. In my opinion, the insurance companies need to look into it, because I'm sure that the surgery that he was recommending would have been thousands of dollars. For essentially $200, the problem was taken care of.

—Kathy H.

work they are not designed to, creating chronic tension. If a person spends long hours in a chair or bed without moving around much, or in an uncomfortable position, muscular tension can develop.

The neck, shoulders, and lower back areas are integral to our everyday functioning. We realize this when we get a really bad crick in the neck or a severe low back spasm. What we physically do, along with the mental stress we often experience, contributes to the epidemic of pain in the neck, shoulders, and back that we see in ourselves and the people around us. Many of us have come to accept this kind of discomfort as "normal," or a sign that we are "getting old," when all we may need to do is move our bodies more, and try a massage.

People also ask, "How does massage relieve the pain and tightness?" There are several possible ways. First, when a muscle is strained from injury, such as picking something up that is too heavy, or from prolonged contraction, as in hours of computer use, a pain–spasm–pain cycle can begin. As the muscle stays contracted it burns more oxygen, and more waste products (lactic acid) are produced. With the contraction, the blood vessels in the area become constricted so the muscle doesn't get enough blood supply. This leads to decreased oxygen and nutrients, which leads to further contraction. Lactic acid levels build which irritate nerves. The tightened muscle also begins to put pressure on surrounding nerves creating pain, numbness, and tingling. Soon the muscle can't respond to nerve impulses coming to it and

---

Two Quick Tips for Relaxing the Neck and Shoulders

1. Imagine a string attached to your head that is being pulled up slowly. Allow the head and spine to rise up, with the shoulders falling. This creates balanced posture with the head over the spine, rib cage lifted, and muscles relaxed. Breathing is easier.

2. Have you ever noticed that your shoulders creep up toward your ears? Most of us hold tension in the upper shoulders for no real reason. Over time, headaches and shoulder and neck pain develop. Take a moment now and tighten your upper shoulders, drawing the shoulders up toward your ears as far as you can. Inhale deeply and hold this "shrugging" position for about two seconds. Now, exhale and let go of your shoulders and arms completely, allowing them to drop as far as they will go. Try it again. Aren't your shoulders lower and more relaxed than before?

As an experiment, try this shrug and release three or four times every day for the next two days. It is often helpful to set your watch to beep every hour at first, and shrug and release when it beeps. You can use this technique while working at your desk, driving in your car, or whenever you feel tense. If you include it as part of your daily routine, it can prevent tension buildup in the neck/head/shoulder area.

instructing it to move (Beck, 1994). Massage increases circulation to the area, carrying off lactic acid, and supplying additional oxygen and nutrients. The muscle relaxes, nerve function returns to normal, and pain is relieved.

Secondly, massage increases serotonin levels in infants (Field, Grizzle, Scafidi, Abrams, and Richardson, 1996) and adults (Ironson, et al., 1996). Serotonin is a chemical secreted in the brain that may interfere with the transmission of pain signals to the brain. Massage may also relieve pain due to the gate theory (Melzack and Wall, 1965). Because of the structure of the nerve fibers for pressure, cold, and pain, the signals for pressure and cold reach the brain before the pain signals. A gate is closed, and the pain signals are not processed. Massage provides the pressure that closes the gate. So it seems that massage helps to decrease the pain while it is healing and relaxing the muscle.

Improved Sleep

Massage is almost magical for putting people to sleep. Some people are snoring within five minutes, and sleep through the entire massage. Some people sleep for 5–10 minutes, and wake up saying they feel like they had a full night's sleep. At least 75% of the people we massage fall asleep for some period of time during the massage.

Sleep is the first thing most of us cut out when we have a lot to do. We think we can get by on a few hours. Have you noticed that there is a big difference between the amount of sleep it takes to simply function through the day, and how much it takes to be creative and enjoy life? Most of us need eight hours of sleep a night to operate at our full potential, and almost two-thirds of adult Americans get fewer than that.

Why is sleep so important? At night while the thinking part of us is taking a break, the entire body repairs itself, especially the immune system. This is why if we don't get enough sleep for awhile we tend to get sick more easily. We also store into memory what we learned during the day. Have you noticed that if you don't get enough sleep, it's harder to remember things? If our sleep is not long enough or we wake up repeatedly, we secrete less growth hormone. Decreased growth hormone causes decreased muscle strength, increased fat, and increased aging. Partial sleep loss for one night results in higher stress hormones (cortisol) the next night. Cortisol lowers overall immune function. Levels of natural killer cells decrease, and these cells destroy cancer cells. With reduced sleep for long periods, we even begin to lose control of our body temperature and metabolic functions (Sobel and Ornstein, 1999).

Very often clients in hospitals can't get to sleep or stay asleep due to tension in the muscles or the mind. Worrying can keep us awake as surely as a crick in the

The Magic of a Foot Massage

Lou is a wonderful nurse who works in outpatient surgery and has been lovingly caring for clients for over 35 years.

"I walked onto my shift the other day and the nurses immediately came up to me, telling me about this lady who was having problems with pain. The nurses always come get me when nothing else works, and ask me to do my magic. I went to talk to the lady. She had had surgery, and the pain medications were not helping her. I asked her if I could try some energy work and foot massage. She said she didn't care. She hadn't slept and felt like she was losing her mind. Her husband was there, and I told him I might be doing things that looked a little strange. He said, 'whatever helps.' My other patients had gone home so I had some extra time. I decided to time how long it took to get her comfortable, so I looked at my watch. I decided to start with her feet. I asked her to go to her favorite, relaxing spot. She said the pain was so great she couldn't even think of a spot. I began rubbing one foot. After one minute I asked her how she felt. She said she was beginning to be able to breathe comfortably. I moved to the other foot. Her husband tapped me on the shoulder. I looked up, and she was asleep. I looked at my watch. It had been three minutes. She slept for a few hours and woke up without pain."

neck. Massage relaxes the muscles and slows the thought train down so we can fall asleep more easily and have a deep, uninterrupted night's sleep. As early as 1900, neurologists used massage for its "tonic and sedative effects to bring about the rest cure" (Scull, 1945).

Massage is very relaxing and pleasurable when applied to the soles of the feet. This is especially true for nurses or anyone who stands on their feet or walks for extended periods of time in their work. If you have a minute or two before bedtime, and a willing friend, a foot massage can send you right off to sleep.

Relief of Constipation

One of my clients is 90 and has had many abdominal surgeries. She has had chronic constipation for years. She no longer feels very steady on her feet, and so doesn't move around much. I massage her abdomen from the lower right corner, toward the head, across the middle, and down the left side, making circular movements or long pulling strokes, with light to moderate pressure. She says that frequently after her massage, she experiences welcome relief.

Clients in healthcare settings often experience constipation as a result of immobility, surgery, and medications. It can also occur if a person is stressed and the intestines become tense. The body eliminates the waste byproducts of digestion, abnormal cells, and toxins we take in—such as pesticides—through the large intestine. If elimination is impaired, various conditions may result, including low energy, arthritis, sinus conditions, skin conditions, and forms of cancer. Massaging the abdomen can also increase elimination by relaxing the intestines and encouraging their natural movement (peristalsis).

In summary, these effects of massage work together to improve physical well-being. Increased circulation of the blood helps to relax the muscles, relieving pain and tension by carrying away lactic and uric acid and bringing fresh oxygen and nutrients to the cells. As muscles in the back and abdomen relax, the intestines move more freely. When the intestines move regularly, tension in leg muscles and the lower back decreases. Relief of pain and tension contributes to a deeper, more restful sleep. As we sleep better, we have decreased sensations of pain. As muscles relax, circulation increases.

MENTAL BENEFITS OF MASSAGE

Most of us have a life that is filled with many details to keep track of. We not only manage our own schedules, but those of our children and family members. Most jobs are filled with more than we can possibly accomplish within the allotted time. Have you ever walked into a room and forgotten why you were there? The mind and brain are ideally suited for the task of managing details, however, they can only handle so much.

Remember your favorite vacation? Your attention was probably on something new, something you don't usually think about. You may have found yourself viewing life in new ways. You may have even noticed your mind slowing down, letting the details slip away. Massage gives us a mental vacation. Some of the benefits of this "mental vacation" are:

- Re-direction of attention
- Relaxed mental focus
- Increased mental clarity, alertness, and creativity
- Modeling mental tranquillity

Re-direction of Attention

Have you ever been intensely engaged in an activity, maybe a conversation with someone or reading a book, and someone comes up and touches you? Touch instantly redirects your attention. It changes the content of your thoughts.

The brain is designed to think. It is very difficult to stop thinking about something. Instead, we must fill our attention with something else. Massage redirects our attention onto something very slow, relaxing, and physical. It is often very difficult for clients to stop worrying about the state of their health or an upcoming procedure. Massage breaks persistent thought patterns, clearing an open space for new ways of thinking to emerge. In most cases, the world of random or worried thinking easily gives way as the mind is filled with the sensations of the muscles being stroked and kneaded. There is nothing to do, nothing to remember, and nothing to worry about.

A one minute shoulder massage between colleagues creates this mental break for nurses. Shortly after the massage begins, conversation usually stops, or takes a very different focus. This re-direction of attention is very important for everyone from time to time, especially those under continual stress. An intentional change of focus improves the health of the body and mind in many ways. (See Chapters 9 and 10 for more information.)

Relaxed Mental Focus

When we have tension or pain in our bodies, our attention is divided, making it difficult to focus on what we're doing. It's easy to become distracted and hard to maintain focused concentration for long periods. When we are mentally stressed, we also tend to have a more narrow view of whatever situation we are in.

During a massage, as our attention is directed into a slower, relaxed rhythm, our mental view releases and expands. We focus with a softer, more open perspective. The act of focusing itself comes more easily. Some people use their time receiving massage to contemplate challenges in their life. As muscle tension and pain dissolve, we can better bring our full attention to the challenges we have to face, and the problems we must solve. Improved concentration enhances our problem-solving abilities. Any activity we happen to engage in can more easily fill our entire attention and receive the benefit of a more open point of view. Some people prefer to wait to think until the massage is over, and they carry this relaxed mental focus into their next activity.

Increased Alertness, Mental Clarity, and Creativity

Mental stress and tension require energy. Have you ever felt like you had to go to bed after working on the computer for hours, even though you didn't move a muscle? When the mind is stressed, we often feel exhausted, mentally foggy, or like we're in a daze. During a massage, as our focus becomes more relaxed, this mental tension releases. Energy levels increase, the fog lifts, and we are more mentally alert.

As we relax and the mental chatter decreases, there is an empty peacefulness. Distractions are gone. In this stillness it is easier to think clearly. From the stillness, we are able to bring about something new, to create, and be innovative. Completely new ideas from within us rise to conscious awareness. One client, an author and lecturer, said she always got at least two million-dollar ideas with every massage she received. A calm, clear frame of mind also enhances our rational, strategizing skills and brings a greater likelihood of success in whatever we do. The mind is more able to analyze and combine information in unique ways. When the mind is clear, it is easier to have a positive shift in perspective on ourselves and on life.

Nurses and clients alike benefit from the shift of perspective that relaxed focus and increased clarity bring. Nurses continually need to be mentally alert and creative in their moment to moment work scenario. Clients whose health is compromised are often mentally stressed. It is difficult for them to focus for long enough, and with an open view, to be able to effectively problem solve. You may have more success helping your clients create strategies that will best meet their needs if you give them a short massage before your problem-solving session.

Modeling Mental Tranquillity

After I have been sitting at the computer for hours, I sometimes begin to notice that what I'm writing no longer makes sense. I remember how it feels to have someone take their palm and slowly iron out the kinks from my lower back to my shoulders. My thoughts shift to how I felt lying on the massage table, and I get a mental break. After a few minutes, when I return my full awareness to the room, the words begin to flow naturally again. Massage gives us a personal experience of mental tranquillity, and since massage is such a pleasurable experience, it is easy to recall the memory of it. If we take a "mental snapshot" during an especially relaxing massage experience, later, when the world around us is in chaos, we can recall the massage. In those moments, recalling that mental model helps us relax wherever we are. The more we practice doing this, the quicker we can bring that feeling back into our daily experiences. Clients can be taught to remember their massage to help them relax before a procedure, surgery, or anytime they feel anxious. Making a daily habit of remembering the massage "snapshot" brings a greater sense of peace that carries over into all areas of life. Intentionally returning to this restful state of mind helps us better connect with our own inner wisdom.

In summary, massage redirects our attention from physical and mental stress and tension to a slow, rhythmical, physical sensation. As the chatter and confusion cease, we are more alert. As we fill our attention with the physical awareness, mental tension releases, our focus expands, and our view opens. In the openness and stillness, the mind clears. Our inner voice can speak, and we can hear it. Creative ideas and solutions to problems arise that we had not imagined. We can take a mental snapshot of how we feel during and after a massage. Then when we experience a difficult situation or must juggle many activities, we can remember that massage. We are suddenly, for a moment, transported to that relaxed place. Just as quickly, we have a mental shift, and our view of the world changes.

EMOTIONAL BENEFITS OF MASSAGE

Very often before a massage, I talk to the client for a little while, asking how her body is feeling, and if there are any areas she would especially like me to focus on. I often see a face with lines of worry and tension in the forehead. The corners of the mouth sometimes turn down. The eyes look exhausted and frustrated. After the massage, the worry lines are gone, the mouth is smiling, and the eyes are soft and twinkly. You will see this in the people you massage also.

Massage changes what a person is feeling. What are feelings, or emotions? They are energy in motion. They are strong and powerful because they are designed to get our attention. To ensure our survival, they strengthen our memories of the situation. We can then remember what feels good so that we can do it again, or notice what feels bad so that we can change it or avoid it. Emotions are designed to get our attention and then move through and out of the body. When we hold on to uncomfortable feelings, or repeat situations that cause them over and over, our health suffers. For more information on how our emotions affect health, see Chapter 9. Movement is growth, health, and life, whether the movement is of muscles or feelings. Therefore, just as massage increases the movement of blood and lymph in the body, it can also increase the movement of emotions in several ways by:

- Helping us feel cared about, appreciated, and loved
- Increasing feelings of safety and openness
- Increasing awareness of feelings and needs
- Providing opportunity for emotional release
- Engendering greater acceptance of self and others

Feeling Cared About, Appreciated, Loved

When we feel cared about we know someone is looking out for our welfare. When we feel appreciated, we realize that another sees who we really are and values us. When we feel loved, we feel that someone believes we are special and is willing to share themselves with us. They are willing to give their thoughts, feelings, and time, and receive those same gifts from us.

Perhaps the greatest benefit of massage is simply knowing and experiencing first-hand that someone cares about you. When we are in need, just feeling cared about can remind us of how much we long to be appreciated, nurtured, and loved. Research tells us that when people feel loved, they have better health outcomes, physically and mentally (Ornish, 1998). (See Chapter 12.) Sometimes it is hard to express appreciation and love in words, especially for someone we don't know well, such as a client. Massage gives us just what we need to share those feelings.

Most species associate slow, repeated touch with caring and nurturing. We gently stroke the face of a newborn as we hold it securely and lovingly. When we hold someone who is in pain, we often slowly stroke their back as they cry. For most people, from the very beginning, and throughout our lives, touch stimulates memories of being loved and nurtured. When a nurse takes the time to give a client her undivided attention combined with the touch of a massage, the client feels valued and loved.

Being the recipient of such compassionate intent enhances self esteem and a sense of self-worth, and these both contribute to a greater sense of control. All three of these, self-esteem, self-worth, and sense of control are important for anyone, and they are especially so for those in need of healing in a healthcare setting.

Increased Safety and Openness

The more we feel loved and appreciated by someone, the safer we feel with them. When we feel safe, we begin to open up. Most of us feel the most physically safe around those we trust not to harm us. Caring touch fosters this trust. Emotional safety is more subtle than physical safety. We often can feel perfectly physically safe with someone, yet would not trust them to treat our feelings with sensitivity and kindness. Emotional safety involves the opening of the heart. It takes an even greater degree of trust because it is here that we are most vulnerable. When we talk about the heart opening what does that mean? As the energy of the body begins to move during a slow, caring massage, the energy of the emotions also begins to move. Emotions affect the heart and solar plexus areas, and movement in these areas begins to dissolve walls. Feelings hidden from sight come more fully into view, and become more available for us to use to reach out and connect. Massage between family members and friends can open up lines of communication that may have closed due to previous misunderstanding. Words and tones are easy to misunderstand. Massage says, "I care about you," without the need for words.

With dogs and cats, after you pet them for awhile, you may be honored with their rolling over. They fully display their heart, their most vulnerable side. You know they feel completely safe when they fall asleep on their back.

When people feel safe enough to open their hearts, they often begin to talk, sharing details about their lives and their feelings and needs. Nurses need ways to open up this level of communication with clients in order to better help them. If the massage releases a stream of non-stop talking, this is also valuable information. We often cover anxiety and fear with seemingly unrelated conversation. You might take this opportunity to ask your client how he is feeling about what is happening in his life.

Increased Awareness of Feelings and Needs

As we begin to open up, we become more aware of our feelings and needs. Very often feelings that are painful are hidden from us. Some of us had childhoods where we were made to believe that our feelings didn't matter, and our needs were unimportant. As a result, we didn't learn to be immediately aware of our feelings and how to effectively express them to see that our needs were met. If we tried to express our needs, we were often ignored. The expression of feelings may have led to uncomfortable consequences. As a result, feelings and needs are often not allowed to surface, whether the feelings are pleasant or uncomfortable.

As massage creates the movement of energy, or emotion, in the body and mind, we may remember thoughts and feelings that we have not had for a long time. Pert (1997) reports that memories are stored in the muscles and tissues of the body, the brain, and every nerve cell. When the muscles are stimulated (as in massage), or we experience a similar situation, we often recall the memories and associated emotions that were stored there in the past. The more we feel our emotions, the more we realize whether our needs are met. According to Dr. William Glasser (1994), we have five basic needs from which all others arise: survival, love and belonging, power and freedom, fun. Power suggests respect or the ability to change our situation. (For more on ways to meet needs, see Chapters 9 and 10.) Ultimately, we are the ones responsible for seeing that our needs are met. Feeling like we have the ability to meet our needs, or have control in life, is one of the most powerful factors for improving immune function and reducing stress (Epel, McEwen, and Ickovics, 1998), and decreasing chances of heart disease (Marmot et al., 1997).

How long has it been since someone asked you, "What do you think you need to heal, or to be happy?" Tears may well up in response to just being asked. We're much more likely to pause and consider a thoughtful reply when we're relaxed and feeling safe and cared about. Most of us know what we need if asked. As nurses, we can ask our clients. In our personal lives we can ask our spouses, friends, parents, and children. We can ask ourselves. And we must listen to the answer. Over her 40-year nursing career, Dr. Helen Erickson (1988) has found that people heal when they get what *they feel* they need to heal. This may not be what we would have ever imagined they would need. One of Dr. Erickson's clients was not responding to treatment. Dr. Erickson asked her what she thought she needed to heal. She started crying, and said she needed to be able to wash her children's clothes, cook for them, and take care of them. She was wealthy and had a maid and a cook. She felt worthless. Her husband said she could have whatever she wanted, and released the cook and maid. She began responding to treatment and got well.

Provides Opportunity for Emotional Release

Once we become aware of stored feelings, massage provides an opportunity for their release.

As we mentioned, a tight muscle sometimes contains stored memories from the past. As the muscle softens with massage, the walls around the emotions crumble. To encourage the continued relaxation of muscles, and health of the body, it is

Nora's Story

For a period of three months, Nora decided to receive a massage every week. For several weeks, during the part of the session when she was having her mid-back massaged, Nora would become very sad and would shed some tears. When asked how she was feeling, she simply said she was feeling sad and that my massaging her mid-back somehow reminded her of her mother, with whom she had a sometimes difficult relationship. The sensations in the middle of her back, she said, reminded her of a feeling, and out of that feeling she saw her mother's face in her mind's eye.

I never really tried to get Nora to talk about her mother. It didn't seem necessary. I just massaged her with a sense of caring and compassion, appreciating her for having such moving feelings and allowing them to come to the surface to be released. It was very touching. After a few weeks I noticed Nora didn't shed those tears anymore, even though I massaged her back in much the same way as I had before. It is an honor just to be present when such a natural movement of healing seems ready to work its way out.

—Jonathan

helpful to let the energy of these emotions move, flow, and release. There are many ways this can happen. Sometimes it is as simple as a few spontaneous deep breaths. Emotions do not even have to come to conscious awareness to be released. Because they are energy, once the energy is moving the constriction relaxes.

Sometimes memories of entire scenes from the past come to awareness with their emotions. Some people sob. Some people take continual, deep breaths until the feelings release. Others begin to talk, expressing anger or other strong emotions, very often coming to an understanding they never had before. People in healthcare settings, especially those in crisis, feel many emotions, including anger, fear, guilt, and resentment. Very often the release of emotion allows healing to occur.

Not all massages stimulate a conscious emotional release, but it is important to know that it can occur. If the person discovers an event that they need more help with than you feel comfortable giving, you can always refer them to a counselor or chaplain.

Engenders Greater Acceptance of Self and Others

During a massage, people feel supported, valued, and cared about. Often recognizing and releasing feelings leads to greater acceptance of ourselves. For these two reasons, after a massage people are able to hold themselves in a gentler place. This acceptance may extend to the myriad situations we find in our lives. In nursing, we often have clients who will not experience physical healing. Massage can contribute to the process of the acceptance that must come.

Massage may help people feel more accepting or loving toward others in their life. Acceptance does not mean condoning hurtful behavior, it means finding a way to understand it, to see it from a different point of view. This kind of acceptance often helps to release old feelings of anger, resentment, and guilt.

Judgments that we hold for ourselves or others are emotions that have become rigid patterns of energy. It is often difficult to feel differently unless we do something out of the ordinary to change that habitual pattern. Massage gently moves that "stuck" energy, allowing old patterns to break up, and the possibility for new patterns to emerge. The period of time immediately after a massage is a most fragile and delicate time, and a very powerful time. It can be a time of new beginnings. The nurse must remember that those first moments after a massage hold great opportunities for connection and healing. As the energy of the heart moves, it is easier to remember loving feelings for others, and to look at situations in a softer and more forgiving light. Mutual acceptance between friends creates a foundation of trust from which we find strength and courage to face the future.

In summary, being massaged in a slow rhythm helps us feel appreciated and loved. We may then feel safe to open our thoughts and hearts to another. As we become more open, we become aware of feelings and needs that usually stay buried. Once we become aware of these feelings and needs, we can choose what to do with them. The movement of energy in a massage presents the opportunity for the movement and release of these feelings. As a result of this mental unstressing, we come to a place of greater acceptance of circumstances in our lives, other people, and ourselves.

MASSAGE, STRESS, AND THE MINDBODY CONNECTION

What would most people say is the greatest benefit of massage? Stress disappears. Continual stress on a daily basis is a contributing factor to almost all illnesses of the body and mind that we know of today. Many would go so far as to say that stress causes most of these problems because it adversely affects the immune, digestive, endocrine, and cardiovascular systems.

The stress response can begin with mental/emotional responses and progress to physical sensations, or it can begin with physical symptoms and end up causing mental/emotional changes. The stress cycle then continues indefinitely, mind affecting body and body affecting mind. (See Chapters 9 and 10 for more detail about stress and the mindbody connection.) To stop the stress, we must interrupt the cycle. Massage interrupts the stress response by changing thoughts, feelings, and physiology, which in turn contributes to all aspects of health.

M. C. works long hours at a computer all day, has a second job, and has a family to care for. Her story one day right after receiving a massage illustrates the benefits for the body, mind, and spirit.

"I never used to be aware of the pain in my body. But after I started getting massaged, I felt what it was like to be relieved of that tension. Even before I have my massage, my body knows it's coming. If for whatever reason I don't get one, I'm so much more aware of all the build-up of tension and stress in my body.

"I've had two physical ailments that have been fixed by massage. One of the reasons I started getting massage was because I had significant headaches twice a week. The doctor had sort of decided that they were tension headaches and gave me a lot of different strong medications for them. They weren't really migraines, but of course they got in the way of me doing a lot of things. I missed a lot of work. After several months of massage, I just sort of became aware of the fact that I didn't have headaches any more. And now I can't even remember the last time I took any Advil. It's amazing.

"I also had a motorcycle accident when I was 14. My knee was badly broken in several places, and I had to have a pin put in it. I basically didn't have any problems until about a year and a half ago. I started to notice when the weather was changing that my knee would hurt. And then it got to be real intense. It hurt a lot and was swollen. My doctor said surgery was what definitely needed to happen. The first massage I had on my knee I really couldn't tell any difference. It felt a little better right after the massage, but then a couple of days later, it hurt again. But after four massage treatments over one month, the pain was actually gone. It's been months now, and it hasn't hurt me again. I'm not going to get it operated on.

"After I get a massage, one thing I notice is that I feel glad to be alive, and I have a lot more energy. Nothing hurts and I feel happy. My family wants to be around me because I'm in such a good mood and very little bothers me. I really have opened up. It's not just about having my muscles loose, my circulation working, and being calm; but I feel opened up so that I'm open to love, or I feel more open to the people around me. They don't annoy me. I can really listen to my daughter and not be in a hurry to get off to do whatever I need to do. It really seems to give me patience.

"After a massage, I feel so completely happy to be in my body that I'm really able to be in the moment. That's another thing. I'm not thinking about tomorrow. I'm not thinking about yesterday. I'm not worried about my mother-in-law's illnesses or the car insurance. I have better focus. My dog likes to be with me after I have a massage because I can really just sit with her and not think about anything else.

The effects of the massage actually last for several days. When we're looking at the budget and where we can cut corners, my husband says, 'Don't cut back on your massage.' Of course, that makes me wonder what I was like before. The longer I get massage the longer those good benefits last. I would never consider not getting massage again as long as I live."

MASSAGE BENEFITS THE GIVER

As we mentioned in Chapter 2, another benefit of massage is that the giver feels better for the giving. Many people over the years have asked, "How have you been able to give massage for so long? Don't you get tired of it?" I think I have enjoyed it for so long because I receive as I am giving. The greatest reward is to see, and hear, the value that my clients receive, each day, with every massage. In addition, I also feel rejuvenated after I give a massage. I am more relaxed than when I began. My muscles are less tense, and my thoughts and feelings are

Firsthand Findings

From our own giving and receiving of massage, and the comments of our clients, we have found that:

1. Massage relaxes tense muscles and makes the whole body feel renewed.
2. Massage is a like a short vacation from stress, and from daily life.
3. The giver becomes relaxed in the giving.
4. Receiving massage creates a memory of relaxation that we can recall when we need it.
5. Massage changes our thoughts and feelings, helping us remember what is really important.
6. Massage can be a way to express love, and help us feel that we are loved.
7. Massage prevents discomfort and fosters healing.
8. Massage opens our hearts, allowing the connection between the giver, receiver, and the Divine to be more easily felt.
9. If we all give and receive massage, it can change the world.

calmer, clearer, and more kind. My view of the world and the people in my world shifts for the better. I am filled with gratitude for the opportunity to help others and connect with them in a way that is meaningful for both of us. As a result, there is very little stress in my work. Even after giving massage for almost 25 years, I still experience these benefits each day. If you add massage to your day, so will you.

In summary, we have shared our experiences of the benefits massage brings to the physical, mental, and emotional self. In addition to these, massage offers a rare moment of true heart-to-heart connection. There are many times in our lives when the future looks dim, whether due to a bad hair day or a health crisis. Uncertainties abound in life. In some ways this life is made of Mystery. Nurses care for clients who are looking for a bright spot in their future. Massage can be a moment to contemplate the meaning of it all, discover hope, and feel the movement of Spirit. The late-night backrub can become one long extended moment of heartfelt listening and being together. Start with a hand massage, then maybe the shoulders, and finally, just two people together in the lamplight, perhaps talking about life, its speed in passing, maybe a regret or two, and some hope. Certain moments have a way of drawing our humanity from our hearts. We can feel its warmth, and its deep power in our lives. Simple moments during a massage have ways of becoming the most priceless and sacred treasures of a lifetime.

RESEARCH STUDIES FOR SPECIFIC POPULATIONS AND CONDITIONS

Now we are going to discuss a second way to gain knowledge—research studies. If you read the body of research on massage, you will see conflicting results. One problem with studying massage is that every person that gives massage does it differently, even if they are doing the same strokes as another person. The order, speed, or depth of the strokes may vary. Two different studies may not even use the same strokes. Field (1998) reported that many of the benefits of massage that she has found are not seen if the massage strokes are light and superficial. So if you see in a study that there were "no significant results," keep in mind that it may be due to the statistical or research method used, the type of massage, the person giving and receiving it, or even the environment.

"No significant findings" as far as the statistics of research goes, may in actuality be very clinically significant, meaning significant on a person to person basis in the practice setting. If you are able to relieve the pain of even one person, is that not significant? Almost all of the recipients in most studies on massage say they feel much more relaxed, regardless of the measurement of the effect on their body. A client feeling more relaxed is as important as a change in a physiologic measure. Even with the above limitations, it is beneficial to review research studies on massage because it helps us realize the wide range of conditions in which it has been effective. In some of the studies you will see a "p" value given. P <.05 means that the results found in the study would have occurred by chance only 5 out of 100 times, indicating that the results were probably due to the treatment.

Tiffany Field, Ph.D., is the current leader in research on the effects of massage. Since 1977 she has been a professor of psychology, psychiatry, and pediatrics at the University of Miami School of Medicine. In 1992, she founded the Touch Research Institute (TRI). There is a branch of TRI at The Southeastern University Medical School in Ft. Lauderdale, Florida, which focuses on the role of massage in prevention and wellness, whereas TRI–Miami focuses on the role of massage in illness. There are twelve paid researchers and many volunteer massage therapists on staff. TRI is the first institute in the world devoted to touch research, and most of it involves massage. All studies done at TRI have control groups, are often double blind studies, and use firm pressure rather than light stroking. Adults receive two massages per week over four consecutive weeks that are 30 minutes long. In studies involving children, the parents do the massages for 15 minutes each night for 30 days.

The best way to gain valuable information through research is to have a control group that does not receive the treatment, and a study group with a consistent treatment that is given to each participant. In all of the following research studies that include T. Field as one of the researchers, the above conditions were met. The other studies may or may not have had control groups and each study probably uses a somewhat different massage technique.

Early Research on Massage

Before drugs and surgery became popular in the mid-1900s, massage was considered a valuable part of healthcare. Research about massage was common in medical literature. From 1813 to 1939, there were over 600 articles reporting research on the benefits of massage in various journals such as the *Journal of the American Medical Association, British Medical Journal,* and others (Collinge, 1996).

In *The Archives of Physical Medicine,* Scull (1945) described physical benefits of massage, citing research studies from as early as 1905. In some of these studies, massage did not increase oxygen consumption, and so did not involve energy loss. These studies also found that massage can facilitate:

1. Enhanced healing of fractures
2. Increased flow of the blood and lymph
3. Increased red blood cell count, especially with anemia
4. Relaxation of muscle spasms
5. Stimulation of the nervous system causing relief of pain and relaxation of the psyche
6. Increased lubricating fluid in connective tissues
7. Increased removal of particulate matter from joints
8. Increased emptying of the colon, prostate, and tonsils
9. Accelerated resolution of pathologic nodules of the lymph system
10. Increased availability of white blood cells
11. Increased dilation of the blood vessels in the area being massaged

Dr. Scull goes on to say that "neurologists have long utilized massage for its tonic and sedative influences." It is our hope that one day soon a visit to the office of a neurologist, or any other healthcare practitioner, will include the option of receiving a massage.

Wood and Becker (1981) provide a thorough account of early research studies on the effects of massage. To mention a few, Schneider and Havens (1915) found that abdominal massage increased hemoglobin levels and red blood cell count in the blood. Drinker and Yoffey (1941) found that massage increased lymph flow by putting a cannula in the lymph vessels of anesthetized dogs and measuring lymph flow while the dog was being massaged. Bell (1964) found that when people received massage on their legs that included deep stroking and kneading, blood flow to the legs doubled, and the effect lasted for 40 minutes.

In the 1960s, nurses began researching the backrub that was a traditional part of nursing care. Kaufman (1964), Sister Regina Elizabeth (1966), and Temple (1967) found that clients who received massage, particularly a slow stroke back massage (SSBM), experienced increased relaxation. Sister Regina Elizabeth was the first to describe a slow stroke back massage with the hands at 60 strokes/minute on both sides of the spine, from head to tailbone and lasting three minutes. Many studies saying they use a SSBM do not follow these steps exactly. Longworth (1982) found that in a non-hospitalized, healthy population, a slow stroke back massage decreased psychoemotional arousal as evidenced by an increased galvanic skin response (decreased stress response), and a significant decrease in scores on the State Trait Anxiety Inventory. Decreased generalized muscle tension was indicated by decreased EMG scores.

Because of its numerous benefits for a variety of health conditions, massage continues to be the subject of research studies today. On July 5, 2001, the *Wall Street Journal* discussed a study on massage published in the *Archives of Internal Medicine* stating, "Massage might be an effective alternative to conventional medical care for persistent back pain" (Charkin, et al., 2001). Fifty-seven years ago, Scull's article in the *Archives of Internal Medicine* mentioned on the previous page reported the ability of massage to relieve lower back pain. Perhaps with research like the study by Charkin, et al., healthcare will once again remember the value of massage. The cycles of life are interesting indeed.

Current Massage Research for Specific Client Populations and Problems

We thought it would be helpful to look at research that addresses some of the problems of clients that nurses encounter to see how massage is helpful in those areas. Studies conducted by nurses in healthcare settings where nurses typically practice are highlighted (for example, **nursing,** is at the end of the study or **nurse** is in the description of the study). These studies include massages that are short enough that a nurse would actually be able to do them in the workplace. The studies by Tiffany Field, even though the massage is longer and more frequent than nurses may be able to do, are important for nurses to know about. If massage is beneficial in these settings, a shorter, less frequent massage may also have similar results. Nurses can be the ones to make these valuable discoveries.

PREGNANCY, LABOR, DELIVERY, AND POSTPARTUM

I have massaged several mothers throughout their entire pregnancy. From the third to ninth month, a woman's body experiences one of the most rapid and dramatic changes it probably ever will undergo. Rapid weight gain and a growing new life put added strain on all systems of the body. Muscles tighten, nerves are strained, joints bear more weight, and hormones flood the mind, creating an emotional explosion. The weight is not distributed evenly, sticking out all in front and putting great strain on the back. Pregnant moms love, and greatly need, massage whether from family, friend, or nurse.

Pregnant women who received massage reported lower anxiety, depression, and stress hormone levels, less pain during pregnancy, less sleep disturbance, and lower prematurity rates than women who experienced other forms of relaxation therapy (Hernandez-Reif, Field, Hart, et al., 1999).

I have had the honor to assist a few friends with the births of their babies, being there from beginning of labor to the birth. Birth is truly one of the greatest miracles of life. While my friends were breathing, contracting, and resting, their backs, legs, necks, and shoulders became very tight and painful. Not much feels good during labor. Massage was extremely helpful in assisting them to relax everything except the uterus, and gave them something to count on and look forward to that was soothing. Having one dependable source of comfort decreases emotional tension, and helps mom know she is not alone. Often the nurse is the one she counts on to help her through this seemingly unending time.

When partners of women in **labor** gave the women a 20-minute massage every hour, labor pain and need for medication was reduced, the women gave birth three hours sooner than women who received no massage, and they had less postpartum depression. They also had lower anxiety, decreased cortisol levels, and spent fewer days in the hospital (Field, Hernandez-Reif, Taylor, et al., 1997). Recall that decreased cortisol levels indicate increased immune function.

Sometimes the baby has been in the adventure of birth for quite a long time in very cramped quarters. When our nephew, Eli, was born, his arm was limp due to a very long labor. Mom, Dad, and I massaged his shoulder, neck, and upper back several times a day. In a few days his arm was working just fine. In parts of Bali and India it is very common for infants to be massaged at least once a day from birth. I was once asked to massage a two-day-old baby. When I started out, he was all contracted, as newborns are, with arms and legs bent. When I finished, in about three minutes, his arms and legs were stretched out completely and he was totally relaxed.

After the thrill of birth is over, mom often begins noticing areas she didn't realize were sore. Also, at this time she needs a little extra tender, loving care. Her world has just changed forever. A five-minute massage is a life saver. Massage is also great for nurses to teach to couples who are pregnant to use on each other, before and after baby.

PEDIATRICS

These days the pressures of life come ever earlier. Children are scheduled so tightly between school and after school activities they have little time for just doing nothing. They begin to experience stress. The body perceives time deadlines and rushing as a threat, and responds with a stress response. I am finding that even children are now getting tight muscles in the shoulders, neck, and back.

Most children love massage. Massage can be given to a child by a nurse at school, in the hospital, in a clinic, or in the doctor's office. Whether they are ill or well, children benefit from the relaxation of muscle tension. When children are anxious and afraid, a gentle massage on the back, head, foot, or hand can help them become calm. The older the child, the more pressure can be applied and still maintain comfort.

So many procedures that children must endure in the hospital are painful, and if they are very young, they may not be able to understand what is happening. All children understand touch. Massage is something the nurse can do, and teach to parents, that feels wonderful. Children's bodies have miraculous healing abilities that are greatly enhanced when they know they are loved. Massage is one very good way to let them know.

Many children enjoy giving massage. The touch of children as they give a massage is so healing because it is innocent and not affected by all the layers of thought that adults have. They are very focused, truly wanting to help. The nurse can teach the children in a family, including the child who is ill, to give a simple massage. This gives the children a new way of relating to each other, and other family members, that is beneficial to all. Treat yourself to a shoulder or foot massage by a child.

In 1985, Field did her first research study in which she divided a sample of healthy **premature infants** in a neonatal intensive care unit into control and treatment groups. As mentioned in Chapter 2, the babies who received massage (through the incubator portholes) for 15 minutes, 3 times a day for 10 days, had a 47% weight gain, greater responsiveness, and left the hospital six days earlier, at a present-day savings of $10,000 per baby (Field, et al., 1986). After one year, the massage group weighed more and had improved mental and motor development over the control group (Field, Scafidi, and Schanberg, 1987). Similar weight gains and signs of decreased stress were found in infants who received massage and had been exposed to cocaine (Wheeden, et al., 1993) and had **HIV** (Scafidi and Field, 1996).

The hippocampus is one area of the brain where memory resides. As you recall from Chapter 1, Modi and Glover (1995) studied very premature, low-birth-weight infants in London and found that massage **lowered cortisol levels** and enhanced hippocampal development in the brain, as indicated by MRI. These infants had **superior memory** performance as newborns and at one year old. In Alzheimer's disease the memory is affected. What if we could prevent it by massaging our babies and each other?

In a study of **full-term infants** of **adolescent mothers,** the infants that received massage for 12 days over a six-week period had lower levels of cortisol, epinephrine, norepinephrine (indicates decreased experience of stress), and greater levels of serotonin (indicates less depression). They had better face to face interaction, gained more weight, and improved on emotional, social, and "soothability" dimensions (Field, et al., 1996).

In 1995, Field found that massage increased **vagal nerve tone** and **insulin hormone secretion** in a group of infants. The vagal nerve is one of the cranial nerves and has many functions, from aiding food absorption to moderating heart rate. In this study she found that firm pressure during the massage produced greater results than did light stroking. Of course the firmness is always adapted to the individual tolerance of the receiver. Using oil in the massage had a greater effect than using no lubricant.

When children with **diabetes** received massage from their parents, the children and parents had less anxiety. After one month of massage, the children's glucose levels decreased from very high (158) to normal range (118) (Field, Hernandez-Reif, Shaw, et al., 1997).

Children were studied with mild to moderate **juvenile rheumatoid arthritis** who were massaged by their parents 15 minutes a day for 30 days. A control group experienced relaxation therapy. The children's anxiety and stress hormone (cortisol) levels were immediately decreased by the massage, and over the 30-day period their pain decreased on self-reports, parent reports, and their physician's assessment of pain (both the incidence and severity) and pain-limiting activities (Field, Hernandez-Reif, Seligman, et al., 1997).

Autistic children study showed little resistance to being massaged. After a 10-day period of massage, they had a decrease in their off-task behaviors at school, a decrease in autistic behaviors, and an increase in "social relatedness" (Field, Lasko, et al., 1997).

Children with **Attention Deficit Hyperactivity Disorder** (ADHD) who received massage for 10 days showed less fidgeting in class, more time on task, and were less hyperactive in class than a control group who had relaxation therapy (Field, Quintino, Hernandez-Reif, et al., 1998). I have been massaging a seven-year-old diagnosed with ADHD once a month for about six months. His mother says that he asks when his massage will be and looks forward to it. After a few minutes of massage, he usually relaxes noticeably, lays very still, and is quiet.

For one month, parents gave their children with **asthma** a 20-minute massage at bedtime. Immediately after the massage, the children had lower cortisol levels and less anxiety. The parents also reported lower anxiety. Over the month, the children had significantly fewer asthma attacks, and significantly improved pulmonary function (Field, Henteleff, et al., 1998).

In a study of children, average age of two and half years, hospitalized for severe **burns,** one group received massage to body parts that had not been burned during dressing changes, and the other group received the dressing change with no massage. Children who did not receive massage had increased facial grimacing, crying, leg and torso movement, and reaching out. The ones who received massage showed minimal distress behaviors and no increase in movement other than torso movement (Hernandez-Reif, et al., 2001).

GERONTOLOGY

I have given massage for 20 years to a wonderful woman who is now 90 and lived alone until one year ago. She says she is still walking because of massage. Massage helps to relieve her constipation, pain in her hip joints, and neck and shoulder pain from muscle tension. As mentioned earlier, massage increases circulation and lymph flow. Often older people have decreased circulation and get less exercise. Muscles get tight and joints become stiff. When the lymph system is working well, the immune system can better do its various jobs keeping the body healthy. Older people also often have dry skin, and massage increases circulation to the skin, helping to improve its condition.

Most importantly, many older people don't receive much touch. Several people I give massage to say their massage is the only touch they get. Spouses are often dead, family may live far away, and some families do not touch very much. Touch is a language we understand even when hearing and eyesight fail. No matter how old the body looks, we are still the same person inside that we have always been. We need touch until the day we die.

Fakouri and Jones (1987) wanted to measure the effects of **nurses** giving a three-minute, slow stroke back massage for three consecutive days to residents of a nursing home who were between 56 and 96 years old. The residents experienced a significant **reduction in heart rate, blood pressure, and skin temperature.**

In a randomized, control group study of 21 institutionalized elderly adults, Fraser and Kerr (1993) found that those who received three back massages over four days had significant decreases on anxiety scores compared to those who did not receive massage.

Massage has been found to be beneficial for people with **Alzheimer's** disease and their **caregivers.** Hand massage (2.5 minutes per hand) was given by trained long-term care **nurses** on an Alzheimer's unit over a period of five days prior to activities that were known to produce agitation. In the people with Alzheimer's disease, there was a significant decrease in frequency and intensity of morning agitated behaviors related to care activities when massage was given, compared with control periods of no massage (Snyder, Egan, and Burns, 1995). Rowe and Alfred (1999) trained family caregivers of people with Alzheimer's disease to give a 30-second to 7.5-minute slow stroke shoulder and neck massage at times when agitation was predicted to occur and at times of unexpected agitated episodes. During week one frequency and times of agitated behaviors were recorded. During week two the massages were given and agitated behavior was recorded, and during week three just the behaviors were recorded. During week two agitated behavior that disrupted the client's sleep (pacing, wandering, and resisting) markedly decreased compared to week one. These behaviors also decreased during the day. A decrease in these behaviors reduces the stress experienced by family caregivers who are able to get better sleep at night and rest during the day. After the massage was stopped in week three, agitated behaviors immediately increased.

Nurses working in nursing/retirement homes have wonderful opportunities to help our Elders receive the touching we all need. We must break the mold of how it has always been done and be creative. What if the families of residents were contacted and asked if they wanted to chip in to hire a full-time nurse, or massage therapist, to give massage to residents? What if all who attended the Elders were taught a one-minute massage for the feet, hands, and shoulders that they could offer to those who were interested?

A Crabbed Old Woman

The body it crumbles. Grace and vigor depart.
There is now a stone where I once had a heart.
But inside this old carcass, a young girl still dwells,
And now and again my battered heart swells.
I remember the pain, and I remember the joys,
And I'm living and loving all over again.
And I think of the years, all too few, gone too fast,
And accept the stark fact that nothing will last.
So open your eyes, nurse, open and see
Not a crabbed old woman.
Look closer. See me.

None of us know for certain where we will be living during our last years. Wouldn't you want to live in a place where once a day you received a five minute massage from? Someone dedicated to helping you feel better through caring touch?

This poem by a 90-year-old woman living in an English nursing home was found in her locker by nurses after her death (Montagu, 1986).

HOSPICE

A few nurses know that it is their calling to care for others as they come to the end of this life. The end of life, just as the beginning, is a passage from one adventure to the next. Those of us left behind feel great pain because we will no longer have our dear one to love and to hold. We often have a hard time talking about dying, yet we want to connect somehow. Massage so beautifully conveys deep love and gentle connection.

Massage was found to be very relaxing to 30 hospice clients who received a slow stroke back massage on two consecutive days. There was a significant decrease in blood pressure (systolic, $p \Leftarrow .0001$ and diastolic, $p \Leftarrow .0001$) and heart rate, $p \Leftarrow .002$, and a significant increase in skin temperature, $p \Leftarrow .0001$, all indicating relaxation. The changes in blood pressure and skin temperature were continuing at five minutes after the massage was over, but not to a harmful level (Meek, 1993).

Refrigerator Wisdom

I am standing upon the seashore. A ship at my side spreads her white sails to the morning breeze and starts for the blue ocean. She is an object of beauty and strength. I stand and watch her until at length she hangs like a speck of white cloud just where the sea and sky come to mingle with each other.

Then someone at my side says: "There, she is gone!"

"Gone where?"

Gone from my sight. That is all. She is just as large in mast and hull and spar as she was when she left my side, and she is just as able to bear her load of living freight to her destined port.

Her diminished size is in me, not in her. And just at the moment when someone at my side says: "There, she is gone!" there are other eyes watching her coming, and other voices ready to take up the glad shout: "Here she comes!"

And that is dying.

—Anonymous

PAIN REDUCTION

Nurses in all areas of practice encounter people with pain. One study showed that massage stimulates the brain to produce endorphins, our body's own morphine-like chemicals that control pain (Kaard and Tostinbo, 1989).

Getting enough deep sleep is vital to pain reduction. During sleep, somatostatin is produced, which decreases pain perception. Substance P (causes pain) is released with deprivation of deep sleep. People with **fibromyalgia** (pain all over the body with no known cause) experience **sleep disturbance.** Massage improves the patterns and depth of sleep. Studies indicate that because of this ability, massage is beneficial for fibromyalgia. Sunshine, et al., (1997) found that people with fibromyalgia who received massage had improved sleep and reduced pain levels. They also experienced reduced anxiety, depression, cortisol levels, stiffness, and fatigue.

Women with **chronic lower back pain** who were massaged 30 minutes, twice a week for five weeks had less pain, anxiety, and depression, compared to a group who participated in progressive muscle relaxation. They also had increased range of motion, improved sleep, and increased levels of serotonin and dopamine (Field, Hernandez-Reif, Krasnegor, and Theakston, 2001). Serotonin and dopamine help elevate mood.

Ferrell-Torry and Glick (1993) found that 30 minutes of massage on two consecutive evenings had significant effects on hospitalized men experiencing **pain from cancer.** The massage consisted of effleurage, petrissage, and trigger point therapy to the feet, back, neck, and shoulders using warm lotion. Both days the massage significantly reduced their pain, $p < .05$, anxiety, $p < .05$, and increased relaxation, $p < .0005$. Heart rate, respiratory rate, and blood pressure tended to decrease from baseline, further indicating relaxation.

A 10 minute back massage was given to hospitalized men and women for pain associated with **cancer.** The group with the greatest level of pain before the massage (men), had a significant decrease in pain immediately after the massage, and the pain level remained the same at one hour, and decreased slightly at two hours. The women who received the massage had a slight decrease, but it was not significant. They started out with a lower level of pain. The medication that was given for pain did not begin to have an effect for more than two hours after it was given. Since back massage had an immediate effect, it could be an effective short-term and interim method of pain relief (Weinrich & Weinrich, 1990).

In a control group study, 262 people who had suffered with **lower back pain** for at least six weeks were randomly assigned to a group who got massage, acupuncture, or self-care education (control). There was a 95% follow up by phone at 4, 10, and 52 weeks, assessing symptoms and dysfunction. After receiving 10 treatments over a 10-week period, the group who received massage improved 33% more than the acupuncture group. The control group was the least improved. The massage group had significantly fewer symptoms, $p = .01$, and dysfunction, $p \Leftarrow .001$, than the control, and also had less dysfunction than the acupuncture group, $p = .01$. The benefits were retained for a full year after the study was completed. At one year the massage group had significantly fewer symptoms than the acupuncture group, p =.002, and less dysfunction, p =.05. The massage group used fewer medications and had overall lower medical costs than the other groups, suggesting that massage may provide a cost benefit for the insurer and employer (Charkin, et al., 2001).

IMPROVED IMMUNE FUNCTIONING AND STRESS REDUCTION

Nurses are becoming more and more interested in psychoneuroimmunology (PNI) and how our thoughts and feelings affect the stress response and immune function. If our clients' immune functions are decreased they have more trouble healing. Massage improves immune system functioning, very possibly due to its ability to reduce the stress response. Many studies of stress and immune function measure cortisol levels (increased stress increases cortisol which decreases immune function).

In a study of people with **chronic fatigue syndrome,** their depression, anxiety, and cortisol levels decreased with massage. Hours of sleep and dopamine levels increased (Field, Sunshine, et al., 1997).

Older men and women who were **well** (average age–65 years) were randomly assigned to a control and experimental group to test the effects of a 10-minute **nursing** back rub, using slow effleurage strokes, on immune function (salivary IgA). Increased IgA indicates enhanced immune function. Only the experimental group (back rub) had a significant increase in IgA (Groer, et al., 1994).

Oncology

Cancer is one of the most frightening diagnoses that people hear, for both the client and their significant others. We are now beginning to wonder if chronic stress plays a role in who gets cancer and who heals. Stress decreases the effectiveness of the natural killer cells (immune cells) whose job it is to detect and destroy cancer cells. Chronic stress elevates cortisol levels which decreases many immune functions, making it difficult for the body to fight invaders from without and mutant cells from within. Some believe that environmental pollutants may be one cause of cancer due to their stress on the immune system.

People with cancer often feel helpless and out of control, which also decreases immune function. Chemotherapy further compromises the immune system. Optimum immune function is drastically needed so that the body can eliminate cancer cells and heal. Massage increases relaxation. The more relaxed we are, the less stress we experience and so the better the immune system functions.

I was asked to give massage to a woman with brain cancer. I saw her at least three times a month for two years. She went through long remissions and recurrences with the accompanying chemotherapy. No matter how awful she felt, how much memory loss, how many headaches, she wanted her massage. She said it always made her feel better. When she was at home with hospice and could no longer talk, I came to give her what turned out to be her last massage. After the massage, although she could no longer speak, she opened her eyes and smiled.

People with cancer need to feel supported and loved, and remember how it feels to feel good. Massage is a wonderful way to do that. Regardless of the severity of the situation, a two-minute massage, very gentle and caring to the feet, hands, and/or face is not harmful, and is very comforting.

One study looked at the effects of a 10-minute back massage for three consecutive days on the perceived well-being of women receiving radiation therapy for **breast cancer.** The women reported less symptom distress, higher degrees of tranquillity and vitality, and less tension and tiredness following the back massage than when compared with the control intervention (Sims, 1986).

Women with **breast cancer** received three, 45-minute massages per week for five weeks. Natural killer cells and lymphocytes significantly increased. They had less anger, anxiety, pain, and depression, and improved body image awareness and well-being (Field, 1998).

A randomized control study of 87 men and women hospitalized with cancer received five minutes of massage on each foot for two nights over three days. The massage was from heel to toe, and included the lower leg to the knee. **Relaxation, pain,** and **nausea** were measured using a self-report visual analog scale. After the massage, the clients had a significant decrease in pain, $p < .01$, nausea, $p < .01$, and heart rate, $p < .01$, and an increase in relaxation, $p < .01$ (Grealish, Lomasney, and Whiteman, 2000).

AIDS

In a study of adults with HIV, regular massage for one month created a decrease in anxiety and cortisol levels, and an increase in serotonin (mood elevator) and natural killer cells (Ironson, et al., 1996).

University students who were HIV positive were recruited from an outpatient clinic and randomly assigned to a massage group or progressive muscle relaxation group. They participated in the therapy twice a week for 12 weeks. They were assessed for depression, anxiety, and immune function before and after the 12 weeks. At the end of the study, the massage group reported less anxiety, depression, and increased immune function including increased natural killer cells (CD56) and CD56+CD3-. HIV disease progression markers CD4/CD8 ratio and CD4 number increased for the massage group only.

White blood cells travel around the body destroying viruses, bacteria, and other invaders to the body. They also provide a front line defense protecting against opportunistic infection. One of the detrimental effects of chronic stress is that the white blood cells, especially T-cells and macrophages, do not do their job as well. Long-term survivors of AIDS report that they intentionally do things for themselves that feel good and are fun. Perhaps massage is beneficial for people with HIV because it interrupts the stress response, and feels so wonderful.

MOOD DISORDERS

In a study of 72 **children** and **adolescents** hospitalized for psychiatric disorders, including depression and adjustment disorders, those who received a 30-minute back rub for five days reported marked reduction in **depression** and **anxiety.** They were also more cooperative, in better moods, slept better, and had lower levels of cortisol and norepinephrine (Field, et al., 1992).

Serotonin is one of the chemicals in the brain that is altered by some forms of antidepressants to attempt to relieve depression and other mood disorders. Massage increases serotonin levels in **infants** (Field, Grizzle, et al., 1996) and **adults** (Ironson, et al., 1996).

Field, Schanberg, et al., (1998) studied **adolescent girls** with the eating disorders **bulimia** and **anorexia.** They received massage two times a week for one month in addition to their therapy session. The control group had only the therapy session. The massage group had less depression, decreased cortisol levels, and their eating habits and body image improved.

PRE- AND POST-SURGERY

Before surgery almost everyone is anxious. The stress response is activated, which compromises the functioning of the immune system. Infection is a great concern in hospitals, especially post-surgery.

In 102 women who had gynecological surgery, those who said they were worried before surgery had greater heart rate and blood pressure during surgery, were harder to anesthetize, and were more likely to experience vomiting, pain, and headache after surgery (Abbott and Abbott, 1995). In 126 people who had back surgery, those who were anxious before surgery had significantly more tension and pain three months later than those who were not anxious (de Groot, et al., 1997).

Since massage is comforting, decreases anxiety, reduces the stress response, and increases immune function, it can be a great aid for clients before surgery. After surgery, massage increases relaxation, promotes sleep, reduces pain, and relieves muscle tension that can be caused from lying in one position for a long time. Increased circulation speeds elimination of anesthesia, and abdominal massage helps to restore bowel function. Thorough foot massage stimulates the reflexology points, aiding the healing of the surgical site and internal organs.

Nixon, et al., (1997) found that when **nurses** gave clients a massage, the clients had a significant reduction in **pain** perception over the 24 hours post-operatively, as compared to a control group.

CRITICAL CARE

We have spent long hours in the intensive care unit with our own relatives as I'm sure many of you have. Nurses, clients, and families in intensive care units need emotional and spiritual nurturing. There is much fear, and stress levels are extremely high. A short massage brings a ray of sunshine to all concerned.

Tyler, et al., (1990) studied 173 critically ill clients in intensive care units. Clients were suctioned and turned. After 15 minutes they received a one minute back massage consisting of slow circular motions. They found a decrease in oxygen saturation and an increase in heart rate, however, the changes were minimal and did not represent clinical significance. Oxygen saturation returned to baseline in five minutes. They believe that for most clients the comforting aspects of a massage, especially for critically ill people, outweigh the risks, but individual assessment is advised.

Lewis, et. al., (1997) also studied the effects of **nurses** turning and giving a one minute massage to critically ill men. They found that if the client had a stable hemodynamic condition, turning and immediately giving a massage was no problem. If the condition was unstable, turning to the right side for the massage was advised. Lying on the left side caused a greater decrease in oxygen saturation. It was also better to wait five minutes between turning and massaging. Oxygen saturation returned to baseline in four minutes.

Job Performance and Work Stress

In a study of the effects of massage on work stress, 26 adults were given 15-minute chair massages in their office twice a week over a period of five weeks. The massage included a deep massage to the shoulders, neck, back, and head. Instead of falling asleep, the workers were energized and more alert. A control group of 24 adults just relaxed in a chair for 15 minutes over the same time period. Before and after the massage the workers were asked to add a series of numbers in their heads. Measurements were taken before and after the sessions. After the 15 minute massages, the subjects experienced: (1) Both groups—increased relaxation, as evidenced by EEG changes; (2) Only the massage group—enhanced alertness as evidenced by EEG changes, lower anxiety levels, lower salivary cortisol levels on the first day only, and computation time was cut in half and accuracy doubled, suggesting that mental skills were enhanced by even a short massage; and (3) at the end of the fifth week period depression scores were lower for both groups, but job-stress scores were lower for the massage group only (Field, Ironson, et al., 1996). In a similar study, Cady (1997) found that workers' systolic and diastolic blood pressures were significantly reduced after the 15-minute chair massage.

These findings are significant considering that the International Labor Organization stated in its 1993 World Labor Report that job stress costs the United States economy $200 billion annually through diminished productivity, compensation claims, absenteeism, health insurance, and direct medical expenses.

Additional research at the Touch Research Institute has found that massage creates an improvement in hypertension, migraine headaches, eczema in children, and multiple sclerosis, to name just a few. The improvements were not only in physical parameters but in anxiety, self-esteem, hostility, positive mood, and body image (Knaster, 1998). The research studies in this section are only a few of the vast numbers of studies that have been done over the last 15 years looking at the physical, mental, and emotional benefits of massage. To say the least, massage is beneficial for a wide variety of conditions. In some of these studies the massage was only performed once and was of short duration, while in others, it was 45 minutes in duration and performed daily for a month. We encourage you to try it in whatever situation you are in, creating the massage routine you are comfortable with and just see what happens. If you discover a benefit not mentioned here, please let us know.

Massage for Other Healthcare Professionals

If you are a healthcare professional other than a nurse you may already be thinking about ways you can incorporate massage into your practice. Physicians, dentists, social workers, dental hygienists, chiropractors, and acupuncturists can either offer clients a one- or two-minute massage, or hire a nurse or massage therapist to give massage to your clients in your office. Having a client who is relaxed before they see you makes any treatment or procedure you use likely to be more effective.

INDICATIONS

After reading this chapter, you may have some ideas about where you think massage would be indicated. Personally, we have found massage to be indicated in almost any situation. Of course, we first ask the receiver if they would like one. If they agree, we have found no situation where the receiver does not benefit from massage on some area of the body, even if for a very short time. Here is where the nurse's knowledge of physiology and the individual's physical and mental state come into play. In some cases, you massage the bottoms of the feet or palms of the hands. In other situations, you just massage the scalp. (See contraindications.) For some people, one minute of massage is all that is needed, while others can use all the time you have.

The reason we believe that massage is indicated in all situations where the receiver accepts your offer, is that massage is relaxing. It feels good. With the level of stress everyone is under these days, massage brings needed relief. And we all can use a comforting touch.

From the numerous benefits of massage already discussed, it seems clear that massage is indicated in almost all nursing scenarios.

- It satisfies the need for comfort, care, touching, and reassurance, especially in high-tech areas, and with children.

- If clients lie in one position for long periods of time, massage can help prevent skin abrasions, encourage increased circulation to extremities and joints, and relieve muscle tension and pain.

- If a person is having trouble sleeping, massage can help to calm the mind and relax the body.

- If family members are feeling helpless and want to do something to help their loved one, you can teach them all, or selected parts of the massage in this book. It is designed to be simple and short so anyone can learn and use it.

- Numbness, tingling, or weakness in an area can be caused from pressure on a nerve from an extremely tight muscle. Massage relieves muscle pressure.

- For headaches, massage the neck, shoulders, and head.

- Massage can help dispel stress and anxiety.

- Massage to the abdomen can help to relieve constipation.

- Massage releases endorphins, the body's own morphine-like substance, to help relieve pain and elevate mood.

- When we massage the feet, we stimulate reflexology points that enhance healing in the corresponding areas of the body. In this way, we can help areas of the body that we cannot touch directly. This is very useful with burns, surgery, fractures, and disease of internal organs and systems of the body.

- Mental and physical tension caused by muscle overuse, or underuse, in workday habits can be eased. This includes any activity sustained for long periods of time, including standing, lifting, reading, driving, sitting at desks, talking on telephones, and typing at computers. Athletes, dancers, musicians, and other performers who practice for extended lengths of time also develop muscle tension.

- When you think a person really needs to talk about a situation, but is holding it all in, massage creates a trusting connection.

With massage we are not attempting to diagnose or cure. We are helping to release blockages in the body, to let information flow as blood, lymph, and energy. The Spiritmindbody can then have the best chance of healing itself.

CONTRAINDICATIONS

There are various opinions regarding contraindications for massage. Some books on massage therapy say that massage should not be done on areas with varicose veins, some say massage can be done near the vein but not on it. Some sources suggest that massage should not be given to people with cancer, some say to only avoid the area where the cancer is (Beck, 1994). Some physician researchers, however, do not believe there is a need for the contraindications about varicose veins and cancer (Field, 1998).

If there is any doubt about whether to massage or not, only work on the feet, hands, and scalp. Unless the client has broken bones, or an infectious skin condition, swelling, or are burned, massage will only help. You will bring comfort and relaxation. If there are contraindications for working on one area of the body, choose a different area that is not affected. The entire body can be relaxed by mas-

---

Until more research is done in the area, these are suggested contraindications:

1. Never put pressure on the spine.
2. Do not massage acutely swollen areas, including joints that are hot, red, or extremely painful.
3. Do not massage an area where there is an infection or rash.
4. Massage very gently when you are near areas of recent injury, surgery, broken skin, or osteoporosis.
5. Massage infants and people who are very frail or extremely ill gently, and for short periods (10 minutes or less).
6. For people in critical care areas, especially with cardiovascular involvement, allow a five-minute break between turning to the side and giving the back massage. The back massage should be only one to two minutes long. With them lying on the back, you can massage the feet and hands, gently, for a little longer.
7. Ask the person if they have varicose veins or problems with blood clotting. Do not massage directly on the varicose veins. This will only apply if you decide to massage the legs.
8. For people with cancer, do not massage the lymph nodes, or any area of known, active cancer.

saging one area. Using your professional nursing knowledge of anatomy and the physiology of the body and disease process, you will probably intuitively know when massage is contraindicated. If you are ever still not completely sure, hold their hand and ask them how they feel and what they need.

SUMMARY

As research continues to confirm the important roles of touching and loving in the healing process, massage will assume the level of esteem in healthcare once given it by Hippocrates. As nurses continue to embrace their roles as healers and primary givers of caring, we hope that massage will regain its original place in the daily life of the nurse. The information discussed in this chapter suggests that massage can greatly improve physical health and emotional and mental well-being for clients, family, friends, and of course, you.

We have now completed Part I, Massage as a Healing Tool. One goal of this section has been to introduce you to a new-found friend, massage. As with any new friend you want to know a few things about them so that you can decide how often you might like to get together. Secondly, we wanted to help you realize how beneficial it is to include massage in your professional and personal life, as both giver and receiver. There are two things that inspire a person to take the time to give a massage: (1) knowing how good it feels because they have received one, and (2) learning about the benefits from hearing personal accounts or reading about research studies. Because we all have so much to do each day, we know that if you are really going to do massage, there had better be some good reasons.

We now continue our journey into massage. The part you've all been waiting for—how to do it. Part II will teach you, step by step, how to give a one- to 10-minute massage that almost everyone will love.

PUTTING THESE IDEAS INTO PRACTICE

1. Take a few minutes and mentally scan your body. Are there areas that would benefit from a massage?
2. Over the last week has there been a persistent thought or feeling that has been stressful to you? If so, consider giving or receiving a massage sometime in the next two weeks and notice any changes in that stressful concern.
3. Recall three clients you are currently caring for. How could each benefit from receiving a massage?

Simple Massage Techniques That Work

INTRODUCTION TO PART II

Part II includes some very helpful background information as well as the hands-on techniques you can use to give a one- to 10-minute massage. We begin Part II by looking at how to prepare the environment for massage, both the external environment as well as your own subjective outlook and approach. Next, we address some of the topics that have come up in classes over the years for final preparation before you begin applying the techniques with practice partners and clients.

Two massage routines are illustrated in detail, each with a chapter of its own. The first, without lotion, is shown with the client sitting in a chair. The second, with lotion, is presented with the client lying in a hospital bed. All of the techniques can be easily adapted for practically any setting or situation. Part II concludes with some final "Practical Considerations" aimed toward enhancing your initial learning as well as your personal practice of massage in the future.

CHAPTER 4

Creating a Healing Environment

Make of yourself a light.
—Buddha

OBJECTIVES

1. Describe at least three primary influences on the "environment" of a massage.
2. Describe two internal maneuvers the nurse can use to create an inner environment that transforms any place into a healing space.
3. List at least four external environmental elements to be aware of before giving a massage.
4. Describe methods for dealing with external environmental factors that are less than ideal.

For 20 years we have maintained a home visit practice. We prefer home visits because most people feel more comfortable and relaxed at home, in their own environment. Home visits have proven to be a great teacher for us, because we have come to appreciate even more deeply the rich diversity of human beings. What "home" is, and what helps us relax, is amazingly different for each one of us. Some of us seem to be most comfortable when surrounded by piles of our most precious possessions, while in other homes there is not one particle of dust, or even a pillow out of place.

Some people need to have constant noise going on in their environment in order to feel comfortable. Others must have several of their most beloved pets on, and under, the massage table because they bring such a sense of love and comfort. We work around the sleeping dogs and curious kitties because we have come to understand that their presence signifies love and healing to their human friend, and of course we get to appreciate a little of that, too.

From all of these rich and varied personal environments, we have learned about, and have grown to appreciate, what things like safety, loving, ambient sound, silence, perfect disarray, and perfect order have to do with "feeling at home." People are a wonderful milieu of expression, each one with a crucial and unique contribution to offer in the ongoing play that we call living a human life. We can draw upon this characteristic richness of expression as we perform massage in the clinic or hospital setting by attempting to recreate an environment we anticipate might be most comfortable for our clients. In home health nursing, we might simply appreciate and learn from the client's personal home space. With friends and family at home, we accept what makes those around us happy, while applying our imaginations to make our own space even richer.

This chapter is about preparing the way, creating the best environment possible for the receiver to receive the greatest healing experience from your massage. The physical space in which the massage is given can be almost as important as the massage itself. But a healing environment can be created practically anywhere, because it includes: (1) the internal environment, or inner thinking and feeling, of the giver; (2) the external environment, including the conditions, people, and activities near and within the physical space; and (3) the interaction between the giver and receiver. It is here, within this coming together of influences that the human connection can be made, and this new, enriched environment contributes greatly to the healing process. Each aspect is important individually, but when all are considered together, they create a synergistic effect that allows the greatest healing to take place. Ultimately, no matter where the massage is given and received, the giver sets the tone. With thoughts, words, and deeds, they create the healing space and carry that healing space with them wherever they go.

We begin this chapter with the internal environment of nurses and how, by observing and influencing their own thinking and feeling states, they generate a personal presence that influences and shapes any physical or interpersonal environment. Next, we look at several key factors in the external environment that can make it more conducive to relaxation and healing. This discussion includes the elements of what might be thought of as an "ideal" environment for massage as well as how to accommodate the environment that appears "less than ideal." Whether or not you ever have the opportunity to transform an empty room into an ideal place for the practice of massage, just considering what might make up this type of environment can be very helpful in accommodating, influencing, or transforming any workplace circumstance.

Since the intention of this book is to not only show how to give a massage, but how to put more heart into your technique right from the start, the information about inner environment presented here is intended to help enrich even your initial hours of learning and practice. A more in-depth discussion of the inner environment will be found in Part III.

Our goal in massage, as in nursing, is to assist the activity of helping and healing to take place, and we assist this most effectively by directing our own personal influence toward that cause. At the same time, it is by preparing our own internal environment that we are able shape our responses to the changing events and people around us. Partly as a result of our preparing for and choosing to influence our interaction with each of our clients, we enable a space for healing to arise between us. Other key influences might include the client's expectations, consciously or unconsciously, along with an element of grace. Where it all starts, then, for us, is preparing our own ground.

SHAPING THE INNER ENVIRONMENT

It really doesn't matter all that much what kind of external environment you find yourself in once you realize that you can generate a healing space with your presence wherever you are. Imagine you are in a crowded emergency room with all the noise, activity, stress, and fear in that environment. Another nurse complains about having a headache and you suggest a short shoulder massage might help. They happily agree.

What can you do to make the external environment "disappear" for a moment as you intentionally engender a feeling of serenity and peace for your receiver? The key is in what you choose to think and feel as you speak and perform the shoulder massage. Your thinking and feeling states affect the expressions on your face, your body movements, choice of words, and the character of your voice. The choices you make in your thinking and feeling also affect the manner in which your hands touch the receiver's body, the application of pressure, and the tempo and rhythm of each movement. Each of these subtle, yet very perceivable factors will influence the receiver's perceptions and their thinking and feeling states as well.

With your intentional thinking and feeling, along with the physical cues and sensations brought about by slow, rhythmical massage, you create a kind of "bubble," or "sphere" of energy, around yourself and the receiver. Whenever two friends are in the middle of a crowd, but have become involved in a deep, personal conversation, you may have heard it said, "They're in a world of their own." The "conversation" between you and your clients begins with what you intend to do for them (helping and healing) and the manner in which you go about communicating that intention through your action. When he or she becomes involved, the two of you connect, and the "conversation" of massage takes on a life of its own. In effect, that is the healing space. Your concerns about the external environment become secondary, and are left behind, as mutual attention becomes focused primarily on your interaction. This mutual attention, infused with your intention to help and assist, generates an interpersonal environment where helping can be given fully and fully received. The gift of healing is invited to take place. And this can be done in any place at any time. For more information on how thinking and feeling affects the giver, receiver, and massage, see Part III.

Since we can directly influence our own personal perceptions and interpretations of events, what might we actually do in order to shape our inner environment before and during a massage? The following is a brief discussion of two strategies for inducing a more relaxed and coherent state within your own mental atmosphere. These strategies include: (1) watching the mind, and (2) shifting states of feeling.

Watching the Mind

The dynamic activity of thinking involves ideas arising to our attention. These ideas are like a continual stream of word-pictures flowing through our mental awareness. We don't often notice it, but we can tune into our own "thought-dreams" and intentionally direct the content of our thinking, thus choosing what we think and, consequently, what we feel. Part of the mind's job is to think thoughts, analyze situations, analyze problems, and formulate potential solutions. It does this automatically, whether we give it a specific task or not. It is our job, then, to direct the mind, to choose the thoughts that we energize with our attention. What we "pay" energy to, in the form of our attention, grows in our experience.

Once we become aware of the content of our thinking we undoubtedly notice that certain trends and patterns occur. These personal "themes of thinking" become habits of thought, and they sometimes take deliberate effort to change. One person may have a recurring theme of, "I'm fat," for example, while another may habitually think, "How many people can I help today?" What kinds of thoughts we tend to think, habitually, is what our experience tends to become and, then, reflects back to us. Since we already influence our thinking and feeling all the time, what we need to do is learn to influence it more intentionally.

One tool for directing our stream of thinking is a technique called "centering." Focusing on breathing is one technique that brings your awareness into the present so you can notice and influence what you are thinking (See Chapters 10 and 12 for more detail). Centering also helps create an inner environment that is most conducive to relaxation and healing. Before entering the room to perform a massage, or just before the massage begins, pause and take 10–20 seconds to center. In so doing, thoughts of your day, your stresses, fall away. The receiver will feel that you are giving him your full attention. Several times throughout the massage you may also choose to re-center, that is, to return your focus of attention to the present.

You may have a meditative practice, or a certain prayer or verse that helps engender this experience for you. If not, here is a process to help you become centered wherever you are.

Centering

1. Focus on your inhale and exhale, take two or three gentle, deep breaths (like a sigh).
2. Let all other thoughts go, and bring your full attention to the receiver and to the moment you are experiencing right now.

It's that simple. Try this two-step centering process whenever you happen to think of it throughout the next three days. Better yet, draw a tiny dot on the back of your right hand and remember to center whenever you notice that dot.

Shifting States of Feeling

Your goal is to intentionally place yourself in a heart-centered feeling state. You can do this by consciously entertaining a line of heart-centered thinking that includes acceptance and appreciation. Practicing mental imagery also shifts what we are feeling (See Chapters 10 and 12 for more detail).

ACCEPTANCE

Acceptance makes us better at helping others because it tends to open our hearts to the moment at hand. This feeling of acceptance naturally extends to our client, the external environment, and even to ourselves. When thinking about the client, the challenge is to accept their words, behaviors, and viewpoint as being perfect for them at this time.

"Perfection" does not only mean that something or someone is "without flaw," it also means that a state of maturing into what we have always had the potential to become is now taking place. Like the ripening of a mango just waiting in its fullness before falling to the ground, we are each in the process of becoming what we were always intended to be. But with human beings, as with human living, the process of becoming "even more" of who and how we are never really ends. And so accepting ourselves, our clients, and the environment around us as being both perfect and flawed at the same time can be a tremendous relief. After all, each is in the process of becoming, and that is perfectly acceptable.

One of the hardest things to accept in this scheme of endless unfolding is suffering, even suffering in its milder form, which we have come to call "stress." But suffering and stress are instructive in the greater scheme of things because they draw out from us both our compassion and our humility. Suffering and stress, and having them to overcome, are both an acceptable part of becoming more human. And before we can assist, we must accept—even embrace—that which we would intentionally help to heal, and accept that greater state of becoming even before we see it with our eyes.

It is said that, "seeing is believing." But sometimes we have to accept a belief in something in our hearts before we can ever see it with our eyes, or help bring it about with our hands. This we can do best through learning, and practicing, acceptance in small, daily things.

APPRECIATION

Appreciation comes from the same root word as prize, price, and precious. It is about recognizing and valuing something and seeing it as the prize it truly is, but sometimes we must see through the outer layers of a thing, or a person, to see the prize within. There is something worthwhile to appreciate in everyone, even if we fail in seeing it the first time we look. Appreciating and accepting each client—just as they are right now—helps us establish that human bond, even if it's only for the few short minutes it takes to rub their back.

You are not going to like all of the people you massage, but you can always find at least one thing to appreciate about them. Focusing on that one thing creates a more accepting atmosphere in which the receiver can feel cared for and valued. Understanding and appreciation are often enhanced by imagining ourselves walking in their shoes for a while. We are all somewhat irritable or demanding when we feel afraid, lonely, or not feeling well. A little appreciation and compassion goes a long way.

Appreciation, acceptance, compassion, and kindness are all expressions of a deeper sense of love. Love, in the highest, truest sense of the word, is a very powerful healing force. Even if we do not especially like the person who needs a massage, we can remember to intentionally love them in that greater sense. This is discussed further and in some detail in Chapter 12.

IMAGERY

Practicing imagery can help us change our thinking and feeling, promote relaxation, and create numerous changes in the body and mind. When imaging, we create a mental picture of what we truly want to experience. We image this state, or condition, in the mind's eye, intentionally including all of the five senses and body movements. Imagery allows us to re-experience something from the past or "pre-experience" something we want to create in the future.

Imagery

To shift your feeling state and create an internal healing environment, remember some place you have been, or some circumstance, where you felt very relaxed and happy. What did you see, hear, and smell? Was there any delicious food? What do you remember that felt pleasant to the touch? How did you feel? Take a moment or two and imagine that place, and that *feeling,* right now.

Encourage your clients to shape their internal environment by showing them how to use centering and imagery. Explain how they can watch their thinking and feeling and shift their feeling state toward enhanced relaxation. If they direct their exhale to a tight or painful area as you massage it, the breath helps the muscle relax. It is very hard to retain tight muscles when we take consecutive, slow, deep breaths. Both before and during the massage, this type of breathing allows you to keep your own body relaxed as well. This helps create smooth, relaxing massage strokes, and allows healing energy to flow. Breathing acts as a cue, but the mental image of relaxation—and recalling what that experience feels like in our body—is an example of using our thinking to induce desired states of feeling.

None of us can control our thinking and feeling all the time. They wander onto what we are having for dinner, or back to the latest argument we had with a friend. But during your moments with a client, whenever you notice yourself thinking these random thoughts, just bring your attention back to the kind of thinking and feeling that benefits the client, and you. Controlling our thinking is a little like catching water with our hands. It's a goal to appreciate, but inefficient at best. On the other hand, shaping or influencing our thinking—and, thus, the way we feel—is something we can reasonly expect to achieve.

INFLUENCING THE EXTERNAL ENVIRONMENT

Any room can be transformed with a few very simple modifications. It is truly amazing what just lowering the lights and lighting a few candles can do.

There are many different environments in which you may want to give a massage. There are those situations where the receiver will be coming into your environment, such as giving massage in your home to a friend or family member. There is also the nurse in private practice who has primary influence over the

Creating an Internal Environment

"I visited a home in August one day to give a massage at about four o'clock in the afternoon. In Austin, Texas, it's about 100+ degrees in August, and it's always humid, and this home had no air conditioning. The evening meal was being prepared over the stove when I arrived. There were three generations living in the same small home, and there was no room large enough in the house to set up my table. Also, there was much lively interaction going on at dinner time.

My client and I had to go back to the bedroom, which had no windows, and do the massage on her bed. There was absolutely nothing I could do to change this external environment. This wonderful woman really needed her massage, too. She worked very hard many hours each day in the kitchen of a restaurant, and her back was really hurting. In a few minutes my clothes were drenched with perspiration. I was climbing around and bending over to do the massage on a regular bed in very small quarters, and I realized I was quickly getting very frustrated.

At that moment she said, "Oh, this feels so good." She said it in a tone that made me realize that all I had been going through was completely worthwhile. Immediately, I remembered to breathe, open up my heart, and let the healing energy of God pour through everything we were doing. My internal atmosphere changed completely. From that moment on, her massage felt as good to me in the giving as it must have felt to her, in spite of the very same circumstances as before. Our acceptance and appreciation for our internal environments completely transformed the limitations of the external things around us.

After we were through, I had the honor of being asked to dinner. Homemade tortillas and tamales were the main course, but the real treat was in sitting around a table of people from six months to 80 years old, all of whom loved each other, all sharing their day. I felt greatly blessed."

—Marsha

décor of her office, and even the school nurse who can shape the room to some extent. A nurse who works in the office of another healthcare provider may also be able to influence the surroundings. In some of these environments you may have the freedom to create the "ideal" external healing space, one in which to practice massage or any other healing modality.

There will be situations where you enter the client's environment, such as home health nursing, and visiting a friend's home, or even hospital nursing. You may have an opportunity to give a massage where both giver and receiver are in a neutral environment, such as at a party, in a classroom, or in the break room where colleagues and co-workers can trade shoulder massage with each other. In some of these situations, you can assess the environment and change whatever is possible and appropriate. You will want to make the surroundings just a bit more

> ### The Healing Room
>
> "On another occasion I went to a home that had very little furniture. It had only two lawn chairs in the living room, a Coleman stove in the kitchen for cooking, and a pallet on the floor for sleeping. The elderly woman was receiving her gift of a massage from a friend, and she led me to the back of the house to a room with only one small table in it. She said, "This is my healing room. Please set your table up in here." I did, and then left the room to wash my hands.
>
> When I returned, the room was transformed by the soft glow of at least 25 votive candles surrounding my table. The scent of incense made me feel like I was in some ancient cathedral in Europe. My client was lying on the table waiting for her massage. I felt great awe and humility as I stood there. It was a moment that was not difficult at all to appreciate, and to accept. I felt honored to be allowed to participate in her healing space."

conducive to relaxation and healing, if possible, in the time you have available. In many of these kinds of massage environments the only change you can make is to your own internal environment.

First we will discuss the "ideal" external healing space, when you do have the time and ability to change the environment. Then we look at what changes, if any, can be made to enhance a variety of situations where you have little control over the external situation.

The Ideal External Environment

When you have the time and freedom to do what you want with the space, you can easily arrange almost any environment with two ideas in mind: (1) eliminate as many distractions and intrusions as possible, and (2) furnish it with the kinds of physical influences that reflect your own personal vision for massage, relaxation, and healing.

THE ROOM

First, prepare the room. Ideally, the room is orderly and reasonably clean. Many clients are sensitive to cigarette smoke, animal hair, dust, mold, and fragrances such as perfume and hair spray. Because we are directly touching the receiver during a massage, we need to consider their needs first. Part of that consideration has to do with realizing that our own presence will be integral to the ambience of the room. In order to create the best healing space possible, client sensitivities must be considered when preparing the the room and all of the elements it contains.

Whenever we receive a massage, we allow ourselves to become vulnerable. Our muscles relax, and we become more sensitive to the world around us. Even our muscular "armor" loosens and sometimes even falls away. We don't want to be surprised by intrusions, so securing the privacy of the room helps the receiver feel that he or she is in a safe environment, one more conducive to letting go. Place a "Do not disturb" sign on the door, and adjust all window shades accordingly. If you have an exterior window, make sure the room is visually secure so that no one can see into the room from the outside.

Be sure you have a sheet or blanket handy so the receiver can be appropriately covered and warm during the massage. If the client agrees, telephones, answering machines, beepers, and televisions should be turned off, or down, so they can't be heard. We are so inundated with noise and having to be constantly "on" and available, that during these few minutes of massage it is important to give the client a little mini-vacation from that hectic world.

SOOTHING THE SENSES

What makes us remember our most favorite, relaxing vacation? The sights we see, the people we meet, the smells, the sounds, and the things we touch that are soothing and comfortable. Experiences are captured by the senses. So when we create our own "vacation spot" for the massage client we should, likewise, address the senses. In addition to the following material, you can refer to Chapter 11 for more detail on light, color, sound, and music and their effects on the body.

Light and Color

Many people are extremely affected by visual input, so what the receiver sees on the walls or on display in the room can truly enrich their healing experience. Displaying artwork with soothing colors and images, photos of nature, including flowers, and generally peaceful images can transport your client's thoughts, and your own, to a place and time that represents peacefulness and fun. It has been found that endorphins are released from the brain at the sight of beauty, creating a feeling of well-being (Justice, 1988).

Lighting greatly affects the feeling or atmosphere of the room. As with the room's temperature, ask your clients if the level of lighting is comfortable for them. A soft incandescent light is preferable to fluorescent lights because the constant flickering of the florescent bulb can be very tiring and stressful (Lieberman, 1991). Whatever type of lighting you choose, be sure your light source does not shine directly in the client's eyes. A room with low lighting usually inspires more relaxation. Natural light from a slightly open window shade might also provide sufficient light for massage, and candlelight always creates a warm, healing glow. Practically speaking, it does not take much light to give a massage because the hands do most of the seeing for us. Your clients will feel most comfortable when the level of lighting is "just right," according to *them*. So remember to ask.

Color is also an important aspect of light. The frequencies of the various colors have specific effects on the body and mind (Lieberman, 1991, Burroughs, 1976, Krakov, 1942, Gerard, 1958, McDonald, 1982). Blues, indigos, and violets tend to enhance relaxation. While green and magenta are overall healing colors, green holds a somewhat greater benefit for the physical body. Magenta, green's complement, is more suitable for balancing the emotions. Red, orange, and yellow are energizing, stimulating the body back to normal levels.

Although we might not normally think about it, color can be added to the healing space in the form of clothing or accessories worn by the nurse (or client). Curtains, flowers, and light bulbs, of course, always bring color to a room. You can affect the environment with the color you choose for painting the walls, the hues of any artwork or wall hangings, and even large pieces of cloth material draped casually over the back of a chair or across a couch. The vivid colors of a prism hanging in a window can add a little magic to the space, as well as provide the body with all of the colors from which to choose for their healing effects. In nature, rainbows always create a sense of wonder and well-being, and have a way of bringing a smile to the heart. So if you have direct sunlight, try using prisms to bring some of that rainbow effect indoors.

Sound and Music

We can also create a healing "soundscape." Generally, the more quiet the room is, the better. If possible, eliminate all sounds of television, answering machines, non-controllable music, and street noise. Sometimes doors and windows can be closed, or "white" noise, like a fan, can camouflage unwanted sounds.

Music often adds a nice touch to a massage, helping both nurse and client let go of distracting thoughts and mentally "float off" into a more relaxed space. If possible, the music should be the client's choice, because all of us feel relaxed by different kinds of music. Music, chosen by the receiver, has been found to bring elevated blood pressure, heart rate, and cortisol levels down into normal ranges (Spintge and Droh, 1992). It might be helpful for you to choose music from a range of various styles so that each selection is a piece, or a collection, that you know to be relaxing. Offer your client a choice from among these selections.

If you have some choice in the music, try selections without words, a slow tempo, and no abrupt changes in volume or tempo. Music has been found to affect the heartbeat, brain waves, respiration, blood pressure, and muscle tension, stimulating or relaxing them depending on the tempo of the music (Goldman,

1992). Have you noticed that when you are eating in a restaurant where fast music is playing you chew faster? A relaxed tempo helps create a relaxing ambience, in general. Many of Mozart's Largos are examples of music that slow respiratory rates to normal and help to create a heart beat of around 60 beats per minute. Also, recordings of nature sounds such as ocean waves, rain, crickets, frogs, and running streams are very relaxing to many people.

The Sense of Smell

In aromatherapy, the essential oils of plants are extracted and used in a variety of ways to facilitate very specific physical and emotional effects. These include relaxation, but also antibacterial, antiviral, vasodilators, and diuretics, with few side effects (Goldberg Group, 1993). What we smell directly affects the part of the brain associated with memory and learning (Steele, 1984), so different aromas can be especially nice in your room for massage. They also create pleasant memories and associations regarding massage and relaxation.

Aromatherapy has been used in France and England for many years. Jane Buckle, R.N., introduced aromatherapy into nursing in England, and has been offering certification courses especially for nurses in the United States sponsored by the American Holistic Nursing Association. There are many excellent workshops in addition to Ms. Buckle's where we can learn to use scents to affect mood and health. Many of us don't realize that when we smell something it is because a chemical is being carried in the air, eventually entering our bloodstream. In this way what we smell, depending on its source, can have positive or negative effects on us physically as well as mentally.

We encounter the use of scents in numerous places in our daily lives, such as body lotions, candles, incense, and potpourri. Clients usually enjoy "sampling" two or three different essential oils to see which one they'd like to have for their massage. A drop or two of essential oil can be added to massage lotion or oil, or placed on a pillow and then covered with the pillowcase. Essential oil can also be put into a small bowl so that the aroma fills the room. Another strategy is placing a drop of oil on a small porcelain ring designed to fit on a light bulb. The heat of the bulb then disperses the aroma into the room. One essential oil that many clients seem to enjoy is lavender. Lavender (lavandula augustifolia) oil in small quantities, and dispersed in these kinds of ways, is very relaxing and healing (Goldberg Group, 1993).

More is not necessarily better in the use of essential oils. A small amount creates the desired effects, so if you use lotion in your massage, be aware of using too much of any fragrance. Health food stores are good places to find lotions that are fragrance free and which contain ingredients that are truly good for the skin.

Some clients will enjoy the smell of incense in a room. Since there are so many different fragrances of incense, try one at home first to see how you like it.

Some can be overwhelming, so before using any kind of incense, or fragrance, in a massage environment, ask your client to smell it first. Many people today are as environmentally sensitive to different scents as they are to mold or dust.

The Sense of Touch

It was through the sense of touch that each of us first felt the warmth and comfort of this world. Throughout our lives, all of the things we touch with our palms and fingers, as well as those things that come into contact with our skin, greatly affect our subjective experience. We humans do not have fur or scales or shells, so everything we touch, and that touches us, greatly affects our experience of comfort, and our healing. For massage to be most effective, the receiver must be comfortable in every way possible.

The temperature of the room is also very important in massage. It is very difficult to relax when you are even the least bit cold, so either adjust the room temperature to about 78–80 degrees or have a couple of blankets ready. Keep in mind that every client will feel slightly cooler while lying down, even underneath a sheet, than when they first entered the room and were fully clothed. Since we all enjoy different temperature ranges, always ask them to tell you if they are too cold, or too warm. A small electric space heater can usually warm one room quite nicely. Try to avoid electric blankets since they have been reported to adversely affect the body's electromagnetic field (Becker and Selden, 1985).

Cold lotion, or cold hands, on a warm back is no way to start a massage, so be sure your hands are warm before you ever touch the receiver. Massage can be given without oil or lotion, with the client fully clothed as described in Chapter 6. If you do choose to use oil or lotion, be sure it is warm. Heated massage lotion or oil begins relaxing the client as soon as it touches his skin. Heating the lotion by opening the top of the bottle and placing it in the microwave for 30 seconds, or heating it in a pan of water on the stove, makes that first contact very soothing. If you are not near a stove or microwave, take a moment to rub the lotion between your palms to at least warm it up a bit.

The purpose of using lotion or oil is so that your hands can glide along smoothly through most muscle resistance without any unnecessary friction or discomfort to the skin. Some people prefer oil, and some lotion, for massage. From the client's point of view, each feels somewhat different on the skin.

Many people prefer oil because it is a completely natural substance with nothing added. Almond, olive, and sesame are commonly used oils. Another advantage of oil over lotion is that you can apply it once and not have to keep reapplying. However, lotion has its benefits as well. Since most lotions feel less "oily," clients don't feel like they have to shower afterward, and lotion does not seem to stain the sheets as some oils do. You will need to read the labels carefully when buying lotions because they are all very different. We generally try to avoid lotions that contain mineral oil if possible because they may feel tacky on the skin, and some say it blocks the pores. Once again, be careful about lotions with scents because some clients are very sensitive to them. Try both oil and lotion and see what you and your clients like best.

Nursing Environments for the Elderly

After a lifetime of work, family, and the concerns of daily life, our Elders deserve an environment that truly nurtures them throughout their wisdom years. Providing care for elders, either at home or in any type of retirement facility, affords an opportunity to envision an almost ideal healing space. Whether an entire area, or just one room, it would be no great expense to incorporate many of the above suggestions for music, artwork, lighting, and color. These would assure that daily living, at least in part, took place in a truly soothing environment. In our wisdom years, we come to more fully appreciate the value of beauty and harmony, and massage enhances the quality of such a life.

LONG-TERM CARE

Nurses who work in long-term care facilities may have an opportunity to create one of the most ideal healing environments. There is usually an exercise or activity room that might be designated as a massage room, or "relaxation room," during certain hours or on certain days. This room could include music, aromatherapy, low lighting, relaxing colors, and even massage. Group rooms or television rooms might be modified to include many of these suggestions, at very little cost, thus creating an ongoing healing environment.

This client population is often one of the most touch deprived of all, and so they may also be one of the most receptive and appreciative, and they would certainly benefit greatly from massage. Massage communicates caring even if the ears don't hear and eyes can't see as well as they used to. Touch makes all of us feel human again. Wherever you, yourself, happen to live when you become an Elder, wouldn't it be wonderful if you could visit the "healing room," and receive a regular massage?

FINAL MOMENTS OF TRANSITION

Each of us will be called, eventually, to leave this world behind. Our personal transition may take place with someone else present, perhaps a family member or two, but for others, that person will be their nurse. Also, there will come those moments in the career of almost every nurse, especially with those clients who are in the final phases of transition, when it seems there is nothing left to do. Even the lightest touch of actual physical massage might be too stressful in that sensitive hour. All that you have learned and felt by touching your clients with your own hands can be communicated, now, only through your heart. In those final tender moments the only changes you may be able to make in their environment will be to become the healing space.

Your appreciation, your inner hopes for the client's peace and rest, and your feelings of support will all become part of the way you make a difference in that room. Simply allowing your client to feel you sympathize with their feelings, and letting them feel the touch of your presence, may be the greatest comfort of all. But most assuredly, in those most exquisite, sometimes very tender moments, if you do rest your hand on theirs—or even if you just rest your arm alongside them on the bed—they will be able to sense your intention and caring. No external environment could ever be more ideal, whatever its conditions, because it holds open the possibility for the most pure of human connection, that of heartfelt touch.

Environments That are Less Than Ideal

We have discussed the ideal situation for massage where the giver has the opportunity to affect the external massage environment. You may have the opportunity to integrate some or all of those suggestions. However, many times we find ourselves in situations that are less than ideal, where we cannot change much about the external environment at all.

WE ARE HERE TO SERVE

We need to be flexible if our goal is to serve the needs of the client. As we mentioned earlier, when we remember to tune in to our own thinking and feeling, we can create a healing environment wherever we are.

During a massage, sometimes cats or dogs may try to jump on the table, or kids come in to ask about plans for the evening. Sometimes babies must nurse. You often have only a few short minutes to give a much needed massage, or perhaps the client arrives late.

There may be many external sounds that you can't control, like loud traffic noises in the street, kids playing in the hall, televisions in other rooms, and stereos next door, or the client's roommate watching TV in the hospital room. If you verbally acknowledge the distraction with the client at the beginning, it becomes much easier for you both to ignore it. The irony of giving a massage "in the midst of things" can actually make the distractions seem funny. Clients have actually laughed out loud at some intrusion right in the middle of their massage. The laughter broke the tension and helped them relax even more. Also, it is not your responsibility to change the things you simply cannot. Tell your client, "Let's let the world be the world and we can have a good massage."

You may find yourself giving massage in the most unlikely of external environments. Over the years we have given massage to dogs, cats, horses, and pigs; and to people of all ages in cars, airplanes, restaurants, and even on a straw mat on a mud floor in a hut in the middle of the Pacific Ocean. Massage eases the cares and worries of all creatures and, as the givers, we must allow for the unexpected in life and realize that a little massage is always much better than none at all. Why should we be irritated or frustrated just because the environment doesn't seem "perfect" to us? Giving massage offers us an opportunity to notice, and let go of, our judgments. We are here to help ourselves and others meet our needs, and every time we remember this simple, undeniable truth, it always points us in the healing direction. What is relaxing can be different for everyone, but the bottom line remains the same: we're here to serve.

WHAT TO DO IN SITUATIONS THAT ARE LESS THAN IDEAL

After reading about what we have called the "ideal" circumstances for massage, you may be thinking, "Well, where I work it is not like that, so how could I ever do massage there?" The answer is, do it anyway. When you see someone rubbing their neck, you can say, "I learned massage. Would you like me to work on that a little?" Give yourself the gift of seeing what happens when you offer to rub the neck of a total stranger. It matters very little where you are, you will be strangers no more.

In the busy hospital, the client's need is the priority

Even though it may not be a private room and it's noisy outside, and maybe the nurse has only 2–3 minutes and the room is freezing. What can you do? Lower the light for a minute and have a blanket ready. Talk to the client about focusing on breathing and using imagery of lying in the sun during the massage for greater relaxation. Be aware of your own breathing and bring your full attention to the receiver. Choose to think only of "healing" for the next two minutes and, if anything else comes to mind, come back to "healing." Choose two strokes you think will be most beneficial to this individual client that can be done in the time available. In all of these ways, you have just created the healing environment. Externally, all you did was dim a light and grab a blanket. But most importantly, you shaped the "conversation," internally as well as externally.

In Specific Medical Settings

Sometimes you'll have 30 seconds for either a hand massage or a foot rub before surgery. A foot rub during chemotherapy could be very relaxing if the client thinks she might enjoy it. For newborns, "massage" might be a one-minute stroking of the back, or simply making small circular movements on the feet of premature babies with a fingertip, or cradling each tiny foot in the warmth of your palm. You might sit in a chair and rock a newborn during a break, holding her close to your warm heart. Your presence is felt by every client, young and old, in any scenario, and this presence touches them, creating safety and comfort, and an opportunity for healing to take place, even "in the midst of things."

If you are a nurse working in a busy clinic, a school, day-surgery clinic, chiropractor's office, or physician's office, while you are with the client for that one short minute, ask if he would like a shoulder or neck rub. Even though you may not ever have more than two minutes to spare, that is plenty of time to help a client relax, and that can help relieve some of the anxiety most people experience when they come for medical care. For us it's a workplace, we go there every day. But for the client it's a "trip to the doctor," sometimes a major event even over a relatively small concern.

You might say, "I'm going to take your blood pressure and pulse and then give you a shoulder massage if you would like one." False high blood pressures are often due to the anxiety of coming to a clinic.

A school nurse can transform her office into a healing space with the addition of pleasant color, and a few small images, chosen specifically because they help make kids smile. Most children love to have their shoulders rubbed, and it doesn't take much of it to help them feel relaxed.

In home health, it is important to remember that most clients are comfortable in their own surroundings, even though they may not seem comfortable to us. So we find the best place, whether in a chair, or on a bed, to give them a short massage. Use as many of the suggestions for the ideal space as are appropriate. At someone's home there may be many distractions, even more than in the hospital. It is important to remember to eliminate any of those distractions that you can, accept any others as just part of the environment, and focus on them and their massage.

When nurses practice massage with each other at work, or with their students during training, the receiver will probably be seated in a chair in either a break room, office, or classroom. There may be people coming and going and sometimes lots of noise. There may also be a general feeling that there is not much time for this sort of thing. In that case, closing a door, turning down a phone, lowering one light, and making the receiver as comfortable as possible, even for a few minutes, may be all you can do for the external environment. When it is impossible to make many external changes, each small change we are able to make becomes symbolic and signifies our willingness to make that time special. Then our attention turns toward the interaction between nurse and the client. And that's really all you need.

> ### *Three Methods for Dealing with the Less than Ideal Environment*
>
> 1. "Accept It." Accepting what we have is always the first step toward making the most of it. We can't control everything around us, but we can shift the direction of our thinking. Focus your attention on opening your heart and moving your hands.
> 2. "Do What You Can With What You Have." In other words, do what you can with what you have.
> 3. "Use It As A Cue" to help you relax. Disturbances are sometimes sent our way as a test of sorts, and can be turned into an inspiration. Any confusion you might notice around you can be viewed as a cue to breathe, relax, and remember what you have come to do. Use everything you notice as a cue to be present and alive.
>
> All of the helping you'll ever be able to do with your massage will start with your own willingness to be present and helpful. Share your warm inner light with a friend in need. Draw them into your own very special "healing room." Few things are ever more powerful than that.

The bottom line when it comes to a less than ideal environment is this: Do whatever you can with respect to more conducive light, sound, privacy, and temperature. But remember that your heart-felt presence can transform wherever you are. You can always give a massage that helps your clients reconnect with their own inner source. There is a place inside of us where we can each feel the goodness waiting at the core of our being. Use your massage to bring your clients back home to their own inner source. That is the heart of healing.

INTERACTION BETWEEN THE GIVER AND RECEIVER

The third aspect of creating the healing environment involves the personal interaction and connection between the giver and receiver. Your interaction is like a "third party" taking part in the healing space.

Entering the Healing Space

We enter any environment in which we offer massage with a degree of respect and reverence. The initial interaction between the giver and receiver can set the tone for the entire massage, and it begins before you ever actually touch the client.

Before you come into their presence, whether they are in their home, their hospital room, or a room in your office, stop for a moment. Take a breath or two and remember something that makes you feel good. Make a point of putting a *smile* on your face. This helps you release stress immediately and feel much more calm and relaxed. Always leave any anxious, stressful, and irritated thoughts outside the door. Because you have shifted your thinking and feeling before entering the room, when you do come in this feeling will immediately uplift the client and charge the atmosphere of the room itself.

Connecting with the Client

Connecting with a client is about "being human together," and coming together for whatever time you have for mutual help and support. Our bonds with each other are far greater than are our appearances of separateness. From this place inside us where we are inherently compassionate and kind, we can connect once again with each client we touch. This heart-to-heart connection creates a circle of giving and receiving that can be healing and uplifting for both giver and receiver. Learn how to make that friendly, heart-to-heart connection with people in a matter of seconds, and practice to improve that skill every day.

SUMMARY: THE ULTIMATE HEALING SPACE

Much more goes on in a massage than one person rubbing the tension out of the muscles of another, and it really doesn't matter where you are physically. What is important is that you have made yourself available for the helping of healing to take place. We *invite* healing to come in and then accept the lightness of having our burdens lifted up off our shoulders. When two or more of us gather together for the betterment of one another, there is much more present than either of us alone. When creating a healing environment, all aspects of the connection between giver and receiver are important, and the externalities can be helpful to the degree that they remind us of what we have come here to do. Our goal is to create a space where each client can let his guard down, where he can allow his mind and body to relax and heal.

When we consider creating a healing environment, we might ask ourselves, "What causes you to feeling most trusting in a situation where you have come to be helped?" If possible, the room is warm, and it feels comfortable, safe. It is generally pleasing to the senses. Most importantly, our client should be made to feel that we are giving her our undivided attention, and that we appreciate and accept her as a good human being.

The more we accept and appreciate even the most seemingly ordinary things that come our way, the easier it becomes to see something extraordinary in the people around us, and especially in our clients. Once we start looking for the extraordinary in even the small things, we tend see it almost everywhere, and so we begin to expect it and prepare for it. Sometimes we have to start the process by seeing it where, just a moment ago, we did not. The practice of massage is an activity that continually places us in moment after moment of acceptance, appreciation, and awe. Becoming more thankful for every opportunity, it is with great honor and awe that we enter into each healing relationship.

Now, with the environment in place, we consider some of the more practical details in the next chapter in final preparation for your practice of technique.

PUTTING THESE IDEAS INTO PRACTICE

Experiment with the exercises below in different external environments, and with your eyes both open and closed.

1. Do you ever notice yourself feeling stressed or anxious? If so, that inner state probably has a physical component that is expressed as physical tension. Where are you most tense right now? Inhale the word "heal" into that physical tension wherever it is, and allow it all to dissipate with your relaxed exhale. Then allow the wisdom of your breath to take over your breathing for about 60 seconds.

Now, notice how you feel.

2. How would you characterize the general tone of your own thinking and feeling states in words right now? Now, choose one word, and one image, that each reflect one of your true aspirations or ideals, and entertain that one word and image together for 15 seconds. Do you notice any changes in your body's subjective feeling-tone as a result?

3. Write the name of a client, friend, or family member on a small card or a piece of paper, someone who you know is in need. Fold that paper into two halves and place it between your palms, resting them in your lap, perhaps on a small pillow. After you become settled and comfortable, mentally visualize that person in word and pictures as "healthy" and "happy." Relax your body completely and allow it to breathe without any effort from you for about 30 seconds. Now, as an internal maneuver, allow this person's personal need to draw your heart's deepest compassion toward him or her.

Do you notice any changes, in feeling or sensation, in your hands?

CHAPTER 5

Before You Begin

Beginnings are delicate times.
—Frank Herbert, in *Dune*

OBJECTIVES

1. Explain how to recognize the natural ability for learning to perform massage.
2. Describe Beginner's Mind and how it can be applied while learning massage.
3. Describe two benefits of learning massage technique by learning routines.
4. Explain how to avoid "falling into a routine" with your massage.
5. Explain why you should ask permission before performing any massage.
6. List at least three "get acquainted" questions to ask a client before their massage.
7. Explain the reasoning behind letting the client lead any conversation during massage.
8. List at least two simple analogies to help clients understand and remember the value of massage.

This chapter contains several key ideas we try to elaborate on during classes and workshops. But the best time to hear about them for the best results is before you begin the actual hands-on learning. In contrast to the previous chapter's concern with environments, this chapter is mainly about the actions that take place there, even during the first learning and practice sessions. We start by addressing one of the most common questions, whether someone may have a "natural ability" for learning to perform massage, and how you might be able to recognize that ability in yourself and others. An honest desire to learn and the simple belief in your own ability will lend themselves to ever greater confidence and success. If you already feel fairly self-confident about your own ability in massage, one of the most rewarding ways to express that confidence is through encouraging others who clearly have potential.

Next, we look at an especially helpful mindset for learning massage called "Beginner's Mind." This elusively simple approach views each client and every massage stroke through the eyes of a true novice. Once you begin to apply Beginner's Mind in learning massage, it can be easily adapted to learning—or re-learning—practically any subject or procedure you might undertake, medical or otherwise.

Mastering a simple routine is one of the best strategies for learning massage. Once you've begun to master the basics of any particular "form," you can then begin elaborating and improvising within that framework. In this way, starting with a good routine helps open the doors to imagination and intuition. The real test of a nurse's massage, however, may not be in the quantity or the complexity of the techniques she uses, but in how well the client can sense her caring intention through the character of her touch. That's what clients refer to when they tell their spouse or physician, "That nurse sure does have 'good hands.'" Learning to bring a fresh perspective to each stroke from the very beginning will assure that your performance of every massage remains fresh and vital for years to come.

Finally, the interpersonal exchange between yourself and your clients, before, during, and immediately after their massage, is truly interactive. And so we enlarge upon that interaction with a few very important things to keep in mind. Primarily, you'll always want to show your client how to let you know if your pressure happens to be "too much." That way, your massage will always help them feel better and relax. We close with some simple, easy to remember analogies that can help you introduce the benefits of a good massage to all your clients, colleagues, friends, and family.

The purpose of this chapter, then, is to help you make the most of your initial forays into learning the actual massage strokes as well as the activity of practicing those strokes with friends. With these ideas in mind—and after taking some time to first read through the routines—you should feel completely comfortable and confident in all of your hands-on learning right from the start.

WHO HAS NATURAL ABILITY?

There are those who have learned how to give a very heartfelt massage, even without the benefit of having ever taken a formal massage class or having read a single book on the subject. That may be because the act of human touch is so natural that the mastery of massage technique, in its most essential form, emerges from some of our most fundamental human instincts. Based on our personal observations, the desire alone to learn how to give massage may be one of the best indicators of natural ability. In other words, if you really want to, that is a good indication that you probably can.

Interest and Empathy

Anyone who is interested in massage enough to read a book or take a workshop should seriously consider giving their potential talents an opportunity to develop. Why? Because the need for massage is so great, and it is all around us. Everyone we know personally could probably use a good massage, and over half of those people will, eventually, become interested enough to give it a try.

You do not need to be a practicing nurse in order to give a good massage. If you are a nurse, but you haven't worked in a hospital or clinic for years, your choice of the nursing profession has already demonstrated that you have a great degree of empathy. Empathy seems to be a very strong indicator for natural ability in massage, especially when that empathy is drawn out further by interest and desire. Can you feel when a client is tired, or worried? Do you feel drawn to help people in need? This is empathy, and it is an indicator of what is needed in learning and performing massage.

DO YOU LIKE MASSAGE?

Enjoyment is one fairly reliable test for anyone who might be wondering if they have what it takes to learn massage: Do you like to receive massage yourself? And if you have never actually received a "real" (professional) massage, does the idea of having a massage hold any appeal for you? If it does, and if you're willing to learn and practice, massage could very easily become a part of your everyday life.

If you can imagine yourself giving and receiving massage, you probably already have the ability to do so. If a friend or another nurse likes the idea of being able to give a massage they, too, probably already have the ability to understand and demonstrate good technique.

"I BET I COULD DO THAT"

Confidence is another of the very best indicators for natural ability in massage. As you watch another nurse give or receive a shoulder and neck massage, you might find yourself thinking, "I bet I could do that." Whenever someone has this kind of simple, instinctive belief in their own ability to learn and give massage, it hints at a potential that shouldn't be taken for granted. Not everybody feels that way. But the only way you'll ever know for sure is by putting yourself in the kinds of situations where that potential ability can develop and grow. Those situations include short classes, workshops, and setting up dates with a friend for learning, practicing, and trading massage.

Be Always on the Lookout

Discovering your own ability to use your hands is probably the best way to recognize it in others. Think of yourself as a "talent scout," of sorts, someone who is always on the lookout for good people who can help others feel better in five minutes or less. Not everyone fits the bill but, occasionally, you'll meet someone and think to yourself, "I'll bet she'd really enjoy a massage." Or, "I'll bet he could learn how to give a great massage, if he wanted to."

If hearing about massage interests you, and seeing one performed is "knowing" it might be worthwhile, then feeling one performed on you is probably the best way of recognizing its value without question. Once we have received just one good massage, we will have no doubt about what its potential value can be. And what most of us need in order to help get us motivated is just a little encouragement. Encouraging others, also, can be a form of self-motivation as well.

In summary, then, regarding natural talent, if you already think massage is a good idea, and you believe you could learn how to give an excellent one if you applied your mind to it, your instinctive confidence is a good indicator that you can. If you have a friend or colleague who you think might have potential, show them what a nice massage feels like and let them decide for themselves.

APPROACHING MASSAGE WITH THE BEGINNER'S MIND

Absolute beginners have two very distinct advantages when it comes to learning massage. First of all, they are never burdened by what they already know. And secondly, because they know practically nothing at all about massage, they naturally view the subject with a completely open mind. This approach of un-knowing and open-awareness has been called "Beginner's Mind," which might be elaborated on as simply forgetting all that we think we know and opening up to the direct experience of perception.

If you already happen to know a little, or a lot, about bodywork and touch, may we suggest that you set it aside for the time being. Consider approaching each new massage technique as if you were looking at the whole subject of massage and touch for the very first time. Assuming the view of a true novice, and in giving up all that we have come to think we already know, we regain a simple confidence and certainty in our approach. Suddenly, we have so much more before us to be learned. Setting aside preconceived notions in favor of simple, direct perception, we are challenged to grasp the essence of each idea, each movement, and each response as if it were an entirely fresh experience. It becomes a possibility that even the most familiar experiences, such as touch, can hold for us certain new revelations; things we haven't ever seen before.

Also, as ultimate beginners, we have little or nothing to prove to anyone else, or to ourselves, except that we're willing to be curious and to learn. One of the greatest impediments to approaching a deeper understanding in any subject, but

Touch Your Hands

Relax for a moment, listen to your body, and look at your own hands through the eyes of a True Beginner.

Turn both of your hands over at different angles so that the light around you can illuminate even their smallest features from several directions. Look at your hands as if you are seeing them, right now, for the very first time. These two hands have been your closest friends and helpers through your entire lifetime. How long has it been since you looked at them? They are the delicate physical instruments through which you reach out, making the finest, most precise of adjustments in your world. They are living extensions of both your heart and your mind.

How do these hands feel? Can you describe that feeling in a word?

Now, rub your palms together in small circles, and feel the friction between your palms. Can you feel their warmth growing?

With the fingertips of your right hand, explore the entire palm of the left. Close your eyes, and run your fingertips along its lines. If your palm could represent a miniature world, what kind of world would it be? What would its terrain be like—its hills and valleys? Now, hold your hands as if they were the most precious tools in the entire world.

Finally, with your palms about six inches apart, imagine that your right palm can extend its ability to sense a few inches farther out than the limits of its fleshy surface. With your right palm, "listen" to your left. Passing the right palm over the left, slowly, to the right . . . then the left . . . , listen and see if you can perceive, or feel, with the right what the left hand is feeling while it is being listened to. Can your left hand feel the sensation of your right hand passing over it? How sensitive do you think your hands could become if you dedicated yourself to the task?

How do you imagine it might feel the very first time you help a client feel better, with nothing more than just these two wonderful hands? The true beginner will always be curious to find out.

especially in massage, might be the mindset of, "Oh, I already know this." In fact, we each know very little when compared to what there is to be known, whether it's about massage, or healing, the effects of simple kindness. We are all novices by nature, and the world is opened up before us whenever we place ourselves in the mindset to see.

Prior knowledge about massage can be very valuable, but it will always be with us, at least subconsciously. Our past experiences provide us with much helpful, supportive background information but, by setting aside what we know—at least to the extent that we can—we reduce the possibility of having what we already know (and what we think about it) divide our attention.

For example, in a massage classroom, mentally comparing and contrasting each new technique with some other technique that we have already learned can easily distract us from devoting our full attention to some detailed explanation or a hands-on demonstration. "That technique is (like/unlike/better than/worse than) the other one (I learned, we used, she did) . . ." etc. In any learning context, each learner's active attention helps support the collective concentration of all the others in the group. Individually, it is hard to be in two places at once without missing something important in at least one of them, if not both. Undivided attention, on the other hand, engaged by curiosity and via direct perception, enables us to learn massage most effectively, and directly, through our hands. Therefore, we urge you to learn and practice all of your massage from the perspective of the Beginner's Mind. Touch each client with a sense of joy and wonder, perceive directly and, with any luck, you will remain a beginner for the rest of your days.

The Destination of Massage

It is no cliché to say that, in giving massage—as well as in learning it, receiving it, and even teaching it—the journey, itself, is its ultimate destination. Each stroke, and every small movement required of your hands, is a complete end unto itself. Of course, motion is ongoing and perpetual, but you will never perform the first stroke in order to "arrive at" the second; or walk through a series of strokes just to "get to the end." That very first stroke is worthy of your fullest and most complete attention, just as helping is an end in itself.

So let each movement of every stroke work its magic in slowing you down, and perform each one of those strokes—not as one more step in a series of small events—but as one extended event that happens to be ongoing and changing slightly as it goes. Realizing that we never completely arrive at any final destination helps us remember that our own arrival takes place as soon as we finally show up. Becoming so fully engaged in the flow of motion helps us shape every nuance of our hands out of direct perception, and to the very best of our ability.

Dwelling on each stroke for as long as it takes to perform it well, is what induces the greatest sensation of relaxation and rejuvenation from the client's point of view. So, from the viewpoint of the Beginner's Mind, there is only one massage stroke, the one stroke you happen to be engaged in right now.

In the role of true beginners, we are compelled to focus completely on whatever we're doing, because we have no idea at all what may be coming next. We are forced by circumstances, and by our own point of view, to be here, wherever we are, before we can even think about wherever it is we might be going. The beginner's dilemma, then, is their deliverance.

Think back to the very first time you rode a bicycle, or to the day you first learned to roller skate. The instant you started thinking about anything else other than the enormous task at hand, you were in trouble! By assuming the perspective of Beginner's Mind, in every massage we look deliberately into the enormous task of what we're doing through ancient, yet very familiar "innocent eyes."

The "destination" of massage—that is, what it is "aiming toward"—is akin to peace, release, vibrant vitality, and deep inner happiness for the client. All of these qualities can only be experienced in the present moment. Otherwise they are simply mental abstractions, something we might wish we could acquire, or have, "someday." Yet peace, for example, if it's a true peacefulness, isn't something to be "had" someday. Peace is lived—today. So is vibrant health—and so is the vitality of healing. It might be said that the beginner's destination is one of perpetual arrival. Therefore, all of our goals in massage are being realized in this present moment, or not at all. And if we are fully realizing them now, their effects will persist in our body's memory for a long time to come. No one can soon forget the massage that brought them back into timelessness, however brief that lingering moment might have seemed at the time.

So if you do happen to find yourself mentally disengaged or distracted while giving a massage, remember Beginner's Mind, and this simple question: "What is *this?*" Distractions, like destinations, tend to fall from view once we're deeply engaged in the moment at hand. And from the perspective of your clients, remember, too, that this beginning is a moment that could just as well go on for a long, long time.

THE VALUE OF LEARNING MASSAGE BY "ROUTINES"

A massage "routine" is a series of massage strokes performed in a logical progression from one body area to the next. To our "left-brained," linear way of thinking, routines provide us with a structure that can be very comforting. The beginning, middle, and end of a routine is familiar, and so it helps us feel like we know what we're doing, where things start and where they will end. With routines we don't need to worry about "What comes next?" because if we just follow along, the routine will unfold in a dependable order every time. To some students, practitioners, and teachers of massage, just the thought of routines may seem rather simplistic and predictable. But for the very beginner, if a good routine provides for some flexibility, it can become an ideal stepping stone for opening up our natural intuition.

While routines may at first appear to be the antithesis of Beginner's Mind—spontaneity versus predictability—the two work together quite well. When our organizing mental apparatus is completely satisfied, it relaxes on deeper levels, and our intuition can peek through the spaces between all the seemingly separate steps. In other words, routines satisfy our need to know what's next so that our intuitive nature is given a chance to emerge. The combination gives us more opportunities for our feeling nature to come into play.

Once you have taken the time to learn the short routines in the following chapter, it will become clear that they were never intended to be rigid, or set in stone. While we strongly encourage you to study and practice them thoroughly during your initial attempts, making sure each client receives the massage he or she needs will always be your priority, not the inclusion, or exclusion, of any set number of techniques. The purpose of learning massage by way of routines is to establish a set of familiar entry points, or "doorways" into the world of technique for helping relieve the effects of tension and pain.

Without some sort of routine to help a beginner get started, it could be easy for most of us to feel a little lost. Telling a student to, "just start wherever you like and then go on to wherever you want," doesn't really provide enough structure for the way we typically think about process learning. "Where should I start? What comes next? What should I include? How will I know when I'm finished?" These are all the kinds of questions someone asks when approaching massage for the very first time, and a good routine provides the answers until we begin to grasp the larger picture. Even advanced students appreciate some structure, especially when its purpose is to foster greater flexibility.

The confidence you'll feel from seeing that you've begun to master a handful of simple steps with good results will relax enough of your mental stress for you to become more attentive to listening with your hands. We suggest you start by becoming completely comfortable with performing all the sub-routines, as outlined, and practice them until you can demonstrate every stroke exactly as described. Then practice with friends, colleagues, and family members. Performing just a few strokes with a sense of comfort and ease can have a noticeably relaxing effect on your client. It's much better to do a half-dozen strokes really well than trying to explore several dozen new ideas before you've had enough time to get comfortable with the basics.

Through learning a series of short routines you'll also begin to re-educate your own neuromuscular system. From the viewpoint of the brain, you are reorganizing more of your synaptic territory into a whole new set of subtle psychomotor skills. Consciously, systematically—and with hardly any stress at all—you will be integrating a fresh level of perception and sensitivity as you engage a whole new array of fine motor movements. Not only are you sending out signals to your hands to "squeeze" or "knead," you are receiving signals back from them of "perceive" and "feel." This heightened kinesthetic sensitivity also helps reorient the logical, thinking mind for something we each already understand very well, instinctively—waking up of intuitive knowing. In short, massage awakens intuition so that intuition starts to make sense. How can you know something you don't really know? You can feel it. And massage illustrates that connection of knowing by feeling for us again and again, not as a "leap" of faith, but as a simple, natural fact. Routines help bridge that connection.

Human Bodies Understand Massage

On the very deepest of levels, human bodies already understand each other perfectly. If we could somehow set aside our cerebral thinking, questioning, doubting, and wondering, our brains and bodies already understand how to give and receive the kind of help a great massage has to offer. You may already know someone personally who has a natural gift for massage, arrived at solely through intuition. They can step aside, in a manner of speaking, and follow along with that flow of instinctive information as it circulates between their hands, muscles, and nerves, and those of their partner's. They "know where to go." How? They feel it. But since most of us need and appreciate a bit more structure in our learning, routines are one way we organize our experience. The patterns we start to notice in what will soon become very familiar can be looked upon as cues and clues, so we can start to interpret this instinctive information as a slightly different way of knowing.

ROUTINES HELP US LEARN

In order to organize our environment and measure our visible progress, we tend to make routines out of almost everything. We develop confidence based, primarily, on understanding our goal and going through the detours of trial and error to achieve it. We stop occasionally to review and reflect on the strengths and weaknesses of our performance so far, consider all the feedback we have gotten and, finally, revise and refine our approach before trying once again. If we had to stop and think this process through every time we learned something new, most of us would just quit learning altogether. Unfortunately, some of us have! But many have learned how to "routine-ize" the learning process itself. We can apply this same skill for making routines in the following manner to learn intuitive massage.

On a "routine" basis, we repeat some given cycle of activity until we feel like we "have it down." Examples are everywhere: driving a car, washing a load of clothes, the several things we each do each night before going to bed, and even putting on our clothes in the morning. We have routine-ized each one of these activities without even thinking about it. So, if we have some process completely organized where do new improvements or insights come from? What is the source of those "ahas!" that reveal to us how to shorten, or enliven, or elaborate on some activity, one we may have even started to take for granted? Often, we run into a "window" of opportunity when we weren't even looking for it.

The spaces between the steps of those patterned activities are where, eventually, our intuitive hunches will have enough room to "pop through." The spaces between the steps of our daily routines are where we "get" a fresh idea for an old problem while we're busy taking a shower. Just as we daydreamed as children while watching the telephone poles fly by out the car window, we get intuitive flashes while passing by the windows that open between the steps of our daily routines. But our mind needs to be relaxed, occupied by some "routine" activity or practice, in order to be able to do it. As a result of all these windows, we tend to continually refine and become very good at whatever we set out to do, whether it's taking a medical history, playing jazz on the violin, or learning how to give a great massage.

Tedium gives way to intuition

Like learning any new motor skill, learning massage strokes may seem a bit tedious in the beginning. The first time we actually walk through our routine, it can take much longer to just read through the written instructions and look over the illustrations than all the strokes will ever take to perform on a client. That's completely normal, and it should be expected. Practicing musical scales also comes to mind. Musicians spend countless hours practicing scales and arpeggios just so they can eventually play and improvise a three-minute piece of music! But what may seem like tedium at first can lead directly into intuition, creativity, and imagination.

Tedium gives way when we intentionally look for patterns and relationships in our new experiences that we've come to recognize and understand in things we have done before. For example, everything you've learned about interacting with clients in ICU will transfer when offering your first dozen clients their three-minute massage. Even though executing the techniques in those first massages might take a little extra effort, the way you initiate interaction, or the way you help a client roll over onto their side, will be practically the same. Noticing these similarities across disparate experiences helps us stay engaged and relaxed, thus opening the possibility for intuitive information to emerge.

PHYSICAL INTUITION

During your first several practice sessions, you might notice that your hands become easily tired. Almost everyone overworks when they first learn massage so that, too, is something you can expect. With this in mind, the more you practice relaxing into your hand movements and assuming equally relaxed body positioning, overall, the easier your massage will be to perform.

By the fifth or sixth practice session, the process of reading techniques from the page and practicing the hand movements—even while talking through each of steps aloud—will start to become second nature.

After a short time, in those fleeting moments between the routine's actual steps, you might get that elusive hunch, or notion, about how much pressure a particular shoulder muscle might like to receive. Exactly how to apply that pressure might occur to you instinctively too, and soon you'll be able to create the kind of physical sensation you want for your client.

Try using what you believe might be the "right amount" of pressure, and ask your partner for feedback. That's how you'll eventually build up your own "encyclopedia" of first-hand knowledge. By deliberately attending to all those details, and repeating movements that may have seemed so tedious for you at the start, you will become much more comfortable with each massage technique and their natural sequence. Then you can step aside, mentally, and let your hands do some of the thinking by themselves. This is where your physical intuition can come into play.

Don't "Fall into" a Routine

Some students, from time to time, have voiced concerns about learning massage through practicing a routine. They fear their massage might become like a "cookie cutter," that is, "one size fits all." This is a worthwhile caution, but it might not present such a problem if we try to explore some of the assumptions behind it and consider some of the possible alternatives.

Human bodies are so unique, that even if you performed exactly the same strokes every time on everyone, the particular needs of each body—and the human character who animates that body and influences its form—would render the net effects of your massage quite different every time. It is practically impossible to do exactly the same massage twice, because even when two physical bodies are almost identical in structure and form, the individual personalities receiving the massage will accept that massage in entirely different ways. For example, our muscle stress naturally resists the pressure of any massage stroke, and our mental/ emotional stresses can influence how easy it is for us to relax and let go. These factors—muscle stress, stroke, pressure, resistance, mental and emotional stresses— each one is unique to the individual, and so will be the subjective effect of every single stroke. So performing the same strokes to the same client a week later would yield an entirely different effect, because the client, and the strokes, would vary over time.

Only if a nurse was, somehow, completely insensitive to all of these human factors (which is most unlikely), could a truly "uniform" massage for all of her clients be a practical possibility. The nuances of a client's personality alone (not to mention shifting themes of thinking and their effects on subjective feeling states), would make all the difference, and these can vary considerably from hour to hour. In sum, each client receives a completely different massage, no matter what you do. Perhaps a greater concern regarding "sameness" might be in the nurse's perception and feeling states.

AN ANTIDOTE FOR BOREDOM

The other part of the fear of "routine" routines is that you might lose interest in "doing the same old massage all the time." When we turn our attention away from the small details in each massage it's much easier to feel bored. So the best antidote for boredom may be in paying closer attention to the details of everything around us, everything we are doing, all the information that is coming through our senses, and how those points of detail are interrelated. Who could possibly be bored with all of those things going on? Losing interest and becoming disengaged are usually the signs of either having lost some degree of focus, or an indication that we have reached some advanced level of mastery of detail and are about to advance to a higher level of organization.

When we master the details of a system or procedure, we experience a need to lift ourselves up into a higher perspective of that system in order to comprehend the greater order in what we're doing. That's why most of us become bored with routine jobs: we have mastered all the details and have intelligence to spare, yet we have nowhere to apply it. Hence, the mind wanders. We are designed by nature to learn and grow.

The antidote for disengagement during massage (spacing out, getting bored, negative thoughts, etc.) is, once again, to pay attention to the details. Deliberately shift your focus of attention onto what you are learning from the client in front of you. Remember that you receive very different input from each human body during a massage in the form of physical sensation and visual information, whether you are aware of it or not. All input being patterned, think of the variations in the information reaching your nervous system through the perception of your touch alone. Then set about figuring out what new possibilities all of this new level of input might represent.

For example, the right shoulder area might be slightly higher and more constricted than the left. So if there is visual asymmetry, you might also look for a correlation in excessive heat somewhere. But if you are preoccupied with thinking that you are bored, you will probably miss many of the subtle details like these, and your mind may wander. This shift in awareness, alone, onto noticing what details you may have been overlooking, will almost always re-engage your interest immediately.

If you ever feel like massage, in general, is becoming "routine" for you, try teaching massage to another nurse. Even if it's only your two or three favorite strokes, listen to what you hear yourself telling that nurse about those strokes and your personal experiences performing them. Paraphrase is the most reliable test of comprehension, it also demands that we think about our thinking processes, which lifts us up into slightly higher levels of thinking about thinking ("metacognition"). You will never be bored if you make an effort to teach something you want to learn.

After only one month of learning and practicing massage you will have received and reorganized billions of bits of valuable information, intellectually and kinesthetically. So you are bound to learn a great deal each time you teach someone else something interesting about what you have learned. Look for that one outstanding family member from among every one of your clients, that special someone who might have some natural ability for massage. Then teach that special family member just two simple strokes. Sharing our interests and enthusiasm with others helps those same characteristics grow and thrive in our own experiences.

Approaching the Classic Form

What is the difference between a well-polished "form" and a well-worn "rut?" Falling into a rut in anything is boring—hollowed out, and as empty of passion as it is of curiosity. But achieving mastery in a classic form keeps us perennially vital and alive. We will eventually get sick of any rut, but of a truly classic form, we will hardly ever get enough!

In the language of jazz, the difference between a competent journeyman performance and the brilliance of mastery may be less about any complex harmonic changes being played, and more about the "groove," the feeling with which we play them. The feeling is what moves an audience to its feet. Like the harmonic changes of "I've Got Rhythm," or "Sweet Georgia Brown," simple "routines" can be practiced, literally, thousands and thousands of times and for countless hours—and they will never be performed the same way twice! Identical as they may appear on their surface, each performance creates a unique set of patterned relationships, feelings, and nuances, and the same applies to other movement-oriented forms as well.

Masters of the many martial arts, for example, such as Tai Chi, Karate, Judo, or Aikido, have been known to practice the same classic forms within their respective disciplines for years, even for a lifetime. Why? Don't they get bored? No. The channeling of their personal vitality through these established forms of physical motion helps bring acute focus to their conscious awareness. Also, by becoming aware of our own personal energy we become aware of universal energy, or "Chi." For masters and students alike, the visible forms they practice might be ancient in origin, but the subtle nuances of performance are always uniquely their own and experienced in the present. Another reason for practicing forms is that through our emulation of those forms, we cultivate inside ourselves a deep and abiding appreciation for the elegant movement of everyday living.

Practicing routines is almost universal, in some manner or another, in every culture and in practically every form of art. Each motion becomes more effortless with practice and, as its practitioner approaches higher levels of perfection, it is as if each sequence or routine were being performed for the very first time. These particular movements you are making in today's practice will never be made again, even if the form out of which they come were to be repeated a million times or more. Once we realize this somewhat enlarged perspective on the practice of forms, a simple, graceful self-awareness becomes its primary aim. Something as simple as walking itself—but engaging in it with consciously focused self-awareness, can be—and is—considered a highly refined form of spiritual meditation.

Through our personal presence we transcend the mere mechanics of "following procedure" and, through our intention, we can bring an element of "soul" into the physical movements involved in any interpersonal exchange. Perform every massage you give with the engaging vitality of that beautiful ballad, "Stardust," along with the graceful presence of the flowing Tai Chi, and you will never find yourself becoming tired of singing anybody else's "same old song."

Toward this end, when the time comes, pick for yourself any three simple massage techniques that appeal to you, personally. Then learn to fill their simple sequence with your own personal version of "Heart and Soul." With practice you will be able to elevate their performance into that same graceful aura of a truly classic form each and every time you perform it.

Finally, remember that the quality of your performance is not dependent upon your solo interpretation alone, because each massage is, in fact, a duet. And since it will always be the same music—that shared vitality—that moves through you both, it is as important to learn when to listen as it is to know how to sing. As a nurse, you just happen to be the partner whose turn it will be, most often, to take the lead. Your opening line is made up of a simple, two-note melody: "May I?" You might come to think of this overture as a "call and response."

FIRST OF ALL, ASK FOR PERMISSION

Before beginning each and every massage, it is appropriate to first ask your client's permission. Most clients will probably take you up on the offer, but some will decline. Either way, asking for permission is where the massage exchange begins. If your client has previously indicated an interest, it is still considerate to ask their permission before actually beginning.

Asking permission is much more than a formality, it is a professional and personal courtesy. Some clients might think it a bit forward, or even intrusive, if you just come up to them and start massaging their shoulders without asking first. So it is appropriate to ask and, then, view their assent as an invitation.

Of course, asking to be invited is a request and, as such, it infers that your offer to help can always be declined. A client in the middle of a migraine headache, for example, may want to sit alone for a moment. Just the thought of having her neck and shoulders massaged during that particular moment might not sound very appealing at all. When you do ask, you should be prepared to receive whatever response the client feels is appropriate, which might not necessarily be the choice you think would be best for them. Ask permission, then listen for and accept their response. The client knows best.

In more informal, non-professional settings, such as with good friends or close acquaintances, asking permission might not always be absolutely necessary. A safe rule of thumb might be, regardless of how friendly you feel toward the other person, it's always better to ask first. In the professional nursing setting, however, you should always ask.

How to Ask

When first beginning your massage work with clients, you may find yourself feeling hesitant to ask. Keep in mind that the request doesn't need to be especially formal, and you can adopt the approach that it's just a friendly offer. Here's one way to proceed. You might ask, "Would you like your massage now? It only takes a couple of minutes." Indicate that a short massage is all a part of regular procedure, if that truly is the case. If massage is something new in your work environment, let the client know that, too. "We're trying out massage for some of our clients to see if it helps them feel better. Would you like to try that?" Be honest and let your own appreciation for the benefits of massage, and how good it feels, come across to the client. The chances are that most clients will accept.

COUNTERING THE SELF-EFFACING DECLINE

Occasionally a client will decline, telling you they "wouldn't want to be a bother." If they sincerely don't want to be a bother, you might tell them that you have just started studying massage as a part of client care, and you were wondering if they might help you get some practice. Presenting your offer from this view will show your clients how they are helping you. After all, most of us could use more practice with our clients. Giving you their permission to perform a massage is in no way a bother to you, because your client is giving you an opportunity to help him. And helping others is always a gift for the giver.

IT'S NOT ABOUT NEED

You are asking if the client would like a massage, not telling them they need one. There is a difference. One is an invitation to enjoy, the other can be easily misinterpreted. They may think you are implying that they are somehow "broken" and you can "fix" them with your massage. As odd as that may sound, and you certainly may not mean it that way, a client who feels depressed, or who is sensing a perceived loss of control in some other area, can certainly view your offer of massage in that light. Make your intentions clear, you don't need to be broken in order to feel better. You have just come to help.

MAKE NO ASSUMPTIONS

Your asking for permission should not infer that your client is about to get a massage (whether he likes it or not). The massage really does need to be partly his choice, because his receptivity plays such a large role in its potential effectiveness. So stop and listen closely to his response. After all, he might not really care for a massage right now, in which case you should offer to stop by again sometime later on. Most clients will be glad to "let you" give them a massage. Asking permission is just another way of respecting the client's freedom of choice, and most of us would probably appreciate the same consideration in being asked.

A MOST REASONABLE REQUEST

You may occasionally notice some hesitation on the client's part. In a case where logic might prove gently persuasive, try asking if she would like to have a short back massage to help her relax and get a better night's sleep. Most of us are sleep deprived, whether we know it (or would admit it) or not. And even a small amount of massage almost always helps us relax, which directly affects our sleep. Just the thought of a good night's rest can often be enough to gently persuade a client or colleague to give massage a try.

Another reasonable approach might be when a colleague complains of tight shoulders, a headache, or sore neck, you might wonder aloud if she's had a shoulder rub lately. If necessary, you can assure, "It only takes a minute." It's reasonable to assume that almost everybody has "a minute." And if anyone, especially a nurse, says, "Oh, I don't think so," you might offer, "Well, if you change you mind, just let me know. OK?" Being just a tiny little bit on the "pushy" side can be justified sometimes when it comes to helping a friend feel better. If you always ask permission with a smile, your offer can hardly seem overbearing.

Keep in mind, too, that most of us have never had a "real" (professional) massage. Others just may not be accustomed to being touched. For a few, it might even seem a little scary. So friendliness is your all-around best approach when asking. Again, it's just a friendly offer.

TODAY'S SUGGESTION BECOMES TOMORROW'S MASSAGE

Sometimes a good idea can take a while to sink in. Clients and colleagues might need to think about it today, then take you up on it tomorrow—or they may take someone else up on the same offer a year from now. The only way you can find out if they're ready is to ask them, and that's why you should always ask before you rub. If you have a good friend who has already enjoyed your massage in the past, and you can clearly see that they could use a shoulder rub, still, ask first.

NEVER TAKE A REFUSAL PERSONALLY

If your offer is genuinely friendly, you have already done a good thing just in offering it. Nothing is for everyone. Not everybody wants to enjoy a big, fresh ripe peach, either, but that doesn't stop peaches from tasting delicious! If your offer is friendly, turning down a massage probably has more to do with something on their mind, it's not necessarily about you.

GETTING ACQUAINTED BEFORE MASSAGE

If you and your client don't already know each other, and they say they would like to have that massage, it's worth spending a minute or so before beginning just to get acquainted. However brief or extended that initial conversation might be, getting things off to a nice start makes the massage more enjoyable for both parties.

Most nursing clients will have already presented with some level of discomfort, either physical pain or some other form of distress. And almost all clients will feel a little anxious about receiving any form of medical care, however minor their condition may seem. Clients who might otherwise be very competent, self-determined individuals will often feel some degree of loss of control over their lives during any type of episode that requires nursing care or a visit with a physician. In more extreme situations, whenever a client is hospitalized or receiving home care, their perceived loss of control, or the inability to make certain decisions for themselves, can become a significant, yet "hidden" stressor. That's one reason it's important to extend ourselves personally to the client and give them an opportunity to discover a new friend. If they know us and like us, they will probably trust us. One good way to garner that trust is through a very brief conversation at the very start.

Just Say "Too Much": The Client is in Control

One of the best ways to help a client feel better and relax at the very beginning of a massage is to show them how they can take an active part in making sure their massage is enjoyable. Let them know they can always say, "Too much." Whenever muscles are tight or sore, sometimes the squeezing or kneading can cause them to "hurt good." That means there is some discomfort but, actually, it feels good. Our massage, though, should never "hurt bad." That means discomfort to the point of wanting it to stop. Pain is not necessary for relaxation. In fact, painful kneading can be counterproductive, however well intentioned it might be. So it's important to let every client know that they are in control of what does and does not feel good to them—and that you want to hear from them. Here is how to let them know they are in control.

Before you begin that very first stroke—stop—and tell your client, "Now, if anything I do actually hurts, just say the words, 'Too Much,' OK?" (Wait until they acknowledge they understand.) "If it's ever a little too hard for you, or if it's a little too deep for comfort, those are the magic words. Right then, you say, 'Too Much,' Okay?"

If a stroke "hurts good," it makes us naturally want to breathe into the area and let go of the tension on the exhale. When your hand pressure hurts "bad," it makes the client want to recoil instinctively, or hold their breath. So if it hurts bad, we tell the client they should say, "Too Much," because this assures them that you're serious about nothing being painful. This puts the clients in control, and that puts them at ease.

If you have an idea that they might not completely understand, there are some additional things you might add as you begin the first strokes. For example, you might tell them, "If you say 'ouch,' or 'that hurts,' or 'you're killing me,' I might think you just like it. But if you say, 'Too Much,' I'll break contact like this (and take your hands off their shoulders for a second to demonstrate). And then we'll start again." Making a client smile is always a plus.

When the client's shoulders are already somewhat tight or sore, the pressure of your hands might make them aware, for the first time, of how sore their muscles actually were all along. The manual pressure of your hands on the client's muscles helps "define" their subjective state of muscle tension in a very unique way. This physical sensation can, literally, be an inspiration, in that it makes your body want to breathe instinctively. So the massage we are learning here will, sometimes, "hurt good," but nothing you do should ever hurt "bad." If the client can understand the difference between the two and, if you will receive a few massages from a friend, you will see the difference, also. If someone ever massages you too deeply—and refuses to stop when you say "Too Much"—you will see how important it is for every client to feel like they are in control of the depth and pressure.

Some clients don't require much pressure at all to help them relax. For example, in some elderly clients just barely touching the shoulders is enough "pressure" to help them feel much better. And that response is all you are looking for. In fact, for some especially frail clients, just resting your hands on their shoulders—and allowing your own body to fully relax for a moment—might be all they need to remind them to let go and relax as well.

Whenever the client thinks the pressure is too much, it is too much. It doesn't matter how much pressure you think the client needs in order "to do him any good," because the extent of pressure you apply should always be the client's call. We respect and appreciate every client's feedback in every massage and we show that appreciation through our actions. So telling everybody about the Magic Words, "Too Much," is one of the best ways to get every massage off to a good start.

Orienting a Client to Massage

Even if the client has never had a massage before, it doesn't take very long to orient someone to receiving a massage, and those preliminaries should be fairly brief. Below is a very thorough list of questions from which you can choose. Since you only want to spend a minute or so on preliminaries, ask only those particular questions that you think will be most useful. The following list is for reference only, and should not be viewed as a checklist. While the questions are presented in a somewhat idealized chronology, items numbered 4, 5, 7, 8, 11, and 12 (marked by an asterisk *) may merit a higher priority and are a bulleted list in the box that follows.

1. "Have you ever had a massage before?"

   If not, you might suggest that it is, " . . . always nice to give someone his first massage, because there's really nothing like it." If he has received massage, ask, "Any specific areas you'd like me to massage today?"

2. "You'll be covered with the sheet, by the way."

   Some clients are modest (regarding the back techniques using lotion) even if they try to act otherwise. This reassures him that his feelings are respected.

3. Tell him the two or three body areas you plan to work on, and ask, "How does that sound, OK?"

*4. "So, how are you feeling today."

   Asking the client directly helps you find any areas to focus on, or avoid. Be sure to look over the chart to see what physical (or other) problems he might be having. If the client doesn't respond with any specific complaints, then try the next question, number 5.

*5. "How about your body? Do you have any particular areas that are sore or tight?"

6. "Any areas we need to avoid?"

   Trust them, they will tell you. But you need to be on the lookout for problematic areas, anyway.

*7. "Be sure to tell me if the pressure's about right—OK?"

   Nice and firm can be relaxing, but it's all supposed to feel good.

   This is a good place to show them what happens if they say, "Too Much" (break contact and start again, but lighter). Even your lightest finger pressure could be painful for some clients. Others prefer a very firm, physical massage. If any client tells you more than once to "go lighter," and you think you're already massaging so lightly that it couldn't possibly be helping, please remember that the pressure this client says he wants is the perfect amount of pressure for him to be receiving right now.

*8. "Feel free to give me any feedback like, 'more here,' or 'slow down there.'"

   Let him know it's his massage.

9. "How it would be most comfortable for you to lay while getting this massage?"

   Considering this client's overall condition, does he think he should sit or lie down for the best massage? If he doesn't know, make an educated guess. If he sits in a chair, be sure he's sitting comfortably, relaxed but not slouched. He might want a table, or the edge of the hospital bed, in front of him so he can lean forward on it, his forehead resting against his folded arms. If he is lying down, ask if he might be more comfortable lying on his stomach, side or back. Position pillows under his ankles if he chooses to lie on his stomach face down; or, when lying on his side, place one pillow under his head and another between his knees.

10. "Feel free to doze off if you like. I won't mind at all."

    You might also add, "Or we can visit, or just lay back and relax. OK?"

*11. Either during or after the massage, remind him, "Be sure to drink some extra water today, OK? So you can get the most good from your massage."

    If he asks why he should drink more water, or if it seems appropriate, let him know that, "Massage stimulates the circulation of blood, so drinking extra water helps the kidneys flush out everything the massage loosens up (like unwanted lactic acid and any other toxins)." Avoid technical jargon when possible and focus on a relaxing sensation throughout all the muscles.

*12. "If you doze off, when I finish I'll just slip out and you can relax."

    Let them know that you can visit later on, if they'd like. Also, suggest something like, "If you can, try not to have much to do afterward, for about 20 minutes." Preferably, even up to an hour, that way he can get the most relaxation and enjoyment out of his massage.

Again, you probably won't ever ask one client all of these questions, so pick and choose the most appropriate. A brief conversation along these lines at the very beginning of a massage is one more thing to help clients feel they have some control over the situation. It also shows that you care about their particular needs and concerns. Additionally, these questions provide assessment information for nursing care, as well as how to customize his massage.

Primary Questions, Before Massage

- So, how are you feeling today?
- Do you have any particular areas that are sore or tight?
- Be sure to tell me if the pressure's about right—Okay?
- Feel free to give me any feedback like, "more here," or "slow down there." Okay?
- Be sure to drink extra water today, Okay?
- If you doze off, when I finish, I'll just leave and you can relax.

How Much Conversation?

Some clients like to chat during their massage, while others prefer to snore! Overall, clients seem to favor enjoying the massage experience slightly more than carrying on an ongoing discussion. But there are always exceptions. After your initial questions, let the client take the lead on any conversation during their massage. Some clients will fall asleep almost immediately, while others stay awake throughout but say nothing at all.

There will be those clients who like to chat throughout their entire massage, but they are the minority. If your client isn't asking questions or initiating conversation, it's probably better to let the silence have its moment. The physical sensation of receiving a massage is a lot of input to take in and digest, so some clients can find conversation distracting. If you were receiving a massage from a nurse who happened to be in a "chatty" mood, how effective do you think that might be? On the whole, honoring the client's personal preferences as indicated by her actions allows her the opportunity to enjoy her massage in the way that suits her best.

A client's level of relaxation during massage seems to be somewhat deeper when there is little or no talking. But for some clients it becomes clear right away that they do need to talk. Their eyes are closed and, since they know you are there to help them, you become a sympathetic ear. She may have some unmet need having to do with sharing her feelings and expressing her thoughts. Or she may want to talk about something related to her condition, or some other issue. Then, too, she may just feel lonely. Receiving massage can help feelings and concerns come up to the surface that she might not have been aware of before she started to relax. Just the experience of feeling cared for in such a vivid way can encourage some clients to feel safe enough to open up and share their stories.

Many clients will tell you about things that have really been bothering them and, as most nurses already know, one of the most supportive things we can do is to listen. Try to listen, not just to the words, but to the tone and inflections underneath them. Let the conversation be mostly a monologue on the client's part, if that seems natural. But also let them know you are interested in hearing everything they have to say. Consider offering your opinion or comment but— almost exclusively—only if asked. One possible exception being if a client were misinterpreting some doctor's order or lab results, etc. In that case, if the client's recollection or misinterpretation of a medical order could result in their potentially causing harm, don't wait to be asked your opinion. But do respond in a comforting, reassuring tone.

Whenever we do talk with a client during their massage we should always remember to speak slowly, and in a relaxed, friendly, supportive tone of voice. Since your client is so relaxed, she may also be equally as open to suggestion. So avoid making any comments that might prove counterproductive, such as, "You sure are tight here." Or, "What have you been doing to make this lower back so sore?" Another favorite we've heard is, "I've never seen shoulders this tight." These particular examples of what *not* to say might seem self-evident, even comical, but we've heard them, and worse. Suffice it to say that we all need to be considerate of the possible consequences any of our casual comments might have whenever a client is very relaxed.

Your initial "connection" through conversation, right at the very beginning of a massage, even if it only lasts a minute or less, can help establish a relaxed, casual atmosphere and start building that friendly trust and confidence. Where you may have begun just a few moments ago as two complete strangers, you now enter into a mutually appreciative and beneficial relationship. Both of you have reason to expect that good things are likely to come out of your next few minutes together.

INTRODUCING MASSAGE TO OTHERS

What if, during their massage, a client happens to ask about its benefits? Sooner or later, a client is bound to look you squarely in the eye and pose a delightfully simple question like, "Why is massage good for you?" or, "Why did you think I needed a massage?" and, "What do you like most about massage?" Most clients won't want or need a long, technical explanation. After all, they're trying to relax and enjoy a massage!

So in order to take advantage of that "teachable moment," it's helpful to have some answers handy that are as simple and straightforward as the question asked.

Having already studied massage at this point, you may be more informed than most people about the many good effects and lasting benefits of massage. But the client usually just wants to hear the headlines. The best headlines are short, easy to understand, and memorable. So here are a few ideas that most clients will be able to relate to right away.

Like an Analogy

An analogy is a figure of speech that makes a vivid comparison. In other words, we want to compare the benefits of massage with another more familiar idea. Using the following four "headlines," you can help your client learn a lot about massage with a few simple comparisons, or "idea pictures." Like postage stamps, these short analogies are intended to "stick in" your memory.

- Massage is like "kneading dough."
- Massage is like "wringing out" the stress.
- The body is like a fiddle, and massage "tunes you up."
- Having a massage is like taking a little "mini-vacation."

These simple phrases are good conversation starters with your new clients. Below are some very brief elaborations, one for each of those phrases to help you better remember them. Once you "get the picture," just memorize a few key words and you can make up your own explanation. The goal is to paint a clear mental picture for your clients in about two to three seconds so they can remember it and, later on, tell a friend.

MASSAGE IS LIKE "KNEADING DOUGH"

The motion of your hands working through the soft muscle tissue makes this analogy especially clear, even tactile. Also, taking the "dough" analogy just one step further, you might need to work out a few of the lumps in some areas. But with a little kneading, everything starts to feel consistent, or "all smoothed out." Most importantly, "Every-body needs to feel kneaded." As you'll see right away, a little humor can go a long way with massage, and massage is ready-made for silly jokes. And sometimes, the more corny or silly the humor, the easier it is to remember.

MASSAGE IS LIKE "WRINGING OUT" THE STRESS

Almost everybody has wrung water out of a towel. And some clients say that after a massage they "feel all wrung out" (a delightful state!). A good massage can be like a few minutes in a nice hot tub: you'll be limp as a noodle! "How can you tell if he's done?" "Well, he just sticks to the chair 'cause he's all wrung out!" How many people do we know who are wound up so tight that they couldn't stand to be wrung out? Well, that's how a good massage makes you feel.

THE BODY'S LIKE A FIDDLE, AND MASSAGE "TUNES YOU UP"

Like a finely crafted violin, all of our body parts are important and designed to work together in harmony. Massage loosens up the tight places, and tones up the loose parts, to help you feel back in tune. So, massage is like a little tune-up.

HAVING A MASSAGE IS LIKE A LITTLE MINI-VACATION

A massage is equal to a whole day at the beach. It's easy to take a three-minute massage vacation, and it changes your outlook, too. Massage does wonders for your point of view.

Word-images in the form of analogies like these can be helpful to hear, especially for the client, or friend, who looks like they could appreciate a few kind words. Talking about massage is also a great way to change the subject, too, should the client's conversation head down the occasional "rough and rugged road."

What we tend to talk about in our idle moments has a great effect on how we greet and respond to our own immediate future. During a massage for the talkative client, try to steer the conversation gently away from idle gossip, pessimistic speculation, explaining past events and "de-stressing chatter."

For example, one favorite topic during de-stressing is the fascinating details of the physical ailments and recent surgeries of friends and family members. Another client detailed a recent shopping excursion to a factory outlet mall. If a client's conversation drifts in this direction during their massage try interjecting a question about the physical sensation of a certain massage stroke. Your intention is simply to draw their attention beyond the familiar day-to-day routine and into the extraordinary experience of the massage. Use one of the analogies above, or anything that occurs to you to draw the client into the present, and onto their physical experience. After all, you can talk about the mall anytime, but the massage is happening now.

Pick an image or two from the list that fits your personal style and memorize it. Maybe use something that seems to fit a particular client's situation or personality. Who knows, you might be placing a pleasant mental picture frame around their image of massage that could last a lifetime. Don't be surprised if they start to associate you, personally, with the experience of feeling good. Years from now, your client might be on vacation somewhere, sitting back and looking out over a grand, beautiful view of the late afternoon sky, sipping on nice tall beverage, and thinking about "that nurse that used to come in a give me those great back rubs." There could hardly be a better way to be remembered.

What's So Great About a Good Massage?

- Massage is like kneading dough.
  "Every body needs to be kneaded."
- Massage is like wringing out the stress.
  "Like a soak in the hot tub, you'll feel like a noodle."
- The body's like a fiddle, and massage tunes you up.
  "You can hear that beautiful music again."
- Massage is like a mini-vacation.
  "It does wonders for your point of view."

SUMMARY

Everything you have learned so far about touch and massage has prepared a strong foundation for using hands-on technique. The next two chapters will help you put this knowledge into action.

PUTTING THESE IDEAS INTO PRACTICE

With pencil and paper, answer the following questions:

1. What three personal characteristics do I already possess that indicate my natural ability for learning, giving, and receiving massage?

2. List two people you already know who you believe could learn massage.

3. Identify one activity you now perform routinely that, with some practice and forethought, could be greatly enhanced by entertaining "Beginner's Mind."

4. List three advantages of learning massage through practicing a massage routine.

5. Identify one activity in which you find yourself feeling bored. List two things you can do in order to elevate your awareness to a higher level of engagement while practicing that activity.

6. For me, personally, is massage more like kneading dough, wringing out stress, a tune-up, or a mini-vacation? How can I remember to entertain this favorite image of massage while learning the first strokes of my new massage routine?

7. Memorize your favorite analogy about massage, the one that makes *you* want to relax.

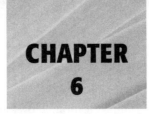

**CHAPTER
6**

The Massage Routine,
without Lotion

But we ought not to consider the organs of the body as the lifeless forms of a mechanical mass, but as the active instruments of the soul.
                                        —Pehr Ling, co-founder of Swedish Massage

OBJECTIVES

1. Perform a "dry" massage, without use of lotion, to the shoulders, neck, head and feet for a client who is seated in a chair.

2. Demonstrate one effective way to find out if the amount of pressure you apply during a massage is comfortable for the client.

3. Taking no more than ten minutes, demonstrate and explain (to a client, colleague, friend, or family member) how to give a relaxing neck and shoulder massage (dry) which they can then perform in 3–5 minutes or less.

INTRODUCTION

This chapter contains a short, yet carefully detailed massage routine consisting of a series of simple strokes, each of which can be performed "dry," that is, without using lotion. These easy to learn techniques will allow you to loosen up the shoulders, neck, hands, and feet for a client who is fully clothed, in a matter of minutes and in practically any setting. Every step and sub-step of the procedure is explained in text and illustrated with photos or diagrams. Don't let all the details confuse you, it's not as complex as it might appear. We have written for the reader who may have received massage but has never given one, as well as for someone who has neither given nor received a professional massage. We believe that nurses will appreciate the option of having *all* the details. The directions, therefore, take more time to describe clearly, in words, pictures, and pages, than your massage will ever take to perform.

Please note that any repetition in this or the following technique chapter is intentional. Since adult readers tend to begin their learning where their interests and needs dictate, you may not read the book in the same order as the pages are numbered. Also, because certain ideas and instructions are so essential, depending on where you decide to start and stop reading, you may run into some already familiar ideas.

This chapter's main goal is for you to understand all of the techniques well enough to feel confident in your early practice with partners. Once you have practiced through the entire routine several times, you should also be able to demonstrate most, if not all, of the techniques for any colleagues or family members who might be interested in massage. For the best results, we suggest that you read the entire chapter first, from start to finish, then practice performing the strokes with a friend.

THREE VERSIONS FOR EASIER LEARNING

As you thumb through the chapter, you will notice we have included three versions of the dry massage routine, Detailed, General, and Brief. The Detailed version contains a wealth of descriptive information and photos. The purpose is to help you clearly visualize each body position and understand exactly how to perform every stroke with your own hands. The anatomical illustrations will help you cast an imaginative eye beneath the surface of the skin as you work. In effect, all of this should help you understand how each stroke might feel if performed on you, yourself, as the recipient. One reader said she could almost see herself giving the massage as she read. Think of the first Detailed version of the routine, then, as a mental "walk-through."

A number of boxes and helpful hints are included throughout this first portion, and the supplemental background, or "asides," they contain are more than parenthetical digressions. They bring to light many of the issues, insights, questions, and answers that have come up repeatedly over the years in massage classes and workshops.

Next, the original routine is outlined again, but this time in a more General level of detail. This General "middle-ground" version includes the numbered steps and lettered sub-steps only, and is intended as a transitional learning tool, one that will help you read the instructions aloud as you continue to practice with partners. After having worked through all of the techniques once or twice using the more Detailed version, you will need far less detail as you begin applying each series of techniques as a continuous set. In fact, too much detail can become cumbersome after you begin gaining some momentum. The General version helps you work unimpeded, without the distraction of having to flip pages and skim over all of those earlier detailed explanations.

Finally, the Brief version lists only the numbered steps themselves. This is for after you start "getting it down." You can just glance back at this one-page "jobcard" for reference to help remind you of what comes next. With a little practice you will soon discover the simple logic behind each sequence of strokes, and be able to move through the entire routine, or any part of it, with ease. Keep an easy rhythm as you move from stroke to stroke with a nice, comfortable tempo in your hand movements, and you are on your way.

After your "muscle memory" has finally absorbed and translated all of the information from the page into first-hand experience, your intuition will help remind you "what comes next." Receiving this same massage from a practice partner will also help educate your hands. Soon, after giving massage and getting good verbal feedback from several partners, you will start developing an intuitive sense for where a client might need massage most. Your goal, as always, is to help loosen and relax the neuromuscular system as a way to stimulate and release the blood and vitality so they can flow freely throughout the body. Inducing circulation by opening up any areas of tension helps alleviate internal stress. It also assists the body and mind when deeper healing is needed, and acts as an aid for more restful recuperation.

PRACTICE WITH A FRIEND

We recommend that you first enjoy a few practice sessions with friends, colleagues, or family members before performing massage on your professional clients. If that's possible, you will benefit from allowing yourself the luxury of several "no-pressure" practice sessions. Give yourself permission to take your time and explore each technique, since being in a hurry to learn massage is somewhat of a contradiction of terms. In those first several sessions, just forget about the clock. Try applying slightly different nuances to the same strokes, or applying either more or less pressure when working on the same body area. For example, experiment with things like applying pressure to the two shoulders separately; your speed or rate of rhythm on the back, or; how soon you should ask for verbal feedback while giving a neck massage. Each of these subtle variations will make an ever so slight difference, both for yourself and for your clients.

Ideally, you and your primary partner might each give and receive four to six massages in your initial practice over several days or weeks. Also, if you know others who are interested in learning massage, you might include one or more sessions with additional partners. But even if you manage to give only three or four massages to your closest friends, if you work patiently, your first experiences with professional clients will proceed with good effect. Overall, you want your first clients to receive a massage that you've already performed comfortably several times and which, according to your practice partners, felt relaxed, smooth, and confident. This is the kind of massage that, even if it only consists of three strokes and lasts two minutes, produces consistently enjoyable results.

GET COMFORTABLE

Whenever you perform massage, even as you are first learning, make sure your own body is physically comfortable throughout. The degree of comfort (or discomfort) you are experiencing, in the way you stand and use your body, will communicate to your client. If you happen to become aware of any physical discomfort during the massage, you can quickly learn to use that discomfort as a "cue" for reminding yourself to relax. Learning to use discomfort as a cue for relaxation during massage will help you learn to use that same cue and response in other circumstances as well, both professional and personal. This works while you are talking on the phone, driving a car, or entering data into a computer just as well as it does during massage. Discomfort is a reminder to relax and enjoy.

TAKE YOUR TIME AND HAVE SOME FUN

Any time we learn a new set of motor skills it can take a while for our hands and brain to coordinate their working together more gracefully. That's certainly true in massage. Those first few friends you work with in the beginning won't mind if you try your strokes several times until you feel comfortable with them. One of the "main things" to keep in mind when learning massage is to let the whole process be, not frivolous, but fun. Massage is work, it's true, and it can be very physical. You are exerting energy and attention to accomplish a task. But it shouldn't feel like "hard" work and, if it does, you're probably working too hard. If so, relax.

Learning massage techniques with a partner, especially somebody who is also interested in learning the same techniques, can give you an idea of how it would feel to receive the very same strokes on yourself. You will always benefit from good feedback but, if your partner just wants to relax and receive their massage—and isn't at all interested in learning how to give one—they still might be able to offer a helpful suggestion or two. Most partners are good for a few minutes of verbal feedback, then they just want to let go and enjoy the massage. For more on giving and receiving detailed constructive feedback, see Chapter 8 on Practical Considerations.

Experiment with Time Limits

In your first session or two of practice make it a point to forget about the clock, you will already have enough to think about. Then, after a few sessions, you can start keeping an eye on how long it takes to perform one or two strokes. If you learn all of the techniques illustrated in this chapter, you will have more than enough techniques to choose from while working on practically any client in almost any situation. Once you consider the client's condition and any pressing needs they might have (such as backache, headache, or neck stiffness), you can quickly pick and choose one or two strokes to start with, and then decide on any others to include depending on how much time you have available.

In your practice sessions, make sure you have a little extra time to spend so neither you nor your partner feels rushed. As soon as you become comfortable working with just one or two of the techniques for a given area—the shoulders and neck, for example—try timing those strokes with a watch or clock. How much time does a "little bit" of massage take on the feet, for example? Then, how much time does "a lot" of massage take on the same area(s). You can decide for yourself how long a "thorough" foot or shoulder massage should typically last. Timing your sessions can help you get a realistic perspective on time. But don't let the clock become a distraction.

For another approach on timing, you could try limiting yourself to spending five minutes on a partner and applying only two techniques. How much more thoroughly can you massage the client's shoulders in three minutes than in one minute? In other words, think about time thoughtfully, but playfully, rather than allowing your massage practice to become yet another thing that gets caught up in a "busy schedule." Experiment with time just to get a general idea of how long it takes to do all of the strokes to all of the areas we cover, remembering that our ultimate goal is to create "a moment" for our clients.

YOUR GENERAL BODY POSITION FOR THE DRY MASSAGE

The "dry" techniques illustrated in this chapter are intended for two people working together with only two regular chairs. Simple folding chairs will do just fine and, if the chairs are not identical, the receiver always gets the most comfortable one. The client, or "receiver," will be seated in their chair at all times. For some of the techniques, you (the "giver") will stand behind the client while, at other times, you will be seated in the second chair facing them. Positioning, as well as indicating when to shift from one position to the next, will be noted and described as we walk though the first Detailed, step-by-step instructions. These techniques can be easily adapted for the client who might be lying down in either a hospital bed or in a regular bed.

WHERE THE ROUTINES START AND WHY

We begin our presentation of the dry massage technique with strokes for the shoulder and neck areas. Most of us think of our shoulders and neck as somewhat distinct areas, but they are intimately interconnected. There are several reasons for starting with this area. First of all, the neck and shoulders are the one particular body area that most of us complain about, and so you will probably receive more requests for massage to the neck and shoulders than for any other area of the body. Second, the shoulder and neck region may be the body area that is most easily accessible for massage. You can rub the shoulders of practically any client by simply standing behind them, and the same will be true for your friends and family.

Third, we start with the neck and shoulders because the muscles in this area always tend to "bunch-up" during a sustained, low-grade stress response. This type of stress is common in the workplace, and so the need for these first techniques is almost universal. Finally, in our own experience, whenever you ask someone where they think they might be able to use a couple of minutes of massage, almost all will say, "Oh, yeah, my neck and shoulders." In fact, you can almost count on it. So the shoulders and neck are where we begin the routine, and we urge you to do whatever it takes to master this one area, even if these are the only techniques you ever learn how to perform.

Some of your client's muscles may be stiff from having lain too long in a hospital bed. Others may be sore from having driven around in traffic clutching their steering wheel. And almost every office has someone who "feels stuck," or "in a bind," from having stared at a computer screen for a couple of hours without stretching. Whatever the case, the slow kneading rhythm of your hands giving a two- or three-minute shoulder rub, then working up the sides of the neck, can lighten up and brighten up even the longest afternoon.

This entire "Dry Massage" routine is so easy to perform that, once you master it, you will be able to "give it away" to practically anyone in almost any setting. It is no exaggeration to say that, with some practice, there may be shoulders that start to relax at just the thought of you walking into the room. That kind of response is an excellent sign that you have been making good progress on your technique.

THREE SHORT "SUB-ROUTINES"

The "dry" massage techniques in this chapter are grouped into three short sub-routines:

(1) Shoulders, Neck, and Head;
(2) Arms and Hands; and
(3) Feet and Calves.

After reading through the whole chapter, start to finish, the first time you work through any of the routines with a partner may appear to take a lot of time. You should expect that to be the case. With just a little more practice, though, it naturally starts to take less time and the sub-routines will begin to feel like a seamless progression. For example, the first sub-routine, Shoulders, Neck, and Head, may take up to 30 minutes to perform the first time you try following the written directions for each technique. There will be some partners who might take as much as an hour, or even more, to work through just the techniques for the shoulders, neck, and head. That's fine, too, since you should never rush through learning the strokes. Others may even be able to trade those same techniques with a partner in less than an hour. Proceed at whatever pace is most comfortable for you.

The second sub-routine, the Arms and Hands, will probably take less time than the first; as will the third, the Feet and Calves. Simply learning to read the instructions while experimenting with the hand movements will become much easier and more familiar as you progress from one body part to the next. You might also find it helpful to try reading the step by step directions out loud, one line at a time. This slows down your thinking and helps you "look into" what you are trying to do.

Take some time learning each one of the three sub-sections, separately, and thoroughly. Then you'll be able to put them all together. Try learning the "form" just as it appears in the book then, whenever you don't have time for the entire form, you can include or exclude whatever steps you like. Once you've learned the first three or four strokes, you'll find that, like most massage strokes in general, they are easy to remember and always fun to give.

MASSAGE TECHNIQUES, WITHOUT LOTION

Below is the "Brief" Outline for the entire dry massage routine. It is included here to give you an idea of where you are headed. Before reading through all the detailed instructions that make up the bulk of this chapter, take just a short moment to look over this "bird's-eye view." It may be helpful to come back to this big picture now and then, over the next week or so, until you have a vivid image in mind of what you are about to accomplish. In a few weeks or, possibly, even in just a few days, this short outline (presented again on one page near the end of this chapter) is all you will need for reference when you perform all of the techniques in order. After those latter practice sessions, this outline will become something you "internalize," and then share with all of your clients and friends.

SHOULDERS, NECK, AND HEAD
1. Loosen the Shoulder Girdle
2. Squeeze and Knead the Upper Shoulders
3. Thumbs to the Upper Shoulders
4. "Thumb Walk" Between the Shoulder Blades
5. Palm Circles Down the Back
6. Knead the Neck
    6.1. "Two-Handed"
    6.2. "One-Handed"
7. Friction to the Scalp

ARMS AND HANDS
1. Squeeze the Arm and Hand
2. Squeeze the Hand
3. Thumb Walk to the Palm
4. Repeat steps 1–3 to the other arm and hand

FEET AND CALVES
1. Squeeze the Foot
2. Thumb Walk on the Sole of the Foot
3. Squeeze the Foot again, as in Step 1, above
4. Squeeze the Calf
5. Repeat steps 1–4 on the other foot and calf

SHOULDERS, NECK, AND HEAD

Position: The client sits in a regular straight-backed chair, or folding chair. Their whole body is turned in the seat at a 90-degree angle from the chair's regular seated position, facing right. In other words, the back of the chair is not directly behind them, it is to one side now, and out of the way. This clears the way for easy access to the shoulders. You may either stand or sit directly behind the client.

1. Loosen the Shoulder Girdle

The muscles of the shoulders and neck attach to several of the bones in the upper body. We like to call this bony structure, as well as the entire muscle mass attached to it, the "Shoulder Girdle" (see Figure 6-1). The anatomy illustration is intended to help you visualize this intricately interlaced network of muscles and bones. As you work over the whole area, kneading the soft tissue, let your hands suggest to the entire structure, "relax now, and let go."

The purpose of Loosening the Shoulder Girdle is three-fold. First, we want the shoulders to become comfortable with being touched and moved around. Secondly, by loosening them, both you and your client will get some idea about how much tension the area is holding. Clients are not usually aware of how much tension is gathered there, but massage brings it to their attention.

Finally, Loosening the Shoulder Girdle begins to undermine some of the general upper body tension and the body's "attitude of holding on." This counterproductive resistance throughout the body is often centered within the shoulders and neck. Loosening the tension in this one area can cause us to become

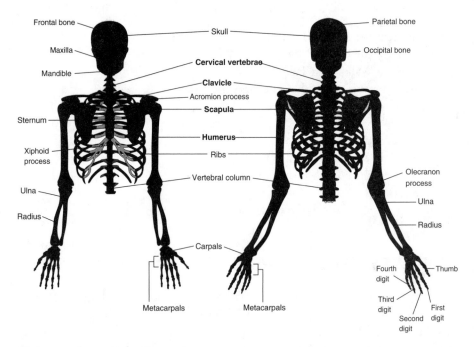

Figure 6-1 The muscles of the shoulders and neck attach to a light and very elegant bony structure. The bones of the "shoulder girdle" weigh very little and are easily moved. As you move the muscles around, most of the resistance you detect will be due to excess tension.

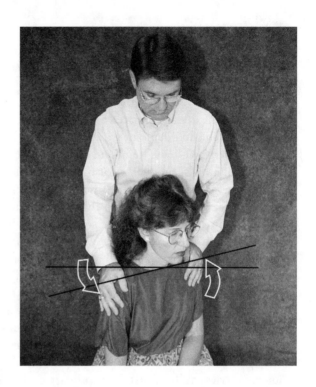

Figure 6-2 Move the shoulders and the upper torso—first to the right, then to the left—to loosen and relax the upper body.

aware of how much we have been holding onto, needlessly, and feel ourselves start to relax all over.

Since this may be your first physical contact with the client, let your personal manner, as expressed through the character of your touch, naturally encourage them to let go and relax. The more relaxed you are, the more comfortable they will feel. Repeating this loosening step once or twice is usually enough.

Loosening the Shoulder Girdle is a short three-step procedure (A through C) as follows:

A. Position your hands on top of your client's shoulders.

Place your right palm on the client's right shoulder blade, and grasp the left shoulder jointly firmly, with the flattened fingers of your left hand around on the front of the joint (see Figure 6-2).

B. Move the shoulders around counterclockwise to loosen them (without the client's help).

Push forward on the right shoulder blade while, at the same time, pulling back gently on the left shoulder joint. This should have the effect of twisting the upper torso around just slightly to the left, with the spine acting like a pivot point.

Do this slowly enough for it to create a relaxing sensation for the client.

Watch and listen for signs of any potential painfulness in the client's shoulders.

Now, let go of the shoulders so that the body returns naturally to its original, face-forward, resting position.

C. Move the shoulders around to the right.

Now, just the opposite: place your left palm on the client's left shoulder blade and grasp the left shoulder joint with the flattened fingers of your right hand.

Push forward with your left hand and pull back with your right.

This should twist the client's torso slightly to the right, slowly, clockwise.

If you sense that your client is holding on, resisting, or "helping you," try suggesting they inhale deeply into the gentle stretch. Ask them to direct their breath right into any of the tension, soreness, or resistance they might be feeling. Then, tell them to let all of their body's tension and holding-on "fall right out" of those same muscle sensations with a relaxed, uncontrolled exhale. If they try to "help" you by twisting their body for you, remind them to let go. Ideally, they should be letting you do all the work. If you let go of their shoulders, but their body remains in that position, it may be a sign they are not accustomed to allowing their body to fully relax and let go. This one simple preliminary movement can reveal a great deal about the client's state of tension and relaxation.

Helpful Hint: For the elderly, or anyone in frail health, always loosen the shoulders very carefully at first. Your primary goal is always to induce relaxation. At the same time, you are assessing the upper body's general state of tension and flexibility. Go easy, and "listen" with your hands.

2. Squeeze and Knead the Upper Shoulders

This one simple technique may be performed by itself, even for several minutes.

A. Rest the heels of your palms on the back side of the upper shoulders.
B. Place your four flattened fingers against the front of the shoulder muscles, so the fingers are opposing the "heels" of your palms (see Figures 6-3–6-5).
C. Squeeze the muscle mass and let go, alternating, with your right hand, then left, etc.

Throughout this entire movement *the thumbs point upward* and never apply any pressure to the body. Also, the fleshy heels of the palms never actually break contact with the shoulders.

This squeezing and kneading motion should not feel like a "pinching" sensation to the client. Make it a firm, pleasant sensation, one that causes the whole area to relax.

Take some extra time to practice this simple movement and become comfortable with it from the very beginning. This squeeze-and-release motion—alternat-

Figure 6-3 Compress and release the fleshy muscle mass of both upper shoulders. Always alternate—right hand, then left hand—using the heel of your palm working against your *flattened* fingers.

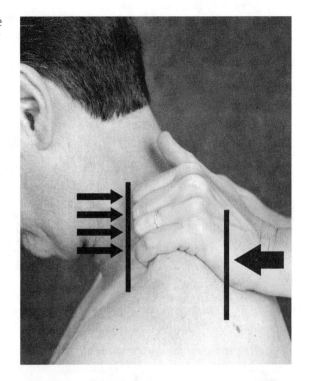

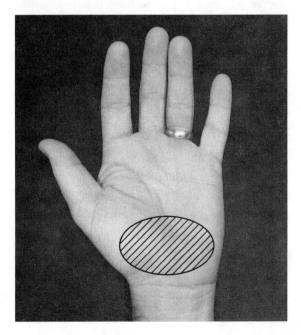

Figure 6-4 The "Heel" of the palm is that fleshy mound next to the wrist.

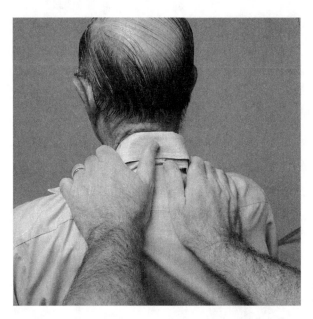

Figure 6-5 Squeeze and knead the shoulders with alternating hands. Note that the tips of the thumbs point upward, because they do not apply direct pressure.

ing with the right hand, then the left, may be the one hand movement you will use most often throughout this massage. The continual, alternating pressure induces a relaxed, back-and-forth rhythmic sensation.

If your client's shoulders are bigger than your own, and your hands seem small in comparison, you might try kneading with both hands on the same shoulder (See Figure 6-9). But if the opposite is the case, that is, if your hands are relatively large but your client's shoulders are small, don't overdo the pressure on this technique. Remember that you are trying to help your client's shoulders feel good, so that may require a different approach than what you, yourself, might prefer. The Golden Rule in massage, then, might be, "Massage unto others the way *they* would like you to massage unto them."

Helpful Hint: How slow is a "slow, alternating rhythm"? When using an alternating motion for squeezing or kneading the muscles, the tempo should be about that of an old, large grandfather clock: "Tick . . . Tock . . . Tick . . . Tock . . ." If you have never heard a grand old clock like that, another comparison might be the rhythm of a kitten kneading on your pillow. If you are a musician, or if you just need a more specific idea on the tempo, try setting a metronome to a slow Largo, or about 40 beats per minute. Don't hurry on this alternating stroke. You are inducing a "letting-go" state of mind by helping this client's body relax.

Why alternate? Feel the difference for yourself. Have a friend or practice partner apply this same movement on you. First, ask them to try this kneading motion simultaneously on your upper shoulders, using both of their hands, and squeezing both of your shoulders at the same time for about a dozen repetitions. Make a mental note of how that sensation feels on your own shoulders.

Next, ask your friend to apply the same amount of pressure but this time using the alternating technique. That is, squeezing back and forth, right hand, then left, etc., for another dozen or so pairs of repetitions. Can you feel any difference? Do you have a preference? After both applying these strokes and receiving them, which approach does your partner feel is probably more effective, simultaneous, or alternating? Our own experience has shown the alternating movement is, generally, much more effective.

Finally, ask your partner to try kneading your shoulders at a noticeably quicker pace. Then kneading them at a slower pace. Which pace seems to make your body want to relax more? Now, if your partner wants to learn this stroke, you can trade places and try the same experiment on them.

Based on our personal experience, with clients and in classes, we suggest a slow, alternating rhythmic motion. Like a rocking chair, or a mother's heartbeat, the quiet rhythm of alternating hands on this one stroke alone can help lull almost any client back into a mild state of relaxation in as little as 30 seconds. We'll use an alternating motion on several other strokes throughout this overall routine.

    D. Gradually cover the entire upper trapezius area in a slow, steady alternating rhythm.

    E. Begin where the neck joins the shoulders, and work out toward the bony ridge of the shoulder blade, until you run out of muscle.

    F. Repeat this sequence to the whole area a couple of times, remembering to alternate, keeping a slow, steady pace.

When your client's shoulders have been holding onto tension (perhaps years of it), they can't be expected to surrender all of it in a minute or two. However, almost any client will feel significantly better from just this one stroke alone. Keep in mind your every hand movement is intended to help this client feel a little bit better.

3. Thumbs to the Upper Shoulders

Now we'll work on the same area, the Shoulders, but this time, more specifically.

CAUTION: Do not apply pressure directly on the vertebrae of the neck or spine.

You will be applying friction with your alternating thumbs (press and release) to the upper shoulder (upper trapezius muscle). But first, let's look at an illustration to help locate some bony landmarks for reference (see Figures 6-6 to 6-8).

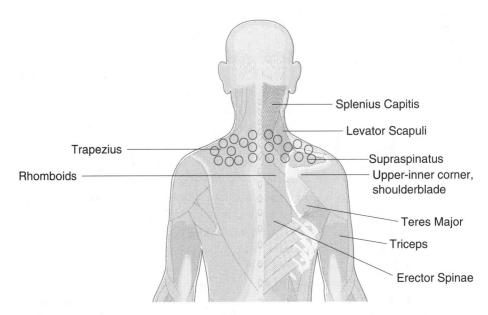

- Splenius Capitis
- Levator Scapuli
Trapezius
- Supraspinatus
Rhomboids
- Upper-inner corner, shoulderblade
- Teres Major
- Triceps
- Erector Spinae

Figure 6-6 Before applying alternating thumbs to the upper shoulders, find the bony landmarks with your fingers, especially the upper-inner corners of both shoulder blades. Focus on massaging the muscles, not the bones.

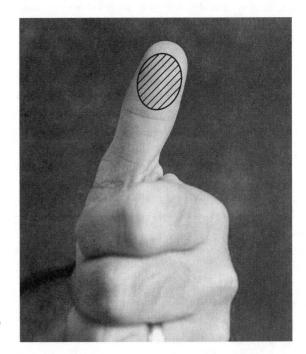

Figure 6-7 The thumb "pad" is that soft, fleshy surface of the last joint, usually thought of as the thumb "print."

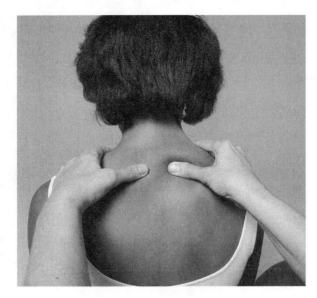

Figure 6-8 Apply alternating pressure with your thumbs into the soft muscles of the upper shoulders. This stroke is slightly more specific than using the heels of the palms, and its moderate pressure can feel very good to the client.

A. Using your thumbs, locate the upper ridge of the shoulder blades (as reference points).

B. Rest your fingers on the tops of the shoulders for support and stability.

C. Apply alternating thumbs to the back side of the upper shoulders.

Begin on the fleshy areas that lie between the spine and the upper bony ridges of each shoulder blade.

Using the pads (the full "prints") of your thumbs—and alternating, right thumb then left thumb—stimulate and loosen the upper trapezius muscle. This will include the slightly deeper levator scapulae muscles on both sides of the spine. Be careful here because some clients may be somewhat tender in this area.

Work from the spine, progressing out (laterally) into the fleshy area. Work across the shoulders, just above the upper bony ridge of the shoulder blade, until you have loosened one "row" of the soft muscle tissue.

Now, re-position your thumbs back near the spine, but slightly higher this time. Repeat this step once or twice until you have gradually worked your way to the very top ridges of the shoulders. Three rows are usually enough to work the area thoroughly (see Figure 6-9).

D. Thumbs to the tops of the shoulders.

Place the pads of your thumbs directly on top of the shoulder muscles near the base of the neck on both sides. Right thumb on the right shoulder, left thumb on the left shoulder, as shown.

Your fingers provide support and stability by resting along the front of the muscle, or against the collar bone (clavicle).

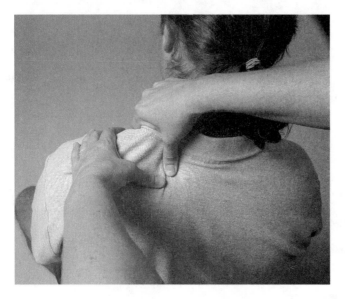

Figure 6-9 If the shoulders are big and your hands are small, use both hands, focusing the work of both thumbs on each shoulder, in turn. Remember to alternate the thumbs' kneading pressure.

Apply pressure downward, with alternating thumbs, and gradually progress out from alongside the neck to the upper bony ridge where the shoulder blade joins the shoulder joint (see Figures 6-10 and 6-11).

Work the entire area in a slow, alternating rhythm.

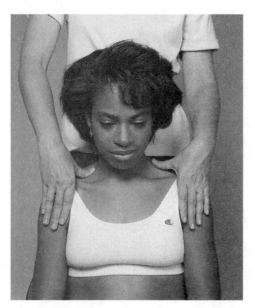

Figure 6-10 If after loosening the shoulder area with general kneading the shoulders are still sore, this technique works well for loosening that uppermost area.

Figure 6-11 Are the tops of your client's shoulders too big for your thumbs to be effective? Instead of using your thumb pads across the tops, try applying a similar alternating pressure using the heels of your palms.

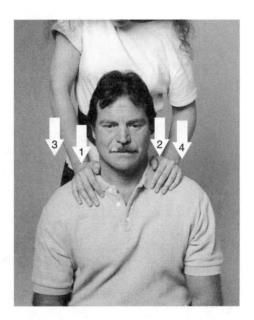

4. "Thumb Walk" Between the Shoulder Blades

Position: Clients get more benefit from this stroke when they can relax the muscles in their backs. Try suggesting that they lean forward in the chair, with elbows resting on the knees. If that feels uncomfortable, they might rest forward against the flat surface of a table, or against the edge of their elevated hospital bed.

Relaxing forward automatically causes the muscles of the upper back and torso to let go and relax, so they aren't pushing back against the pressure of this "walking" stroke. If the client feels more comfortable sitting upright, this stroke is still effective (see Figure 6-12 and 6-13).

A. Begin by resting the pads of your thumbs on opposite sides of the spine, just below the seventh cervical vertebra (C-7).

Locate the seventh cervical vertebra, the lowest vertebra in the neck. This bone usually protrudes somewhat beneath the skin on the upper spine, about where the neck meets the shoulders.

B. Apply a "walking" friction to the rhomboid muscles.

Using your alternating thumbs, press directly into the muscle mass.

Move the tissue in a direction slightly up or away from the spine with each contact, or "step," of the walking motion.

Your finger pads maintain contact with the body for stability and support throughout the entire stroke. Re-position the fingers as you go, allowing them to follow along with the walking movement of the thumbs.

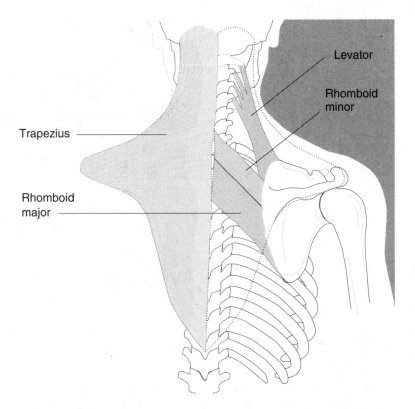

Figure 6-12 Systematically "walk" your alternating thumbs all over the rhomboid areas as indicated. This is a natural gathering place for tension, and it becomes sore from hours of holding the shoulders erect.

C. Re-position your hands as necessary.

The right thumb stimulates the rhomboid muscles on the right side of the spine, and the left thumb stimulates those muscles on the left side.

D. Work the entire area between spine and shoulder blades.

When you reach the muscle area about level with the bottom tips of the shoulder blades, re-position your thumbs out, just slightly closer to the shoulder blades.

Then "walk" back up and all around the designated areas, moving the fleshy mass with each "step" of your alternating thumbs.

If time permits, and you sense that the lower areas of the back need additional attention, you might try walking the thumbs all the way down into the upper lumbar and lower back. Explore the area for tension as you "walk."

This stroke stimulates and loosens an area of the body that is almost always unnecessarily tight. The muscles alongside the spine are sometimes actually sore

Figure 6-13 The fingers of both hands make a firm contact, "grounding" on the client's body, while the thumbs "walk" up and down, systematically softening the muscles.

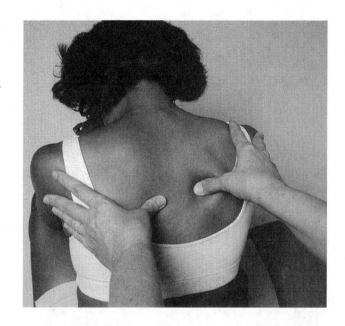

to the touch, so ask the client for feedback on the amount of pressure you are applying as you work.

5. Palm Circles Down the Back

Now use the palm of your dominant hand to make circles all over the client's back.

Position: From where you have been standing (which was directly behind the client), re-position slightly and stand at the client's side, facing their back.

For example, if you are right-handed, stand to the client's left, so you can use your right hand to make the palm circles. If you're left-handed, stand to the client's right, and make the circles with your left hand.

The client can remain relaxed forward, if desired, as in the previous thumb walk stroke. Or, if they think they would feel more comfortable sitting upright, that's fine, too, as long as their torso is generally relaxed and not stiff or rigid.

Rest your other (non-dominant) hand comfortably on the client's shoulder closest to you. This is just for stability and support, and to help reinforce a friendly, comfortable contact with your client. Your own body posture, your sense of physical comfort, and your hand movements should all work together. Let your body language suggest to your client that it's perfectly okay to relax and enjoy the massage. This technique, especially, seems to lend itself to conveying that type of message.

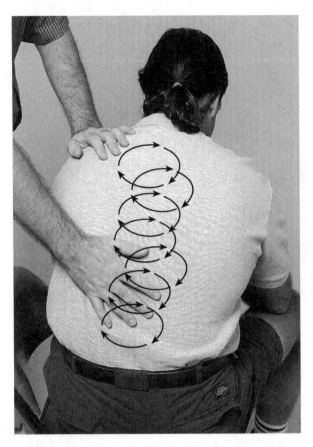

Figure 6-14 The "Palm Circles" are very simple, yet extremely beneficial. Stimulate the entire back, especially down and alongside the spinal muscles. For some clients this may be the only stroke you perform when you have only 30–60 seconds to spare.

The instructions below are for making circles with the right hand (see Figure 6-14). This is one of several strokes that can help you become more comfortable with using your non-dominant hand. After you become comfortable using your dominant hand, try making the palm circles with each hand in turn. This is just to let you experience any differences in how the movements feel to both yourself and your practice partner.

A. Place your right hand on the client's upper back.

Place your right palm near the one large vertebra (C-7) that protrudes beneath the skin between the shoulders. This vertebra marks where the base of the neck ends and the thoracic spine begins.

B. Make palm circles down the spine.

Make large, clockwise circles with the palmar surface of your hand and fingers, covering the spine and the areas immediately next to it along both sides of the back. Work gradually all the way down, making sure to include the lower back.

The diameter of the circles should be about the same as the length of your own palm, but it's not necessary to be exact. Bigger or smaller circles are okay, and you can even vary the size as you move along. The object is to make a sensation that induces relaxation in all the muscles.

   C. Continue the palm circles all over the back.

Palm Circles for Every Body!

The "Palm Circles" technique can be performed almost anywhere, and almost anyone can learn how to give it. It looks so simple, but don't make the mistake of underestimating its effectiveness. The motion and contact of this stroke has a way of making the whole body want to let go. That effect, alone, can start to undermine a great deal of the held-in muscle tension, not only in the back, but in other areas as well.

The clockwise motion coupled with the pleasant sensation of contact stimulates and, in effect, "stirs up" the energetic tension that's held within the muscles all across the back. You can pause to concentrate this "unraveling" motion more specifically over any areas that feel unusually tight, "stuck," or sore as you go over them.

If the client asks you to "scratch that spot," try flexing (or curling) your fingers slightly so that your finger tips (rather than just the softer palms and finger pads) are now making primary contact on the back. A few seconds of this fingertip contact, by all of your fingers circling a small area at once, can then be alternated with the more soothing sensation created by the flattened palm. Your circular motion is a somewhat more systematic approach to that old familiar request to "scratch my back." Be careful, though, if you have long fingernails. Some clients may enjoy that more pointed sensation, while others may not.

You might try beginning with your palm, then "stir-up" any specific tension across the back with the fingertips. Finish it off by "smoothing out" the area down the back with long, gliding strokes with your palm. Again, one of the best ways to perfect this stroke may be to receive it yourself from several partners.

Palm Circles are also a good exercise for helping develop your physical intuition. Try this: after working over the whole back, see if you can return to that one specific area that feels (to you) like it could use a little extra attention. Maybe it was especially warm, or cool, or "prickly" to your touch. Or maybe you just have a hunch that, "If my back felt like this spot feels, I'd want it rubbed (or scratched) right *here*!"

With enough practice, your hands will learn to recognize and go straight to, and dwell on, the "good spots" for a few seconds. Trust your hands, and ask for feedback: "Is *this* a good spot . . . ?" You may be surprised at how quickly you start finding some of those "good spots" on your own.

After covering the whole area down the mid-line of the back, re-position your right palm just above either of the shoulder blades.

Make another spiraling line of palm circles down that side of the back, then down the remaining side. You have now systematically covered the whole back at a relaxing pace.

Ask your clients where on their back they might appreciate a little more of this pleasant friction. You can always return to concentrate on any part of the back at the client's request since it only takes a few seconds extra.

6. Knead the Neck (Two Methods: 6.1 and 6.2)

NOTE: Next are two methods for massaging the neck "dry" (designated Steps "6.1" and "6.2"). Here is the difference:

In Step 6.1, you will massage up the neck using both of your hands at once, and you will not support the client's head.

In Step 6.2, you will massage the neck with the thumb and fingers of your dominant hand only, and you will support the client's head with your other hand.

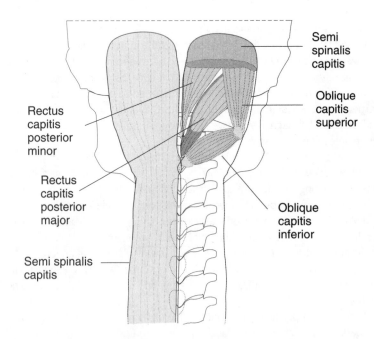

Rectus
capitis
posterior
minor

Rectus
capitis
posterior
major

Semi spinalis
capitis

Semi
spinalis
capitis

Oblique
capitis
superior

Oblique
capitis
inferior

Figure 6-15 The muscles of the neck can almost always use some massage. They work continually to keep the head poised on top of the spinal column, except when we lay down for rest.

By learning both methods you can choose whichever one feels best to you and for the client. We begin with the first method, Step 6.1, letters A through H.

CAUTION: When massaging the neck, do NOT apply direct pressure on the carotid arteries. These are located slightly toward the front of the neck. If you practice these two techniques as described you should have no problem with the carotid arteries. That's because your contact will be focused on the muscles along the sides of the neck, not the front.

6.1. Knead the Neck, "Two-Headed"

Position: Stand next to the client's left shoulder, facing their neck.

A. Ask your client to let their neck relax forward.

B. Move any hair off the neck and out of the way.

C. Your hand placement "straddles" the neck.

Your points of contact are the "sides" of the neck.

With your palms facing down, place your two thumb-pads (prints) side by side on the side of the client's neck closest to you.

Then, line up the index and middle fingers of both your hands, forming your finger pads into one continuous row, running along the far side of the neck.

D. Begin at the bottom of the neck.

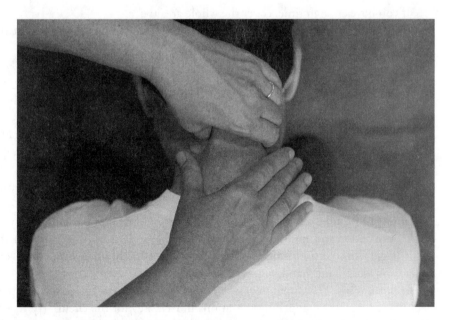

Figure 6-16 The muscles up along the sides of the neck respond well to kneading. If the client's skin seems especially dry, or sensitive, apply just a spot of lotion to the area to help reduce the friction.

The kneading pressure of this stroke is directed *into* the neck muscles. Your two thumbprints (on the near side) are working against the pressure of the four fingerprints (on the other side).

E. Knead the neck muscles, alternating.

Begin at the bottom of the neck, and apply a press-and-release motion, alternating your hands.

Inch your way gradually up the neck muscles as you knead in toward the spine.

Create a continual rhythm—right hand, then left, etc.—never actually breaking contact with the skin as you inch along.

F. Re-position, gradually working up the neck.

Your fingers and thumbs should work together, creating a very pleasant, rhythmic sensation for the client.

Knead just slightly higher with each motion, and gradually work your way up the neck toward the head.

Generally, you will have worked from the base of the neck (closest to the shoulders) up to the base of the skull, that is, just beneath the bony occipital ridge.

If you have enough time, cover the whole area twice.

(NOTE: The next two sub-steps, "G" and "H," are identical to those at the end of Step 6.2, the "One-Handed" version.)

G. Allow the client's forehead to rest in your left palm.

H. Apply thumb and finger friction under the occipital ridge (see Figure 6-17).

Using the thumb and fingers of your right hand, make very small circular movements to stimulate and loosen the muscle tissue just underneath the occipital ridge.

Begin near the ears and inch along inward, from both sides simultaneously, toward the center line of the neck or spine.

Your thumb rides along underneath the ridge on the (left) side closest to you, while your index and middle fingers do the same underneath the ridge on the other (right) side of the spine. Stabilize the client's forehead, lightly, with your other (non-dominant) hand.

Helpful Hint: The upper neck is a key area. Receiving massage to the upper neck can create very compelling sensations in that area for the client. Try receiving it and see for yourself. The intricate muscles in the neck, coupled with the degree of tension usually stored there, can experience some very unique physical

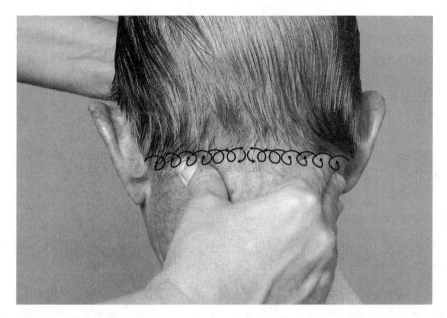

Figure 6-17 Apply thumb and finger friction to the neck muscles just beneath the occipital ridge. Make very small rotating circles with your thumb and forefinger, working gradually inward toward the spine.

sensations while the sub-occipital area is being stimulated and loosened. Client responses will vary, all the way from the inability to let go of the neck to that of delight and appreciation.

Some clients may prefer less pressure than you, yourself, might enjoy or feel is needed. Others might ask for slightly more pressure than you would feel comfortable applying. For that reason, the neck is another body area where it is especially important to ask each client for feedback. While the amount and the depth of sensation should always be aimed to suit the particular client, you should never apply so much pressure that you feel unsure or uncomfortable. This technique, like all the others, should feel very comfortable in the giving as well as in the receiving.

To fully appreciate the subtleties of this technique in this very important area, have several partners perform this whole sequence of strokes on your own neck. That way you can see for yourself how it feels first-hand and your own technique will improve as a result.

OPTIONAL, BUT RECOMMENDED: You can also perform this stroke from both sides, especially if it feels as though your thumbs are applying more pressure into the muscles than your fingers. Because of the way the hand works, the thumb may feel more focused, or stronger, when working from this position into the upper neck. Especially while you are learning, re-position your body and try approaching this stroke on the neck from both sides. Most clients will appreciate the extra work.

6.2 Knead the Neck, "One-Handed"

This is the second method for massaging the neck "dry." Some clients prefer this "one-handed" approach because you support the weight of their head continuously. This allows their neck muscles to be more relaxed throughout (see Figure 6-18).

Position: Same as in 6.1, standing at the client's left side, facing their neck.

A. Allow the client's forehead to rest comfortably in your left palm.

Now, using only one hand, apply a kneading motion to both sides of the neck.

If you are left handed, of course, you can position yourself, standing at the client's right side, allowing the forehead to rest in your right palm. If that's the case, just follow the instructions accordingly. The sequence below assumes that the left hand supports the forehead and the right hand kneads the neck.

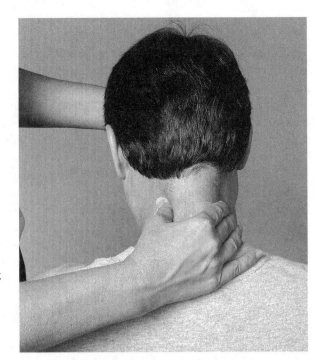

Figure 6-18 If letting the neck relax forward without support (as in Step 6.1) is uncomfortable for the client, support the head with one hand and apply this "one-handed" approach.

B. Move any long hair out of the way.

C. Squeeze and knead the neck with your right hand.

Begin by placing your right hand at the bottom of the neck.

Your thumb rests on the side of the neck closest to you, while the pads of your first two (or three) fingers rest on the other side of the neck, opposing your thumb. The single working hand "straddles" the neck.

Apply the kneading pressure to the neck. With a fluid, squeeze-and-release motion, your thumb on one side works against the opposing fingers on the other. Neither the thumb nor the fingers ever break contact with the skin as they knead.

D. Work your way up the neck, gradually, to the base of the skull.

Knead into the soft muscles, exploring as you inch your way up along the sides of the neck. Your intention is to remind those muscles that letting go feels much better than holding on.

Remember, just a small spot of lotion, if needed, can reduce friction on the skin.

E. Apply thumb and finger friction under the occipital ridge.

Apply the same small circles with your thumb and fingers into the muscles that lie just beneath the occipital ridge. This is exactly like you did in the "two-handed" method, Step 6.1.

F. Repeat as needed.

Helpful Hint: Loosening the neck helps to ease many headaches. Just loosening the muscles beneath the occipital ridge has helped ease many headaches. Relaxing the neck with a brief massage has a way of releasing general tension, some of which may have been stored, not just in the neck, but also in the shoulders, the head, and the facial muscles as well. Loosening the muscles beneath the occipital ridge can also be helpful for easing eyestrain.

One reason the neck can become tight is in the way we carry our head. Simply put, we tend to sit and walk with the tip of the chin slightly elevated, unintentionally. In order to raise the chin, we must flex the muscles in the back of the neck. Although "chin-up" is a good attitude to assume, figuratively speaking, flexing any muscle continuously—especially without moving and stretching it—will eventually cause it to become sore. To counter this old habit, try becoming aware of relaxing your neck while driving.

After having our neck massaged, it can also be helpful if we intentionally allow both our jaw and chin to relax and drop downward ever so slightly. You will feel the neck muscles let go, which will also allow the head to rise ever so slightly.

The cushions between the neck vertebrae no longer need to be compressed. Interestingly enough, this opening up of the occiput and jaw also tends to free the diaphragm muscle and the whole lower rib cage, so we breathe more freely. Another good time to practice allowing your neck and jaw to relax is while giving a massage, or even while you are already relaxed, such as when reading a book.

Try Using Your "Other" Hand

Being "both-handed" (ambidextrous) can be an advantage in massage. The majority of us are right-handed, but massage is one "low-risk" activity where you can experiment with using your non-dominant hand. Especially while practicing the techniques with friends, using your "other" hand can be like discovering it anew.

Relax both of your hands (and your whole body) and let your instincts come into play as you massage. It's true that you might feel a little less control over the fine motor skills and detailed movements when you first use your "other" hand. But at the same time, you might also gain a fresh appreciation for using the entire non-dominant side of your body. You'll be actively waking up a slightly different part of your brain and neural system, and the person receiving your massage won't be able to tell much difference, if any at all.

7. Friction to the Scalp

First of all, always ask permission before stimulating the scalp.

In fact, ask your client's permission before even touching their head and hair. Some clients just simply do not want their hair "messed-up," under any circumstances. For others, it could be one of the most relaxing parts of their massage.

Helpful Hint: Always begin with a light touch on the scalp. Personal differences are important when it comes to what we like in massage and the scalp area is one where we should pay special attention to the client's preference. For example, some clients prefer their scalp massage to be quick and vigorous, while others prefer it to be done very slowly. Occasionally, clients will enjoy a good, firm pressure on the scalp, but others—elderly clients, for example—often require a much lighter approach.

Each client's preference is determined by what feels most comfortable and pleasurable to him or her. So, once again, we are reminded that the client's preference may be quite different from our own. Since the head and scalp are such personal areas, make it a habit of asking for feedback before you start stimulating the scalp. If they request, gladly omit the area entirely.

Position: Stand behind the client, who remains seated in a chair.

Depending on your client's need and preference, you can use either one hand or both when stimulating the scalp. For the two-handed approach, you might suggest that the client allow their head and neck to relax forward (as detailed earlier in the neck massage). This way you'll be able to use both of your hands on the scalp at the same time.

For the single-handed approach, stand to one side and support the client's forehead in your (non-dominant) palm (see Figure 6-19). Then, stimulate the scalp with your free hand. Both types of hand movements discussed below work with either approach.

A. With your palm(s) facing downward toward the head, and your fingers and thumbs slightly bent . . .

B. Let your thumbs and finger pads rest comfortably on the scalp.

C. Stimulate and move the entire scalp by moving your finger pads in either small circles or short, back-and-forth friction movements (see Figure 6-20).

D. Re-position your hands continually as you gradually cover the entire scalp.

You may break contact with the scalp in order to re-position the finger pads on different areas of the scalp.

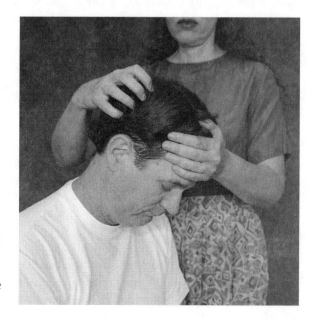

Figure 6-19 Support the client's forehead with your left hand and, while using the finger pads of the right hand, apply friction to the scalp. Ask for feedback to make sure the client enjoys the sensation.

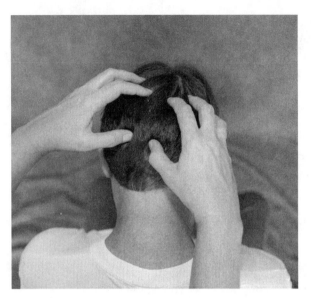

Figure 6-20 With the client's neck relaxed forward, apply finger pad friction to the scalp using both hands. Your fingers should be slightly arched, yet flexible.

Helpful Hint: Heads to watch out for. Work carefully on the scalp of children and the elderly—and anyone else whose hair is either fine or thin. The head and scalp can be extremely sensitive, especially if a client is ill. But the same can be true for some clients even when they're robust and healthy. Clients who are either bald, or balding, often really appreciate a vigorous scalp massage, while others do not. Ask first. A good scalp massage, one applied with sensitivity and care, can be very pleasant and very relaxing for the client.

ARMS AND HANDS

1. Squeeze the Arm and Hand

Position: With your client seated in a chair, sit or stand facing either of the client's arms. While working on the arm, it should be neither bent at the elbow nor resting in the client's lap, but hanging freely by the client's side, completely relaxed.

A. Knead the upper arm.

Place both of your thumbs against the back side of the deltoid muscle at the top of the arm. All of your fingers rest together on the front side of the muscle, so they can work against the pressure of the thumbs.

Squeeze and knead the soft deltoid muscle, alternating with your right hand, left hand, etc. (see Figures 6-21 and 6-22). The hands never fully break contact with the arm.

Continue this rhythmic motion, working downward, into the biceps and triceps muscles along the length of the upper arm. This kneading sensation is almost always very pleasant for the client.

Knead the muscles all around the elbow joint, both just above and below it. This may be another area storing some hidden tension and soreness, so take it easy, especially at first. Clients may occasionally ask you to repeat the upper arm and elbow areas, since most of us hardly ever realize how much tension and soreness can be stored there.

B. Knead the forearm and wrist.

Continue the squeezing and kneading movements, alternating, down through all of the muscles in the forearm and wrist. Take your time and explore these areas. Time permitting, gently work out any pockets of soreness you might discover. Some may be quite tender.

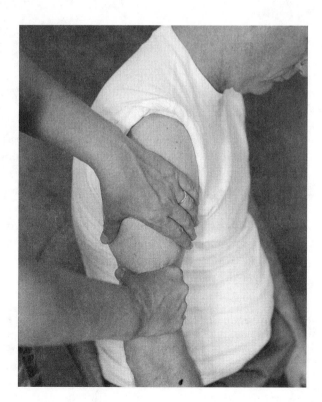

Figure 6-21 Squeeze and knead down the upper and lower arms with thumbs opposing fingers. Use an alternating motion.

Figure 6-22 Because the muscles of the arm do a lot of work, they seldom rest, so they store a lot of tension. They also respond well to a good, thorough kneading.

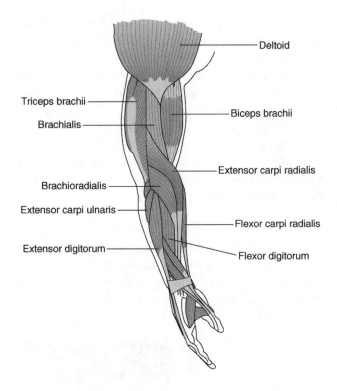

Deltoid

Triceps brachii

Biceps brachii

Brachialis

Extensor carpi radialis

Brachioradialis

Extensor carpi ulnaris

Flexor carpi radialis

Extensor digitorum

Flexor digitorum

C. Squeeze the hand briefly, alternating.

D. Repeat steps A–C, to the other arm.

Helpful Hint: We suggest that you become comfortable with working on the arms, as outlined here, by going back and forth from one arm to the other. That is, first, massage one arm, then the second arm; followed by going back to the first hand, then the second hand. This takes about the same amount of time as completing the arm and hand of each side in turn. But because you go back and forth from one side of the body to the other, the overall effect can be especially relaxing for the client. However, if you prefer, try massaging each entire arm and hand, together, in turn, and see which approach you prefer. If you have a chance, be sure to receive it both ways, too.

2. Squeeze the Hand

There will be occasions when you just don't have enough time to massage both the hands and arms. If you only massage the hands, just position your two chairs facing each other, and work on each of the client's hands in turn.

Position: Seated in a chair, now facing the client.

A. Position the client's hand palm down.

Using both of your hands, grasp the client's hand, with your fingers under their palm.

B. Knead the hand to loosen.

Knead the hand using an alternating motion, working generally from the wrist area toward the fingers (see Figure 6-23). Remember to be careful with very young hands, the hands of the elderly, or with any hand that appears sensitive, painful, or frail.

Your intention is to stimulate the soft tissue and the flow of blood, and to cause at least some slight movement in all of the bones and joints throughout the hand. This encourages the tiny, intricate muscles and tendons to relax and let go of any tension.

Helpful Hint: Whenever we are ill, or in the middle of some particular stress, just having our hands massaged can cause our whole body to open up and relax.

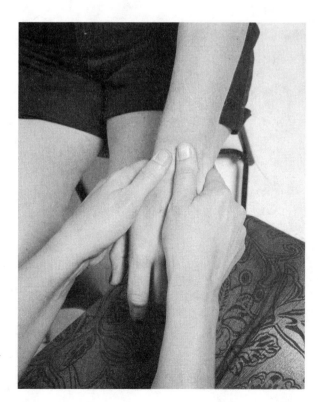

Figure 6-23 You can loosen the hands in almost any setting and help a client or friend feel better, even when you have only a minute or two.

Hand massage helps us to "let go of our grip" on life, and allow ourselves to receive the help of a friend. In fact, hand massage embodies quite elegantly that sweet, simple act of giving and receiving. The spirit of the technique, on those occasions, is less concerned with the completion of a few detailed strokes. It's more about reaching out and connecting with a friend. Learn to give a nice, friendly hand massage and you will always be ready to lend a helping hand.

3. Thumb Walk to the Palm

A. Turn the hand over, palm up.

B. Apply alternating pressure to the palm, using alternating thumbs.

Using the pads of your thumbs, stimulate the fleshy palm by applying a press-and-release motion. "Walk" your thumbs all over the palm's soft surface (see Figure 6-24).

Begin near the wrist and "walk" out (toward you), to the base of the fingers.

Create a continuous, alternating, press-and-release action with your thumbs to the palm.

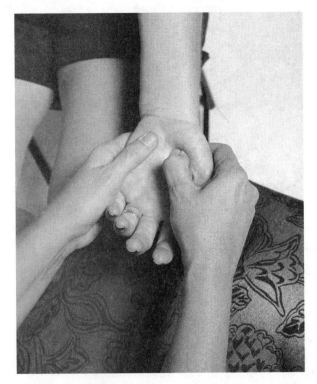

Figure 6-24 The Thumb Walk, when applied to the palm of the hands, often causes the client's entire body to relax.

If you happen to have fingernails (even if you think they're "not very long"), you might cover the client's hand with a lightweight cloth or towel. This avoids the unpleasant sensation of sharp contact so the pressure-and-release sensation will always feel comfortable on the palm. Again, practice giving and receiving this stroke with a friend until you feel comfortable giving it and have experienced how pleasant it feels.

4. Repeat steps 1 through 3 to the other hand.

FEET AND CALVES

Position: Nurse and client are seated in simple chairs, facing each other.

The following, like most of the techniques in this book, can be easily adapted for the client lying in a bed. For clients in a bed, adjust your body position and approach accordingly so that your own body remains comfortable as you apply each stroke. (See the body positioning in Chapter 7 for the foot massage with lotion.)

1. Squeeze the Foot

A. Squeeze and loosen the heel and ankle.

With one hand, lift your client's foot up about 12 inches off the floor. Support the heel of that foot in your other palm.

Then, using both hands, knead all around the entire heel area in general (see Figure 6-25).

Stimulate and loosen the areas, including those around and behind the ankle and up the lower part of the achilles tendon, just above the heel.

B. Take the foot comfortably in your hands.

Hold the foot firmly by placing the heels of both your palms on the top of the foot, and positioning your hands back near the ankle.

Line up your finger pads underneath the foot so that your fingers form two parallel rows up the middle of the fleshy sole (see Figure 6-26).

You should now have a firm, but comfortable grip on the main body of the foot.

C. Squeeze and knead the entire foot.

Apply a stimulating press-and-release action to the whole sole of the foot.

Plant the heels of your palms firmly on top of the foot for stability. The finger pads of each hand work as a unit, apply their alternating pressure underneath (see Figure 6-27).

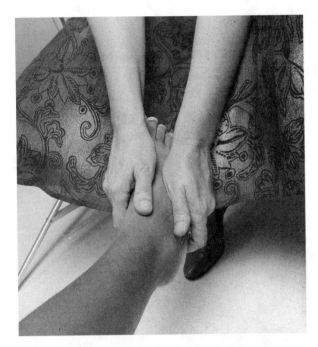

Figure 6-25 Grip the foot firmly, but comfortably, using the amount of pressure you think the client will most appreciate. Squeezing tension out of the foot with alternating hands releases a general sense of relaxation throughout the whole body.

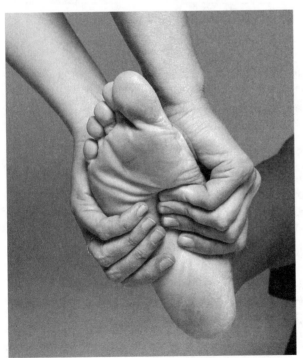

Figure 6-26 With each hand in turn, stimulate the sole of the foot thoroughly with your alternating finger pads. Apply a slow, rhythmic squeeze-and-release pressure into every area. Use caution with clients who are elderly, frail, or recovering from serious illness or surgery.

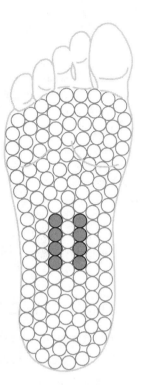

Figure 6-27 Stimulate every square centimeter of the sole, working from beneath the heel to the base of the toes. The darkened ovals indicate the relative placement of all eight finger pads.

Alternating hands—right hand, left hand, right hand, etc.—inch your way up the middle of the sole. Squeeze and release repeatedly. Be sure to include that area of the sole extending along the base of each of the toes.

Now, re-position your hands back toward the heel, and work up again. This time, knead that part of the fleshy sole out and along underneath its outer edges.

The heels of your palms are still following along on top of the foot, never fully breaking contact as your fingers knead their way up the sole.

Helpful Hint: Is help possible for ticklish feet? Ticklish feet can sometimes result from having been poked, pinched, or tickled when we were children. Yet it seems a shame to think of faithful feet never experiencing a good massage. The question is, would the client be willing to spend a minute or two to see if the ticklish reflex can be reduced or eliminated?

The ticklish foot reflex seems to be related to tension held in the pelvic area, the area that automatically flexes, or recoils, to draw the foot back from a stimulus. Hold the foot firmly between your palms, and suggest that the client take a few relaxing breaths, allowing the foot, leg, and hip areas to relax from the pelvic area. Then, slowly apply a firm, squeezing pressure to the foot, sustaining it for just a few seconds at first. If the client can feel the urge to recoil, remind him to inhale into the muscles' physical urge to flex and draw up. Then let the breath—with all of that tension—fall out with the exhalation. Repeat this cycle of stimulation and release as many times as needed all over the foot until the whole complex relaxes as much as possible. This is an exercise in gentle patience, because it does take some time. So the client needs, first, to be interested enough and willing for it to help in order for it to be effective.

Continue the foot massage and repeat the same process to the other foot. Some clients with extreme ticklishness may need several trials, and a lot of patience on their own part, in order for their feet to be even touched, much less thoroughly massaged. Others will be amazed that all it took was a minute or two on each foot and now they can enjoy a real foot massage for the first time. Also, if your client is sensitive or uncomfortable about their feet being massaged directly, for whatever reason, all of the strokes for the feet can be performed with them wearing their socks.

2. Thumb Walk on the Sole of the Foot

A. Rest the client's right foot on your left thigh.

Lift the client's right leg, placing your right hand behind the knee for support, and lifting up their foot with your other hand underneath their heel. Their leg should be fully relaxed. (Practice this a couple of times.)

Rest their lower leg (calf) down on top of your left thigh, so that it supports the leg's weight at a point somewhere above their ankle. To avoid any discomfort, try to minimize hyper-extending ("straightening out") the client's knee joint.

This positioning allows the client's entire leg to relax more fully while you apply the thumb walk to the sole of their foot. Ask for feedback about the positioning, making sure the client is comfortable.

Helpful Hint: If this positioning proves to be too uncomfortable for the client's knee, you can either omit this stroke, or perform this entire foot massage sequence with the client lying down. Place a pillow under their knee for support, if necessary.

B. Stimulate the sole of the foot with alternating thumbs.

Beginning on the heel's fleshy mound, stimulate the sole of the foot by "walking" the pads of your thumbs over the entire area.

In this position, your fingers rest on the top or sides of the foot, providing the stability and positioning for the "walking" pressure of your thumbs into the sole (see Figure 6-28).

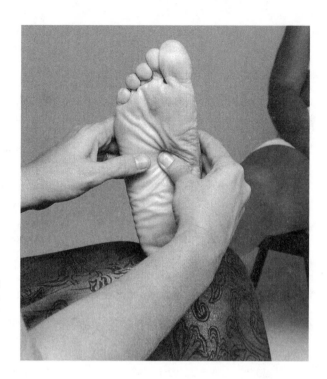

Figure 6-28 With the client's lower leg resting on yours, stimulate the sole of the foot with your "walking" thumbs. Be sure their knee is relaxed and comfortable, that is, not hyper-extended.

Work the whole sole of the foot thoroughly and systematically, gradually reaching the area just under the base of the toes. Re-position your fingers from time to time, following the action of the working thumbs underneath.

The motion is, once again, press-and-release, left thumb, right thumb, establishing a continual rhythm. (This is a stroke most clients will let you continue for a while.)

For additional information about the benefits of working on the foot, see the section on reflexology at the end of this chapter.

Helpful Hint: Practice both giving and receiving this Thumb Walk to the Foot and, if possible, with several partners. The best way to improve a technique is to know what it feels like by receiving it yourself.

3. Squeeze the Foot Again, as in Step 1, Above

A. Gently, but firmly, "wring" the remaining tension out of the foot.

Use both hands, as before, alternating, right, left, right, left, etc. Squeeze the remaining tension from the heel, through the sole and out the toes. The foot should now feel thoroughly stimulated and "wrung out."

At the beginning of your work on the foot, that first initial squeeze was to loosen it up. This worked out the "road tension" and helped reduce any initial resistance in the foot.

Next, the Thumb Walk stimulated and loosened most of the deeper tension more specifically. This is the held-in tension that gathers over time around the small bones, joints, tendons, and the intricate muscles inside and throughout the foot.

Now, at the end, this second squeeze is aimed at "wringing out" all of the tension that's been "stirred-up" in the process.

If you ever happen to leave out this second and final squeeze, the client's foot might tend to feel "full," or "incomplete," when the massage is over. A nice, firm kneading at the end makes the client feel like the foot has been fully addressed. It now feels "complete." In class, we like to say "it's cooked."

B. Set the foot back down onto the floor.

Lift up the client's leg, as before—from behind the knee and under the ankle—then set the foot down comfortably onto the floor.

Some Feet Can Be Delicate

In elderly clients and children, remember that the bones and joints of the foot might be much more sensitive or frail than those of a strong, healthy adult. Therefore, be very mindful of how much pressure you apply. Use your own experience and intuition but, most importantly, find out by asking them. Your direct questioning, coupled with their verbal feedback, is the only way to find out what your client feels is good for them, and how much pressure is just right—not "too much." It's much better to massage a foot too lightly in the beginning, and have the client ask for more pressure, than to ever cause your client any actual pain.

4. Squeeze the Calf

CAUTION: Contraindication—Any history of problems with varicose veins or blood-clotting would indicate that squeezing or massaging the calf muscles should always be avoided. *Varicose veins and clotting problems are contraindications for massage to the legs.* Most of your healthy clients will probably not have varicose veins. However, it's far better to be safe than sorry. Ask your client about varicose veins and any history of clotting problems, AND CHECK VISUALLY for varicose veins, before massaging any part of the legs.

A. Lean forward in your chair, and rest the heels of both of your palms on the client's upper shin bone (tibia) just below the knee.

Allow the flattened fingers of both your hands to rest just behind the leg. Here you'll feel the fleshy (gastrocnemeus) muscle of the upper calf.

B. Squeeze and knead the meaty muscles on the back of the calf.

Alternate, right hand, left hand, etc., with flattened fingers. The heels of your palms, planted firmly on the front of the upper shin, provide stability and resistance for the kneading action of your flattened fingers (see Figure 6-29).

C. Work gradually down the calf, from just below the knee to just above the ankle.

D. Repeat this process, A–C, to the calf if needed or desired, time permitting.

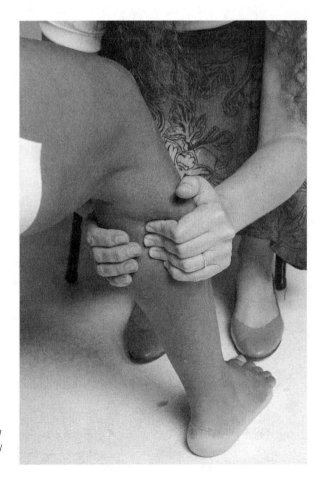

Figure 6-29 Squeeze and knead the calf muscles with both hands, alternating. Start just below the knee and work down gradually to just above the ankle.

5. Repeat Steps 1–4 on the Other Foot and Calf

This is the end of the Detailed "dry" massage routine. What follows is a less detailed, or "General," version of the same routine. Now, you can refer back to this Detailed version for study while you are practicing on friends and integrating all of the background information.

GENERAL DRY ROUTINE OUTLINE

The entire detailed "Dry" Routine—Shoulders, Neck, and Head; Arms and Hands; Feet and Calves—is abbreviated below in a more General form. All additional commentary, notations, boxes, and helpful hints have been omitted leaving only the numbered steps and lettered sub-steps. After you have studied and practiced the above fully-detailed routine a few times, the following more streamlined version will allow you to work through the procedure while turning fewer pages.

As suggested earlier, practicing with friends, colleagues, and family members helps you become comfortable with the natural "flow" from one technique to the other and from each step into the next. After you have studied the Detailed routine, you might have a friend talk you through this more General version by reading all of the sub-steps for each step out loud directly from the book before you perform it. Then, even after you have begun practicing with clients, you might still want to keep a printed version of the (final) Brief outline handy for quick reference.

Let each client know that you are learning something new that you hope will help all of your clients. Whenever you are having fun learning massage, your client will probably enjoy it, too, and appreciate an opportunity to "help you out."

Shoulders, Neck, and Head

1. Loosen the Shoulder Girdle

   A. Position your hands on top of your client's shoulders.

   B. Move their shoulders around counterclockwise to loosen them (without the client's help).

   C. Move the shoulders around clockwise.

2. Squeeze and Knead the Upper Shoulders

   A. Rest the heels of your palms on the back side of the upper shoulders.

   B. Place your four flattened fingers against the front of the shoulder muscles, so that your fingers are opposing the heels of your palms.

    C. Squeeze the muscle mass and let go, alternating, with your right hand, then left, etc.

    D. Gradually cover the entire upper trapezius area in a slow, steady alternating rhythm.

    E. Begin where the neck joins the shoulders, and work out toward the bony ridge of the shoulder blade, until you run out of muscle.

    F. Repeat this sequence to the whole area a couple of times, remembering to alternate, and keeping a slow, steady pace.

3. Thumbs to the Upper Shoulders

    A. Using your thumbs, locate the upper ridge of the shoulder blades (as reference points).

    B. Rest your fingers on the tops of the shoulders for support and stability.

    C. Apply alternating thumbs to the back side of the upper shoulders.

    D. Thumbs to the tops of the shoulders.

4. "Thumb Walk" between the Shoulder Blades

    A. Begin by resting the pads of your thumbs on opposite sides of the spine, just below the 7th cervical vertebra (C-7).

    B. Apply a "walking" friction to the rhomboid muscles.

    C. Re-position your hands as necessary.

    D. Work the entire area between spine and shoulder blades.

5. Palm Circles Down the Back

    A. Place your right hand on the client's upper back.

    B. Make palm circles down the spine.

    C. Continue the palm circles all over the back.

6. Knead the Neck (Two methods: 6.1 and 6.2)

    6.1. Knead the Neck "Two-Handed"

    A. Ask your client to let their neck relax forward.

    B. Move any hair off the neck and out of the way.

    C. Your hand placement "straddles" the neck.

    D. Begin at the bottom of the neck.

    E. Knead the neck muscles, alternating.

    F. Re-position, gradually working up the neck.

    G. Allow the client's forehead to rest in your left palm.

    H. Apply thumb and finger friction underneath the occipital ridge.

  6.2. Knead the Neck, "One-Handed"

    A. Allow the client's forehead to rest comfortably in your left palm.

    B. Move any long hair out of the way.

    C. Squeeze and knead the neck with your right hand.

    D. Work your way up the neck, gradually, to the base of the skull.

    E. Apply thumb and finger friction under the occipital ridge.

    F. Repeat as needed.

 7. Friction to the Scalp

First: Always ask permission before stimulating the scalp.

    A. With your palm(s) facing downward toward the head, and your fingers and thumbs slightly bent . . .

    B. Let your thumbs and finger pads rest comfortably on the scalp.

    C. Stimulate and move the entire scalp by moving your finger pads in either small circles or short, back-and-forth friction movements.

    D. Re-position your hands continually as you gradually cover the entire scalp.

Arms and Hands

 1. Squeeze the Arm and Hand

    A. Knead the Upper Arm.

    B. Knead the forearm and wrist.

    C. Squeeze the hand briefly, alternating.

    D. Repeat steps A–C to the other arm.

2. Squeeze the Hand

    A. Position the client's hand palm down.

    B. Knead the hand to loosen.

3. Thumb Walk to the Palm

    A. Turn the hand over, palm up.

    B. Apply alternating pressure to the palm, using alternating thumbs.

4. Repeat steps 1–3 to the other arm and hand

Feet and Calves

1. Squeeze the Foot

    A. Squeeze and loosen the heel and ankle.

    B. Take the foot comfortably in your hands.

    C. Squeeze and knead the entire foot.

2. Thumb Walk on the Sole of the Foot

    A. Rest the client's right foot on your left thigh.

    B. Stimulate the sole of the foot with alternating thumbs.

3. Squeeze the foot again, as in step 1, above

    A. Gently, but firmly, "wring" the remaining tension out of the foot.

    B. Set the foot back down onto the floor.

4. Squeeze the Calf

    A. Lean forward in your chair, and rest the heels of both of your palms on the client's upper shin bone (tibia) just below the knee.

    B. Squeeze and knead the meaty muscles on the back of the calf.

    C. Work gradually down the calf, from just below the knee to just above the ankle.

    D. Repeat this process, A–C, to the calf if needed or desired, time permitting.

5. Repeat steps 1–4 on the other foot and calf.

THE DRY ROUTINE, IN BRIEF

Below is your most brief version of the full dry routine. After you have absorbed all of the details, hints, and directions from the Detailed and General versions—but still feel the need for a visual prompt to remember the order of the steps—you can refer to this single page. Keep the more detailed outlines handy until you thoroughly understand the logic behind the sequence of steps, and the order of the sub-steps have become second nature.

You have probably already begun to look at the whole dry routine as a "unity," which is important. You will be able to pick and choose which strokes to use according to time and the client's need but, for now, try learning the routine as "one piece," and view it as a complete whole.

With time and practice, you should be able to perform all of the strokes listed in the Brief Routine in about 10–15 minutes, more or less. That statement may seem overly ambitious or even unlikely at first, but the whole routine, its steps, and all the hand movements will look quite different in a month or so of reading and practice. Remember, too, please don't rush through any of it in the beginning, neither the steps nor the sub-steps. It's not how many massage strokes you know, or include, that helps your client most, or how quickly you can hustle and get through them. It's how you perform each stroke that counts. Rather than to try to rush through seventeen strokes in order to "get everything in," it will always be much better to perform three strokes with a feeling of genuine caring and kindness.

Our client will never be concerned all that much with our repertoire or whether or not we "get it all in" or "leave any out." He just wants to feel better. And he will probably feel a lot better if he feels like we're enjoying what we're doing while we're working on him. It's easier to enjoy giving a massage when you feel like you have all the time in the world, and feeling that way doesn't cost a thing. That attitude comes across to the client, too. So if we assume the right outlook and have a good attitude, three minutes work with nice, steady rhythm can be about all the time anybody would ever need. Don't rush, it's not a contest. It's a massage! Enjoy.

SHOULDERS, NECK, AND HEAD

1. Loosen the Shoulder Girdle
2. Squeeze and Knead the Upper Shoulders
3. Thumbs to the Upper Shoulders
4. "Thumb Walk" between the Shoulder Blades
5. Palm Circles Down the Back
6. Knead the Neck

6.1. "Two-Handed"
6.2. "One-Handed"
7. Friction to the Scalp (Ask first)

ARMS AND HANDS

1. Squeeze the Arm and Hand
2. Squeeze the Hand
3. Thumb Walk to the Palm
4. Repeat steps 1–3 to the other arm and hand

FEET AND CALVES

1. Squeeze the Foot
2. Thumb Walk on the Sole of the Foot
3. Squeeze the foot again, as in Step 1, above
4. Squeeze the Calf
5. Repeat steps 1–4 on the other foot and calf

SUMMARY

You now have both the knowledge and the practical tools to help people feel better just by using your hands. You are also now ready to start practicing with friends and colleagues. Think of what you will soon be able to do when you have just 60 seconds to help a client feel better. Imagine if you had five whole minutes! The possibilities are many and the limitations are very few.

The next chapter builds on what you have learned here. In it you will learn to perform the massage with lotion, which will always be a real treat. Keep in mind, the massage you learned in this chapter, without lotion, requires neither privacy nor any extra tools whatsoever. All you need are your hands, maybe a chair, and a desire to help. And even the chair can be optional.

PUTTING THESE IDEAS INTO PRACTICE

1. If one of your friendliest colleagues knew every technique illustrated in this chapter, which three of those techniques would you most enjoy receiving right now? On a sheet of paper, write down the names (and page numbers) for those three favorite strokes.

2. Which two body areas, out of all the body areas that we covered in the "dry" massage, would you most like to master and be able to perform for your

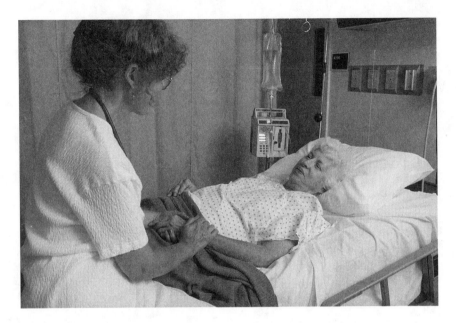

Figure 6-30 In many nurse–client interactions there is often that brief instant where two people meet and connect. Massage helps us turn that connection into a very special extended moment.

clients and friends? Write down the names of those body areas and the page numbers for the techniques that cover them.

3. What are the names of three friends who you think might be happy to let you practice your "dry" massage techniques on them? Write those names on that same sheet of paper.

4. Now . . .

(A) Re-read the sections on your "favorite" strokes for the body areas you listed above in question 1; and

(B) Re-read all of the strokes you listed in response to question 2; then

(C) Set up a time with each one of your three good friends to help them learn how to master those very same strokes—on you. Demonstrate on them, first, by reading each step of the instructions right out of the middle, General routine. Then, read the same instructions aloud for them as they try it on you.

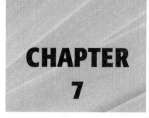

Massage Routine, with Lotion

Memorizing melodies, scales, and chords gives courage to one's imagination.
—Jerry Abersold, "How to Play Jazz and Improvise"

OBJECTIVE

1. Demonstrate how to apply massage techniques with lotion for the Back, Shoulders, Neck, Hands, and Feet.

The main objective for this chapter is to help you learn how to perform and demonstrate a brief massage using lotion. The main content consists of a body of techniques for the back, shoulders, neck, hands, and feet. We begin with a few ideas to keep in mind while learning and beginning to practice these strokes.

The chapter on Practical Considerations, immediately following this one, can be viewed as a companion to both this and the previous "dry" technique chapters. Practical Considerations will help you prepare for the road ahead as you begin to practice with friends and colleagues. It will also discuss in detail how to begin timing your massage so you can select which techniques to apply for good effect when you have as little as one minute with a client.

Time should not be one of your primary considerations in the early stages of learning. However, after reading this and the following chapter—and practicing on several friends—you should be able to give a pleasant massage with lotion lasting anywhere from as little as one minute up to about fifteen minutes, or even longer. If you have only three or four minutes for a massage, you will soon be able to respond to a client's particular needs without feeling rushed.

As in the previous chapter, most of the additional commentary, the "Helpful Hints," and the information highlighted in boxes are ideas we have repeated in classes, many of them in response to students' specific questions and comments. Our goal for you as you read along is for you to feel as if you have two instructors sitting beside you. This is "the whole story" about how to perform each stroke for the best results on a client or a friend.

Repeat Each Stroke

Repeat each of the strokes several times when first getting acquainted with the hand movements. This repetition helps you become familiar with the physical sensations of giving the massage as well as those of encountering and addressing the resistance you will notice in the client's muscular system. Repetition also provides your practice partner with additional time to reflect on what they are feeling as you work and, hopefully, they will be able to offer some helpful verbal feedback. The best verbal feedback is always aimed toward helping your technique become even more effective and more pleasurable to receive. (We will elaborate on good verbal feedback in the following chapter.)

After your initial period of learning and practice, whenever you massage a client, try applying a stroke, then repeating it at least once again, maybe even twice. In addition to helping your movements become more natural and fluid, your client becomes familiar with the feel and rhythm of the relaxed repetition and that, itself, is naturally comforting. In those instances when you want to extend the length of a massage, the same strokes can always be repeated an additional time or two for good effect.

Constructive Time Limits

The main consideration about time while you are learning is simple, don't wear yourself out. It can be tiring to massage someone for too long at one stretch, especially in the beginning. Therefore, after you have begun to learn the logic of the routine and start to feel fairly comfortable with all of the strokes, try limiting most of your practice massages to about 15 minutes or less, or up to 20 minutes if you feel inspired. This might seem fairly short to someone who already enjoys regular professional massage, which can last 60 to 90 minutes. But giving a massage is more physically taxing than receiving it, and limiting yourself to giving the shorter massage can be much more effective while learning. First of all, it will be easier to complete a "whole" massage. Secondly, since it's less likely to be tiring, you will be inclined to practice more often. And finally, your client will almost always want more of your massage, even if you give them an hour. So you shouldn't worry about giving them all they want or need because, practically speaking, you probably couldn't do that anyway! Just remember to honor your own limitations regarding physical stamina and mental concentration and quit while you still have energy to spare.

A massage of just five to ten minutes can be a wonderful addition to most clinical settings, regardless of how much time you have available. Even one to three minutes is enough time to help almost any client relax. Use your own intuition. For more information on timing and making a quick plan for each client, see the following chapter.

Suggested Learning Strategy

We suggest you read through the whole chapter before practicing on a friend. Picture each hand movement as you read along, and pause for a moment to look over each one of the photos and illustrations. Not only will you engage more fully all the associated details, but this first read-through also helps you form a mental "big picture" for learning the routine as a whole. Then when you do begin practicing with a friend, having visualized the whole process beforehand, you will already have a feel for each stroke and how it fits into the routine's overall flow.

If you are fortunate enough to have a partner who is also interested in learning massage, try working through just one sequence of the routine at a time, the shoulders for example. Then switch roles and receive that same sequence. Actually feeling the sensation and the subjective results of each hand movement— while it is being applied on you—will make your own massage that much more sensitive, effective, and enjoyable from the very beginning. For your partner, having just received those very same techniques will give them a better idea of how they want to make them feel when they perform them on you (and their future clients).

THREE OUTLINES

Once again, if you happened to skip the previous chapter, you will have three outlines for the "with lotion" routine. The first time through includes all of the details, including summaries of many of the parenthetical discussions we have had in previous classes. You will also find the Helpful Hints, which are detailed explanations designed to give you a more complete mental picture or insight into the hand movements and other related issues. For the most part, it will take you longer to read the detailed instructions for a sequence of strokes than it will to perform the actual hand movements. The background information should provide you, first, with additional insight into giving your massage and, secondly, with an effective aid to memory.

The second outline contains only the numbered steps and lettered sub-steps for each technique. These are exactly as they appear in the first outline, but with all of the details omitted. When you have read the (first) detailed routine and are ready to practice, this abbreviated version will save you a lot of time because there is nothing extra. Finally, the chapter ends with a brief outline including only the numbered steps for each of the body areas. That final outline can become a "job card," something tangible to keep handy so you can refer to it once you have reached the middle stages of mastering the overall sequence.

This chapter focuses on learning the actual hands-on procedures and techniques for what we have found to be: (a) the areas that hold the most tension; (b) the techniques that help induce the most relaxation, and; (c) on the body areas that are requested most by clients. And to help you get started with a bird's-eye view of the entire routine for the back, shoulders, neck, hands, and feet, what follows is a brief preliminary outline showing only the numbered steps. Take a moment, before reading the detailed portion of the chapter, and study this brief outline to get a clear mental picture of the entire "with lotion" routine. This is a sequence of strokes that will be easy to learn, effective for relaxation, and helpful for all of your clients and friends.

THE MASSAGE WITH LOTION

THE BACK

1. Apply Lotion
2. "Palm Circles" Covering the Back
3. Friction to the Rhomboids
4. Knead the Shoulders
5. "Rotating Thumb Friction" to Muscles Alongside the Spine
6. Heels of Both Palms Up the Back
- OPTIONAL: Petrissage the Neck
- OPTIONAL: Apply Friction to the Scalp

THE SHOULDERS

1. Alternating Palm Effleurage Between the Shoulder Blades
2. Rotating Thumb Friction to the Shoulder Area
3. Effleurage Around the Shoulder
4. Repeat to the Other Shoulder

THE HANDS

1. Squeeze the Palm While Applying Lotion
2. Rotating Thumbs to the Palm

3. Squeeze the Hand Again
4. Repeat Steps 1–3 to the Other Hand

THE NECK

1. Apply Lotion to the Neck
2. Apply Alternating Friction to the Shoulder and Neck
3. Repeat Steps 1 and 2, to the Other Shoulder and Side of the Neck.
- OPTIONAL: Friction to the Cheeks
- OPTIONAL: Friction to the Temples
- OPTIONAL: Effleurage to the Forehead

THE FEET

1. Apply Lotion to the Foot
2. Knead the Foot Thoroughly
3. Apply "Stripping" Friction to the Sole
4. Apply Rotating Thumbs to the Sole of the Foot
5. Squeeze and Knead the Foot (again, as in Step 2)
6. Repeat Steps 1–5 to the Other Foot

Getting Off to a Good Start

Your massage with lotion should be easy to give, pleasant to receive, and provide unmistakable therapeutic value for every client. Make it clear to each one of your practice partners that, since you are learning something new, you would welcome and appreciate any feedback. Since you will never be able to receive your own massage, whether or not you tend to "agree" with their views, opinions, and preferences, all of their comments should be considered and taken to heart.

After listening to all of their input, let them know that you genuinely appreciate hearing what your massage feels like from their point of view. Good verbal feedback will be a major factor in making continual improvement right from the beginning, and the more you actively encourage good feedback, the more of it you are likely to receive. Eventually, with study and practice, giving a good massage will become so second nature as to be almost effortless.

BACK MASSAGE

In order to give you a clear overview of our very first sequence, here again is a list of the six main steps (and two optional strokes) included in the Back Massage.

1. Apply Lotion
2. "Palm Circles" Covering the Back

No Forceful Pressure to the Spine

Caution: Do not apply direct manual pressure onto the spine itself.
We begin the back massage with a small yet very important caution. Since massage addresses the soft tissue throughout the body, your entire massage should be aimed toward relaxing the muscles, not the bones.

Although you will include the skin and fleshy areas around the spine whenever you massage a client's back and neck, you should be careful to avoid direct, forceful pressure to the bony spinal vertebrae, themselves. Forceful pressure applied directly to the spinal column might prove to be quite painful for your client. Spinal manipulations should only be practiced by medical professionals who have been specifically trained to perform them.

This does not mean, however, that you should be overly cautious, or self-consciously lift your hands up off the body, so that you never actually touch the area around the spine, far from it. The skin and muscle tissue in those areas does need stimulation and clients do enjoy having all of their back massaged, but to avoid the risk of any potential harm during your massage, just remember that you should never apply direct or forceful manual pressure directly onto the body's bony structure, and especially that of the spine.

3. Friction to the Rhomboids
4. Knead the Shoulders
5. "Rotating Thumb Friction" to Muscles Alongside the Spine
6. Heels of Both Palms Up the Back
• OPTIONAL: Petrissage the Neck
• OPTIONAL: Apply Friction to the Scalp

Position: The client is lying on their right side in the elevated bed, facing away from you. Stand at the right side of the bed, facing the client, who is properly covered with only the back exposed. Curtains are usually drawn, also, out of respect for the client's comfort and sense of privacy.

NOTE: Throughout the massage with lotion, the client should be fully covered with the sheet and, possibly, a soft blanket. To ensure the client's warmth and sense of privacy, the only areas that are ever exposed should be those particular areas that are being massaged. When you complete one body area, be sure to cover it before proceeding to the next.

1. APPLY LOTION

Practice applying just enough lotion to cover the back, from the shoulders down into the lower back. Getting just the right amount may take a few tries, but

Why Demonstrate with the Client Lying in a Hospital Bed?

Each of the "with lotion" techniques, along with the nurse's body positions, are probably much easier to understand and adapt after having seen them demonstrated on a hospital bed. Some other settings for giving massage might include clients who are lying in a regular bed at home, using a professional massage table, or even massaging a member of your family informally while they are lying on a palette on the floor. (We will mention each of these later.) But learning the techniques and body positioning for these settings first—then trying to adapt them for the hospital setting—could prove much more challenging than simply beginning with the elevated bed.

Thousands of nurses have already been trained to work with clients who are lying in hospital beds, so there is prior familiarity, and almost any client who is confined to a hospital bed could benefit from a brief massage. From a purely "common sense" perspective, any massage routine intended for use by nurses should certainly be presented clearly, and specifically, for the hospital bed.

There is one more important reason. The members of a client's family may not be accustomed to dealing with hospital beds, especially in their home. It would be unfortunate if the unfamiliar presence of an elevated bed kept any client from having a much-needed massage from a family member during recuperation. Therefore, for those family members who express an interest in learning to give a short back rub for their loved one once they return home, illustrating the techniques for the elevated bed might help eliminate just one more reason for any hesitation or reluctance.

you can always towel off the excess and try again. Your first partners probably won't mind, because the physical sensation feels so good.

Start with an amount of lotion in one palm about the size of a half-dollar, then spread that lotion evenly across the surface of both palms. The hands should "glide, not slide." You can always add more lotion, but only if needed.

A. Place the lotion on the client's upper back.

With lotion in your palms, rest the edges of both hands on the client's upper back, near the base of their neck.

B. Now move the lotion slowly back and forth, left and right, across the shoulders with your hands.

Only the edges of your palms and little fingers are making contact. As you move the lotion across the shoulders a small amount should be allowed to cover the skin.

C. Draw the lotion down the back with both hands (see Figure 7-1).

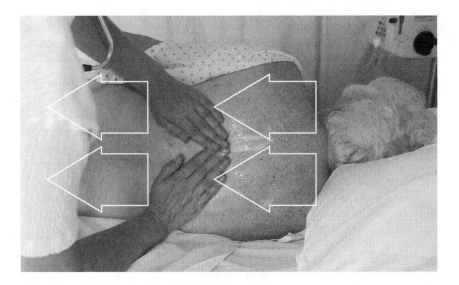

Figure 7-1 The sensation of having the lotion applied down the back can set a relaxed tone for the client's entire massage. Note that the client is covered except for those areas being massaged.

As you draw the lotion down the back, toward and into, the lower lumbar area, leave behind just a moderate amount of lotion on the surface of the skin.

This is one continuous movement—relaxed, comfortable, and relatively slow.

When you reach the lower back, there should be enough lotion on the back for you to proceed right into the next stroke, the Palm Circles.

Applying Lotion is Part of the Massage

Applying lotion is an important part of each massage, and it should never be performed in a rushed or incidental manner. The skin is a very perceptive living organ, and this movement is the opening sensation for the client's entire massage. With a relaxed, easy approach we can influence their expectations for what lies ahead. As you start to gain confidence in your massage techniques, applying the lotion can become like an opening stanza of sorts for the pleasant interlude that is about to follow.

You will become more skilled in applying lotion as you experience, repeatedly, having lotion applied to your own back. In those first few seconds, in your role as the receiver, identify the subtle qualities of touch, tempo, and pressure that you, yourself, really enjoy. Then, bring those same qualities and nuance into your own approach each time you make that very first contact with the client's skin.

2. "PALM CIRCLES" COVERING THE BACK

When working on almost any body area, start by applying the more general strokes first. This is especially important on the back, and Palm Circles is a very relaxing general stroke (see Figure 7-2).

The continuous motion of the Palm Circles helps the back become accustomed to being touched and receiving massage. Its circular rhythm also encourages the neuromuscular system to let go of most of its superficial tension right from the start. About halfway through this step many clients will let go a nice sigh of relief.

A. Begin by placing the hand you are most comfortable using at the top of the client's spine.

Note: Since most of us are right-handed, we illustrate here accordingly, with the client lying on their right side. If you happen to be left-handed—and the client needs to remain lying on one side or the other throughout the entire back massage—you might consider having them lie on the left side. Applying the Palm Circles with your dominant hand may be more comfortable for you (although that may not be the case in all circumstances).

During this stroke your other hand may rest comfortably on the client's shoulder, arm or hip, acting as an "anchor" of sorts. If that contact seems "too

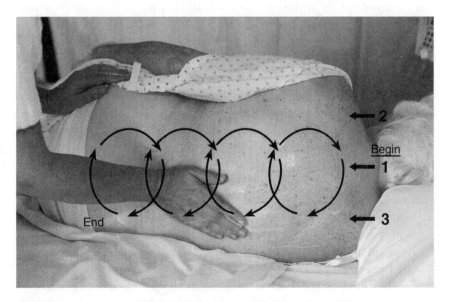

Figure 7-2 Cover the entire back with three slow passes of Palm Circles, working downward each time. This may be one of the most pleasant and important strokes you can use on the back, especially when your time is limited.

familiar," or inappropriately casual in any massage, your hand can just as easily rest on the surface of the bed.

B. Make clockwise circles with your relaxed open palm, progressing down the spine, and into the deep lower back.

The circular pace should be relaxing and comforting, neither too quick, nor too slow.

Ask yourself, "What tempo would I prefer if I were this client?"

The very center of your palm makes continual circles that are about equal to or slightly greater in diameter than the width of your own palm. Slightly smaller or larger circles can be equally as effective.

The entire back seems to appreciate this stroke, especially the lower back if it is either tired or sore. Your intention is simply to cause the client to relax.

C. Re-position your palm back up near the top of either shoulder.

Now, work the circles down that side of the back, all the way to the bottom. Take your time.

D. Repeat this step, now, down the other side of the back.

Continue until the entire back has been covered with Palm Circles.

Time permitting, re-visit any areas that seem to need a bit more attention.

The key to performing this stroke—as in virtually every other massage technique—is to let yourself imagine how it feels *to them* as they receive it.

Since your client might like a slightly different pace or pressure than you, yourself, be sure to ask for feedback.

3. FRICTION TO THE RHOMBOIDS

With this stroke, apply a firm friction up and down both pairs of rhomboid muscles, which are located between the shoulder blades. Use both of your hands, simultaneously, with the fingertips of all eight of your fingers forming one line, which is generally perpendicular to the centerline of the spine. The direction of the stroke is parallel with the spine.

Note: If you have long fingernails, use the "pads," or "prints" of your fingers on this stroke, not the tips. This avoids the risk of causing unnecessary discomfort or actually scratching the skin along the back.

A. Place both of your hands on the tops of the shoulders as close to the neck as possible.

B. Apply friction by pulling down, directly across, and over the rhomboids (see Figure 7-3).

Slightly flex the fingers of both your hands and hold them together firmly.

Apply a fairly firm "raking" motion with the finger pads, pulling and dragging them down the muscles along both sides of the upper-middle (thoracic) spine.

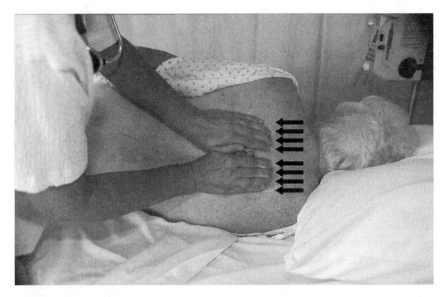

Figure 7-3 Fingertip friction to the rhomboids is a two-part, back-and-forth motion that "strips away" tension from the area between the shoulder blades. Begin the pull-down with fingers slightly flexed, applying pressure with your finger pads.

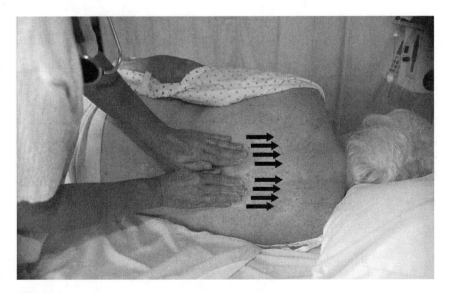

Figure 7-4 Straighten the fingers for the return up. This steady friction to the area—pulling down, with a forward return—uses the pads of all eight fingers in unison. Apply a moderate pressure, with an easy, fluid motion back-and-forth.

The heels of both hands maintain a comfortable contact with the client's body to provide stability.

Position your hands so the finger pads of the right hand drag down firmly over the muscles just to the right of the spine, while the pads of the fingers on the left hand drag down the same area on the spine's left side.

    C. Begin the "return" portion of the stroke at about the midpoint of the back, toward the bottom of the rib cage.

This time the finger pad friction is pushing up and into the rhomboids, toward the head, back to the starting position (see Figure 7-4 and 7-5). With practice, this raking motion will become very easy to perform. To make this continuous back-and-forth motion even more fluid, try imagining that you are drawing long, slender "figure-eights" into the soft muscle tissue beneath the skin. This stroke opens up the entire upper back (see Figure 7-6).

    D. Repeat this short stroke 3–4 times.

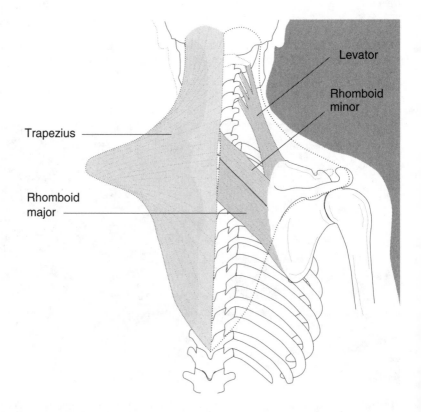

Figure 7-5 These deeper "intrinsic" muscles contract, or flex, to draw the shoulder blades up and back. Stripping off the tension here helps relax the shoulders, chest, and neck.

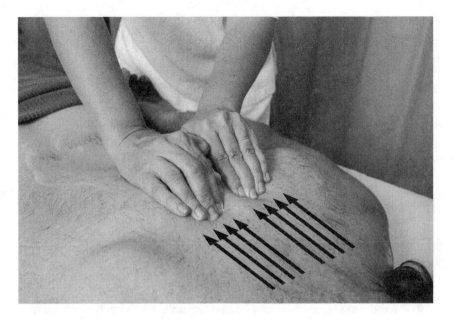

Figure 7-6 If the client can lay comfortably in a face-down position, applying this stroke to the rhomboid area can be easier and more effective. A pillow beneath the chest and abdomen reduces the amount of strain on the neck.

4. KNEAD THE SHOULDERS

This detailed sequence is almost identical to step 2, "Squeeze and Knead the Upper Shoulders" in the "dry" routine. In the sequence below, however, you are now using lotion to reduce the friction of the hands as they work directly on the skin (see Figure 7-7).

A. Rest the heels of your palms on the back side of the client's upper shoulders.

Place your right hand on the right upper shoulder and your left hand on the left, as indicated.

B. Align your four flattened fingers against the front of the shoulder muscle, positioned so the fingers are opposed the heels of your palms.

C. Squeeze the muscle mass, then release, alternating, right hand, then left, etc.

Your hands maintain contact with the muscles throughout the stroke.

D. Gradually cover the entire upper trapezius area using a slow, steady alternating rhythm.

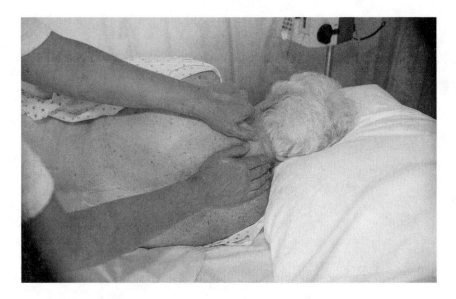

Figure 7-7 An easy stroke to perform, kneading the upper trapezius area with alternating hands helps relieve one of the primary gathering places of physical stress from lying in bed.

Rather than ever "attacking stress" with force, our aim is to encourage relaxation. This stroke, then, is less like a "demand" to relax and more like an *invitation* to let go. Let every movement of your hands communicate that friendly intention.

E. Begin where the neck joins the shoulders and work out toward the upper bony ridge of the shoulder blade until you run out of muscle mass.

Try to make this alternating sensation one of the best things that has ever happened to your client's shoulders.

F. Repeat this sequence to the area a couple of times, remembering to alternate, and keeping a slow, steady pace.

Helpful Hint: Very tense shoulders? "Rome wasn't built in a day." So don't feel like it is all up to you to get rid of 100% of your client's shoulder tension in their first two-minute massage. If tight shoulders happen to be the client's main complaint, it could take several short massages to feel significant relief. Your goal should always be simple, that is, to help this client feel better right now. A little help for just a couple of minutes is much better than no help at all, and sometimes the results can be a pleasant surprise.

5. ROTATING THUMB FRICTION TO MUSCLES ALONGSIDE THE SPINE

We now apply a technique we call "Rotating Thumb Friction" (RTF) to the Erector Spinae muscle "groups" (see Figure 7-8). For the sake of clarity, there is a specific pair of muscles called "erector spinae," but we are using the term here in reference to *all* of the intrinsic muscles that interlace up along both sides of the spine. These two "groups" of muscles make up a complex but elegant network which, when working in concert, not only hold the spine erect, but help us flex our bodies from side to side. Needless to say, this whole area truly deserves, and greatly appreciates, a good massage.

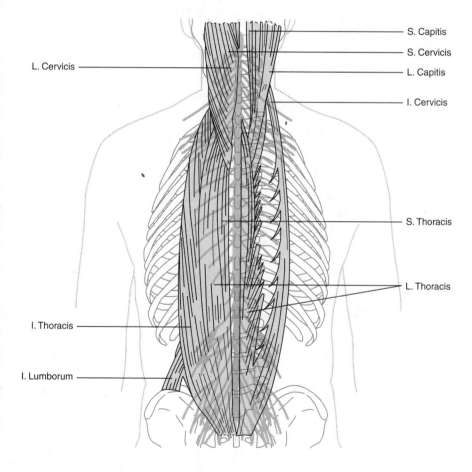

Figure 7-8 The Erector Spinae "Groups" consist of a number of muscle pairs. These interlace and overlap, and are visible as two long bands of muscle running up along both sides of the spine from top to bottom.

The RTF technique has been dubbed "the garden-tiller" by some students, because of the way the two thumbs work together in a continual rotating motion (see Figure 7-9). While it generally stimulates the muscles for relaxation, it is also especially good for searching out and relieving "pockets" of tension and soreness. It also draws circulation to the many small areas and helps "wake them up" when they have become chronic and, possibly, "desensitized" due to years of strain, pain, or overuse.

Describing and illustrating the RTF technique does require some time and detail. But once you understand the simple hand movements well enough to apply it, you will find the RTF easy to adapt for almost any muscle group in the body.

For many of your clients, due to time restrictions, you may need to limit the amount of time spent on the RTF technique, or even omit it entirely. Certainly

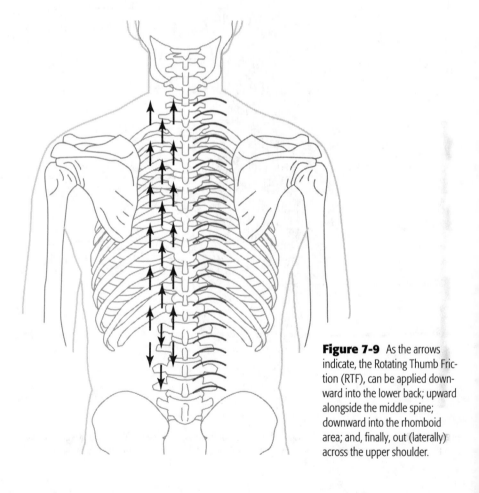

Figure 7-9 As the arrows indicate, the Rotating Thumb Friction (RTF), can be applied downward into the lower back; upward alongside the middle spine; downward into the rhomboid area; and, finally, out (laterally) across the upper shoulder.

any back massage can be effective and appreciated without including this or any other particular technique. However, if another nurse or practice partner ever performs the RTF technique on you, the physical sensation alone will convince you of its value. The generally consistent yet varied muscular "terrain" of those muscle groups alongside the spine provides an ideal area for learning this very versatile "seek and soothe" massage technique.

If the client is able to lie on each side, in turn, you may begin by working on the muscles along the "higher" side of the spine (the side of the back most easily accessible, as shown in Figure 7-10).

After you help the client turn over, so they are lying on their other side, work up along the other side of the spine. If the client is unable to lie on both sides, each side of the spine may be massaged in turn without the client moving at all. Adjust your approach accordingly. In either case, both of your thumbs are working together on the same side of the spine.

The following is a step-by-step breakdown—in "verbal slow-motion"—of exactly how to perform the RTF technique. Once you have carefully learned this stroke, it will always be much easier to perform than its detailed written description might suggest (Figure 7-11).

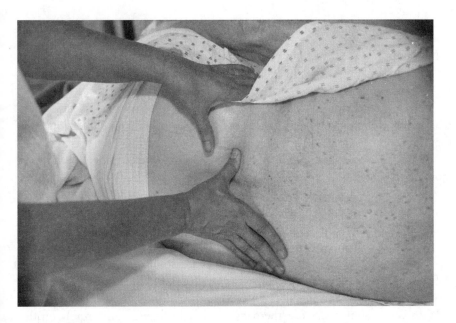

Figure 7-10 The muscles of the lower and middle back respond well to being explored and loosened with the Rotating Thumb Friction (RTF). When time is limited, this stroke may be viewed as optional.

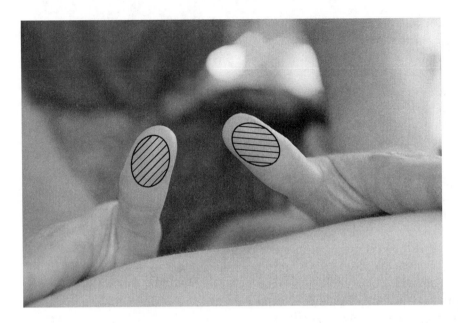

Figure 7-11 For the RTF technique, make direct contact with the client's skin using the pads, or "thumbprint" areas of both thumbs.

Note: Applying this technique to the back will take some additional practice time in order to perform it thoroughly. Take your time while learning it, but avoid overworking your hands, wrists, and thumbs (and your back). To avoid "wearing out" your thumbs, apply only a moderate pressure. It will always be much better to encourage the soft tissue to loosen by using your subtle *intention* rather than trying to force it with only your physical strength.

You might easily spend 20–30 minutes on this one stroke alone, but you will seldom have that much time. Remember, during a typical 5–10 minute back massage, you may have only a minute or two to apply this stroke, either very generally, or to some specific muscle area on the back. So learn it thoroughly, and extensively, but apply it sparingly.

A. Rest your hands on the client's lower back, and position both of your thumbs on the muscles along one side of the spine.

Begin in the lower back, just above the sacrum, near the bottom of the lumbar spine. You will be working all the way to the top of the shoulder.

With your palms open, rest the pads of all eight fingers comfortably on the client's body. (If you have even moderately long fingernails, make sure your finger pads are resting on the client's back, not your nails.)

Your thumbs should rest, almost touching each other, side by side on the skin.
B. Start the motion with a small friction stroke, using your right thumb, by moving it forward on the skin.

You are applying pressure downward with the thumb, and into the soft tissue just below the surface. At the same time, you are pushing forward (away from you) into the skin.

This single short movement should be only about one-half to three-quarters of an inch in length.

C. As the right thumb finishes its short stroke, lift it up just slightly off the skin, and begin an identical short movement on the skin with the left thumb (Figures 7-12 and 7-13).

As each thumb lifts up off the skin, the other thumb begins sliding underneath it onto the skin.

D. Repeat the movement until the motion of both thumbs becomes rhythmical, cyclical, and continuous.

The tiny circular movements of both thumbs working together explore, stimulate, and loosen the muscle tissue beneath them.

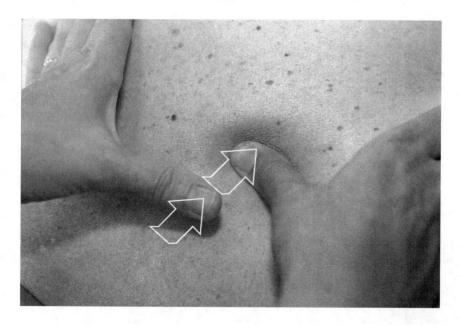

Figure 7-12 The Rotating Thumb Friction begins as two very short strokes, one with each thumb, in turn. As each thumb follows the other, continuously, a rotating movement is created. The effect will become that of a small, neuromuscular "tiller."

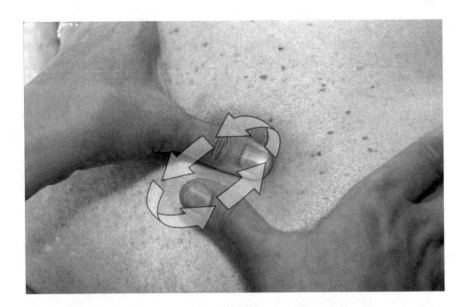

Figure 7-13 The RTF motion feels like a small, persistent motor moving along on the skin. With a light-to-moderate pressure, it loosens the soft muscle tissue just below the surface.

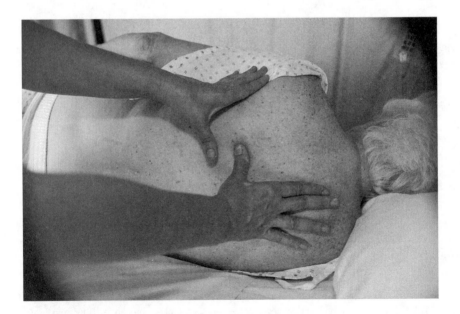

Figure 7-14 Rest the fingers of both your hands on the client's body in support of the rotating thumbs. This technique is especially well-suited for exploring the muscles throughout the mid-back area.

With just a little practice, this technique becomes almost automatic and effortless.

E. Guide the whole movement through the muscles, gradually, continually re-positioning your hands (as needed, for support) along the back (Figure 7-14).

This somewhat specific stroke is effective for locating sore areas in the muscles of the back. Its rhythmic sensation is unique in encouraging almost any tension to gradually let go. As mentioned, the RTF can be applied to just about any other body area as well.

Exploring the RTF Technique

In a typically brief massage, the RTF applied to one side of the back might take as little as one minute to perform. Although one minute up one side of the back would require moving along at a fairly moderate pace, the client should never feel like the RTF is rushed.

If you plan to massage the back for as long as 15 minutes, the RTF technique might even be "featured," including up to four or five minutes of the detailed work up each side. This would be enough time to explore the back muscles in fairly thorough detail. In those cases the RTF technique has proven very beneficial. At some point in your initial practice you might even devote most or all of one session to trading this technique alone. (Begin and end with the more general strokes, as usual.)

Once you have begun to master the RTF hand movements, try "putting your eyes into your thumbs," so to speak. Slowly assess the subtle character of the muscle tissue just beneath the skin as you move along. "Listen" with your hands for how the texture and temperature of the muscles tend to vary as you progress out of one part of the muscular landscape and into the next.

The muscles just beneath the skin in one area, for example, might feel decidedly "thick," even hard, or slightly cool to the touch. Then, in just the next couple of inches, those same muscles might feel uncharacteristically soft, noticeably warmer, or unusually tender to the pressure of your touch. Some part of the back might "feel like it would like to be scratched." Make a mental note of any noticeable changes like this, especially inconsistencies between one side of the back to the other. For instance, you may also notice that several areas feel noticeably hot to the touch on one side of the mid-back but not on the other side. By contrast, a corresponding area on the second side of the mid-back might be of an entirely different texture and character altogether than that of the side you massaged first.

In even more subtle terms, you may notice that some particular area feels "vacant," as though it might be almost numb. You may get the impression this

continued

area has been "cut off," so to speak, from that warm vitality you can so easily feel in the tissue just above, below, and all around it. You are now starting to gather information for future reference about how muscles feel to your touch "from the inside out." This personal encyclopedia of experience, over time, will help you learn how to "go straight to the good spots," and know instinctively what to do in order to help encourage those areas to open up and relax.

Remember, too, that you can gather even more information with just a casual question or two. For example, if a muscle area seems especially warm to your touch, ask your client how that area feels from their point of view as you massage it. Find out if the sensation feels any different than the area just above or below it. Maybe it does, and maybe it doesn't—perhaps the client can't tell any difference one way or the other—but you can. The way to find out is to ask. Your client might volunteer, even without prompting, that one particular area is, indeed, extremely sore when you touch it. Make another mental note that, "this is what a sore area feels like." Or, "this is a sore area that I didn't notice, and that I can't feel." (See Chapter 8 for more on giving and receiving detailed feedback.)

CAUTION: Remember, we should never cause a client pain. From their viewpoint, your massage should only "hurt good," that is, if it even hurts at all. So whatever you do, do not overdo this RTF stroke. And don't let anyone overdo it on you, either.

Prolonged RTF with its detailed and specific work into muscles, especially when those muscles are already sore and tight, can result in even more soreness for the client after the massage is over, or on the following day. For some clients this soreness might feel very therapeutic at the time, but that will not be the case for everyone. It is far more helpful to give the client too little of the specific work (and run the risk of their wanting more) than giving them too much of a good thing and having them feel real pain or be unnecessarily sore the next day.

Also, working too deeply for too long can tire out your own thumbs and wrists. After some practice, and when the RTF is done properly, neither your thumbs nor wrists should feel very tired at all—certainly not painful. "It doesn't need to hurt bad to do you good" applies for the giver of massage as well as it does for the receiver.

If your hands do hurt or feel worn out after the RTF, try working the soft tissue with less forcefulness. Give up on ever trying to "make" a client's muscles let go, or "fixing" all of their painful areas through your hard work. Try viewing your rotating thumbs as a way to *encourage muscle tissue to soften and open up. This slight shift in your approach still helps infuse the cells with increased vitality and circulation, but that result comes more readily out of a sense of ease and enjoyment. The primary purpose of the RTF, like the rest of your massage, is to help your client relax and feel better. Even if your technique may seem a little more effortless from your point of view, their capillaries will continue to relax and your client will still appreciate your massage.*

F. Repeat steps A–E to the muscles up and along the other side of the back.

6. HEELS OF BOTH PALMS UP THE BACK

Position: Stand at the same side of the bed near the client's hip, facing their head. Make sure your own body is as comfortable as possible.

We now effleurage, or glide, up the back muscles using the palms of both of hands. The hands glide in parallel, making one long, slow stroke up the muscles along both sides of the spine simultaneously. Now that the RTF has "churned up" the muscle tissue alongside the spine, this general stroke gives the entire area a deep sense of completion.

A. Place the palms of both hands on the sacro-iliac area (the very bottom of the lower back).

Your right palm rests on the muscles along the right side of the spine, while your left palm rests in the corresponding position on the left side. The fingers also make contact.

B. Lean some of your upper body weight into the heels of your palms.

C. Allow your hands to glide slowly, simultaneously, up the long back muscles (Figure 7-15).

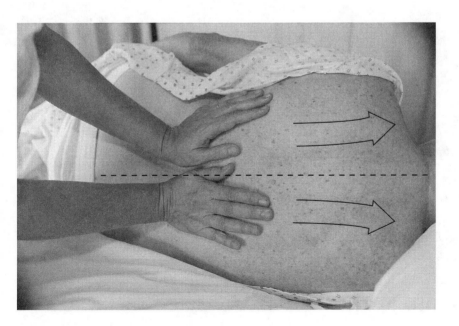

Figure 7-15 Both palms glide up, slowly and firmly, alongside the spine. This slow stroke up the back gives a sense of completion and finality to the whole area.

Apply a slow, gliding pressure to the long band of muscles on both sides of the spine, until you reach the tops of the shoulders.

Once again, do not apply any pressure directly onto the bony spine itself.

D. Complete this stroke by kneading the shoulders, using the alternating motion. (See Figure 7-7.)

This gives the shoulders and the back a sense of completion at the end of each long, gliding stroke up the back.

E. Repeat the entire stroke at least once.

If your client is able to lie face-down, this stroke may be able to accommodate slightly more pressure from the weight of your upper body (Figure 7-16). Frail clients, of course, will always need less pressure overall, and far less on the back near the spine. Ask your clients for feedback on the amount of pressure and what feels most comfortable for them.

You may also have occasion from time to time to perform a short back massage for a client or friend while they are lying on a "pallet" on the floor (Figure 7-18). Many who practice massage professionally actually prefer working on the floor, especially those who follow the Asian traditions. The strokes you are learning to perform here can be easily adapted to working on the floor, but it may take

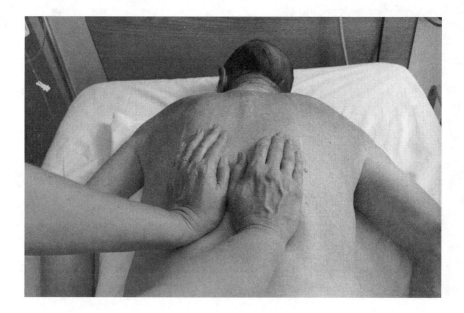

Figure 7-16 With the client lying face-down, glide the palms of both hands up alongside the spine. When you reach the top, knead the shoulders, alternating.

> ### Home Health Setting and the Bed of Regular Height
>
> Most clients will not have an elevated hospital bed in their home, so home health nurses may be called upon to perform massage for a client lying in a regular bed. Figure 7-17 illustrates relative body positioning. Notice how the client is lying with her body situated at an angle with respect to the foot of the bed. The nurse can then sit close to the client's body from either side. It may seem more comfortable to effleurage one side of the back at a time, as indicated, then switch sides. Also, note how the pillow is positioned lengthwise under the client's torso. With the client's head facing one side, the pillow reduces the acute angle on the neck and helps relax the lower back as well, making lying face-down much more enjoyable.

some practice. Keep in mind that whenever a client senses that you are comfortable, it reassures them and helps them to relax as well. If you are ever uncomfortable while giving a massage, with the client lying on either type of bed or at floor level, simply pause and re-position your body with ease and comfort in mind. For more detail on working at floor level, and instructions on how to assemble everything you'll need for working with a pallet on the floor, see Chapter 8.

• OPTIONAL: Petrissage the Neck

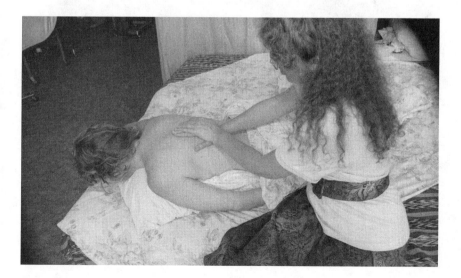

Figure 7-17 Sit comfortably alongside the client when working at standard bed height. Re-position as needed in order to apply each stroke effectively, and for your own physical comfort.

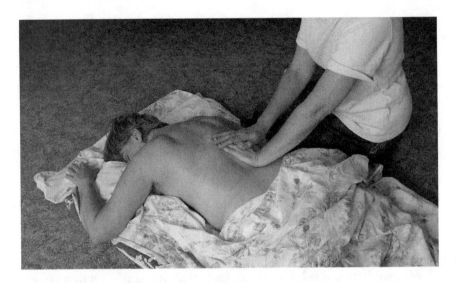

Figure 7-18 For clients lying at floor level you will have better access for some of the strokes while either kneeling or sitting on a pillow, whichever is most comfortable. Performing massage on the floor can also be a great workout for agility and body flexibility.

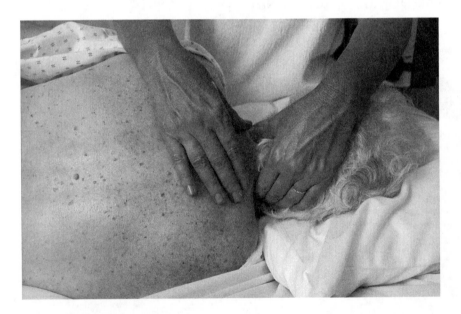

Figure 7-19 Loosen the client's neck with a brief kneading whenever she turns her head or shifts sides. Make sure the pillow is supporting the head comfortably.

Your client's neck can become tight or uncomfortable from lying either face down or on one side for an extended length of time. Use this optional stroke anytime you work on the client's back (client lying in any position).

Both before and after the client repositions their head so that it is facing in a different direction, petrissage or knead the neck. The technique is similar to that illustrated in the "dry" massage.

A. Petrissage both sides of the client's neck with your thumbs opposed your fingers.

Begin at the bottom, or base, of the neck nearest the shoulders.

Apply pressure with the pads of both thumbs, opposing the pads of the index and middle fingers of both hands aligned up along the other side. Alternately squeeze and knead the soft neck muscles inward, toward the spine, inching upward.

Work your way up to the area just beneath the base of the skull.

After the client turns to face the opposite direction, you may apply this same stroke from the other side as well. This whole stroke should take only a few seconds.

Note: Those parts of your hands that are not making contact are relatively relaxed. This technique is practically identical to the stroke you performed on the neck during the massage without lotion. The only difference being that the neck is now slightly turned toward you rather than facing directly downward (Figures 7-20 and 7-21).

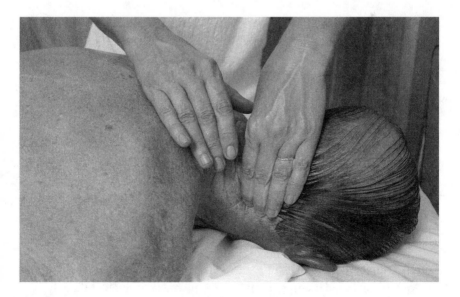

Figure 7-20 With the client lying face-down and a pillow supporting his upper torso, loosen the neck by kneading it both before and after he turns his head.

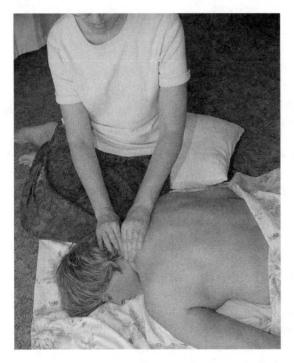

Figure 7-21 When working at floor level, make sure you can sit or kneel comfortably for this important stroke without reaching or straining.

B. Apply friction, using your thumbs and fingers underneath the Occipital Ridge at the back of the skull (Figure 7-22).

This is a slightly more specific stroke for helping loosen the neck muscles just beneath the occipital ridge. Use it, also, after your client has been lying on one side for some time. The friction contact slides along under the ridge (from lateral to medial).

• OPTIONAL: Apply Friction to the Scalp (Figure 7-23)

Some clients enjoy having their scalp stimulated while others do not, so ask the client before beginning. In general, very fine or thin hair may indicate a sensitive scalp. Be sure to remove any lotion from your hands before touching the hair.

A. Flex your fingers slightly.

The fingers of your dominant hand should be slightly flexed so that the pads of your fingers and thumb can all make contact with the scalp at the same time.

Note: If you have fingernails of even moderate length, make sure to use the pads of your fingers, not the tips. Even short fingernails, if applied directly, can irritate the scalp and cause discomfort. Using the prints virtually eliminates that possibility.

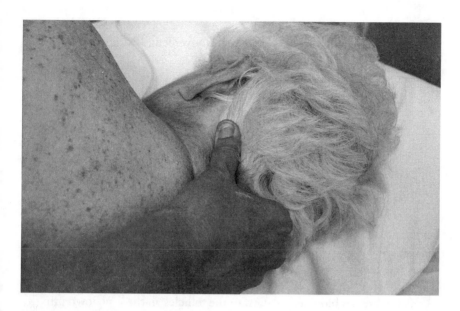

Figure 7-22 Apply a gentle friction to the neck muscles just beneath the bony Occipital Ridge at the base of the skull. With thumb opposing fingers, apply the friction toward the centerline, working gradually toward the spine.

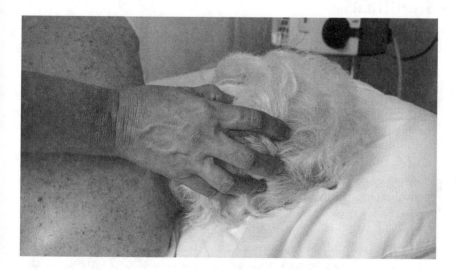

Figure 7-23 Ask permission before stimulating any client's scalp. With the finger pads of your dominant hand, apply enough pressure and rhythm to "wiggle" the scalp just slightly all over. This pleasant sensation helps many clients relax even more.

B. Stimulate the scalp thoroughly

You can use either a short back-and-forth movement on the scalp, or small, continuous circles.

With your finger pads, apply just enough pressure to move the scalp ever so slightly on the flat bony surface of the skull. Avoid pulling the hair. Ask your client for feedback about speed and sensation.

Depending on whether the client is lying on their back, face down, or on one side, you might try stimulating the entire scalp using both hands at the same time.

Or, if you stimulate each half of the scalp in turn, use one hand to lift the client's head just slightly up off the pillow for more access. Your free hand will then be able to stimulate the portion of the scalp that's now accessible.

Ask yourself, "If I had hair just like this, what would feel best to me?" Begin with that approach in mind, then ask the client, "How does this feel?" Listen for their answer, even asking again, if necessary.

Thirty seconds can seem like a long time to stimulate the scalp, because that would amount to 15 seconds on each side of the head. "Thorough" scalp stimulation means it increases blood circulation to the follicles all the way down into the root of each hair. Whatever approach you take to stimulating the scalp, just make sure your client thinks it feels good, too.

THE SHOULDERS

Since chronic tension tends to gather in the shoulders, this will be one area of primary complaint for most clients. Therefore, shoulders merit special attention. Add to this the fact that practically everybody enjoys a good "shoulder rub," and it becomes clear why being able to address the shoulders fairly well in a relatively short amount of time is a valuable skill to have.

Although the "shoulder girdle" includes parts of the neck as well as the front side of the upper body, the following sequence focuses on the tops and back (superior and posterior) shoulders, and it can be included as just one part of an overall back massage. On the other hand, if the shoulders happen to be the number one area of complaint, these strokes alone might make up the sum total of a much-appreciated "back" massage.

The amount of time spent on each of these strokes will be determined both by your client's need and the amount of time you have available. For example, a rather long 5- or 10-minute back massage might consist solely of massaging the client's shoulders. However, applying the following three-step shoulder sequence, first to one shoulder, then to the other, need not take more than about two minutes altogether if that happens to be all the time you have.

Three Steps for the Shoulders

The following is an overview of the order of strokes in this sequence for the shoulders, followed by the purpose of each stroke.
1. Alternating Palm Effleurage Between the Shoulder Blades
2. Rotating Thumb Friction to the Shoulder Area
3. Effleurage Around the Shoulder
4. Repeat to the Other Shoulder
The Purpose of Each Step
1. Alternating palm effleurage loosens the whole area
2. Rotating thumb friction explores and loosens the soft tissue more deeply
3. Effleurage around the shoulder gives the area a sense of completion

Since you may use this sequence a great deal in your own home, we illustrate and describe it here with the client lying on a bed of regular height. It can be easily adapted for the higher hospital bed by lowering or removing the bed's headboard, whenever possible. If that proves impractical, help the client re-position her body with her head resting at the foot of the hospital bed so you can have better access to the shoulder areas. If the client can neither reposition, nor lie comfortably face-down, have her lie on each side, in turn, and perform the same strokes on one shoulder at a time. Adapt your approach as necessary, because this sequence will always be well worth the effort.

Position: The client is lying face-down in a bed of regular height. Her entire body is positioned diagonally, that is, headed into one corner of the bed at a 45-degree angle (as shown in Figure 7-24). The client rests her head as closely as possible to the very corner of the bed, with a pillow placed lengthwise beneath her upper torso. Position the pillow's upper edge down far enough beneath her torso so that its upper edge puts no pressure on her throat.

Position your own chair with its front edge making direct contact with the corner of the bed. You should be directly facing the client's head.

1. Alternating Palm Effleurage Between the Shoulder Blades

Apply an alternating effleurage, using your palms, to the area between the shoulder blade (scapula) and the spine (Figure 7-25). This is the area of the rhomboid muscles.

With the client facing right, focus on the left shoulder first (or vice versa).

In other words, if you are satisfied that the client's neck is comfortable (and does not need to be turned), you can begin with the shoulder the client is facing away from.

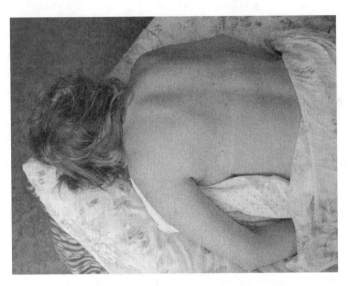

Figure 7-24 Help the client position herself on the bed with her body at a 45-degree angle into one corner, as shown. Her head should be as close as possible to the corner's edge.

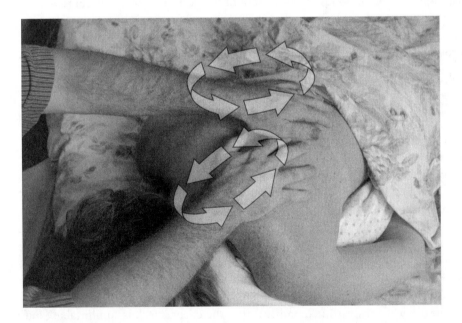

Figure 7-25 When you want to take some of "the weight of the world" off a client's shoulders, use Alternating Palms to the whole area. This is the first step in a three-step sequence.

A. Begin at the upper shoulder, next to the spine.
B. Apply a short, gliding stroke with one palm, down through the rhomboid area.
C. Follow up with the same stroke, using your other hand.
D. Repeat continually, allowing a relaxing, alternating rhythm to develop between the two gliding palms.

This open-handed rhythm of the two alternating palms should be gentle, yet firm.

The motion of this stroke is similar to that of the RTF technique. Except that, now, the surfaces of both alternating palms are making contact with the body, rather than just the pads of the thumbs.

The palms, along with the relaxed fingers of both hands, follow along over the body's contours, making full contact. However, the heels of the palms exert the primary pressure against the client's body. That pressure should be light to moderate. As always, you might ask your client for some feedback about the pressure.

2. Rotating Thumb Friction to the Shoulder Area (Figure 7-26)

A. Apply Rotating Thumb Friction (RTF) to the Rhomboid and Levator Scapula areas.

The rhomboid muscles (major and minor) contract to draw the shoulder blade toward the spine (Refer to Figure 7-5).

The levator scapula muscles, anchored on the upper-inner corner of the shoulder blade also attach to the vertebrae in the neck. These muscles are often very sore, sometimes even tender to the touch. A moderate amount of massage to this area helps loosen the whole shoulder area.

B. Apply RTF to the upper trapezius.

Continue with the RTF around the corner of the shoulder blade. Work the uppermost part of the fleshy shoulder (trapezius) muscle thoroughly. Then continue outward (lateral), along and above the upper ridge of the shoulder blade (Figure 7-27).

Keep in mind that the other shoulder will probably need and appreciate an equal portion of time and attention.

3. Effleurage Around the Shoulder

A. Begin by resting your hand on the area where the shoulder meets the neck (Figure 7-28).

B. Glide your palm out, over the top of the shoulder.

From near the neck, glide out toward the shoulder joint, with your whole hand relatively relaxed.

Your fingers should contour along the surface of the shoulder, with the fleshy palm making the primary contact with the body during this first one-third of the stroke.

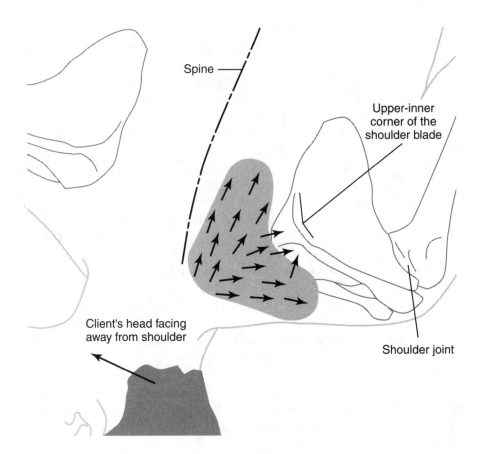

Figure 7-26 First, locate the upper-inner corner of the shoulder blade for reference. Then apply Rotating Thumb Friction systematically to the soft tissue (shaded area). The arrows indicate the general direction of the short RTF strokes.

C. Fingers around the shoulder joint.

Continuing the stroke, let the inner surfaces of all your fingers glide around the deltoid muscle (at the uppermost part of the arm), and then begin the stroke's recovery underneath the shoulder joint (Figure 7-29).

The soft (posterior) surfaces of the fingers should slip around, under the shoulder joint, and your knuckles will momentarily touch the sheet.

D. Recover up to the neck.

Recover this stroke to the starting point. With your flattened fingers gliding up against the front edge of the shoulder muscle (Upper Trapezius), let the

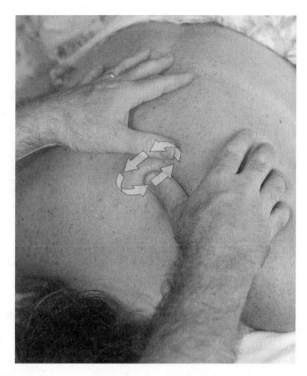

Figure 7-27 Apply the RTF technique between the shoulder blade and the spine (as shown), working around the upper-inner corner of the shoulder blade. Then, work along above the blade, and out across the top of the fleshy shoulder until you run out of muscle.

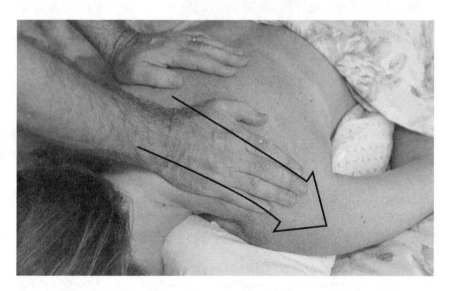

Figure 7-28 This starting position is the first of three illustrations for one continuous motion. With just a little practice, this stroke can be applied in a relaxed, fluid manner.

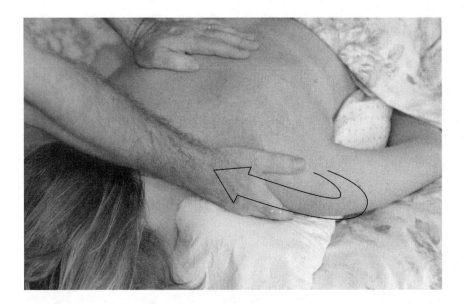

Figure 7-29 The palm rides across the upper shoulder out to the shoulder joint. There, the flattened fingers glide together, around the fleshy deltoid muscle, enclosing the uppermost part of the arm.

motion slow down for an instant at the base of the neck near their original position (Figure 7-30).

Your palm remains in contact with the client's body throughout this very pleasant, fluid stroke.

E. From the original starting position, repeat this stroke at least once or twice.

This entire stroke is really very simple, and can become so fluid that its repetition feels to the client like one, continuous, circular stroke.

As you connect the end of one cycle to the beginning of the next, this sensation helps bring a sense of completion and finality to the entire shoulder area.

Remember, now, to petrissage the client's neck for a few seconds before she raises her head and repositions, facing the opposite direction. She will now be facing the shoulder you just completed. After turning the neck—if it still appears to be stiff or uncomfortable—you might petrissage it again, briefly, after the re-positioning is complete.

4. Repeat Steps 1 through 3 to the Other Shoulder

Let's briefly review the 3-step shoulder massage sequence. Remember that using the palms for an alternating effleurage loosens up the whole shoulder area. The rotating thumbs then explore and loosen the intrinsic muscles more deeply.

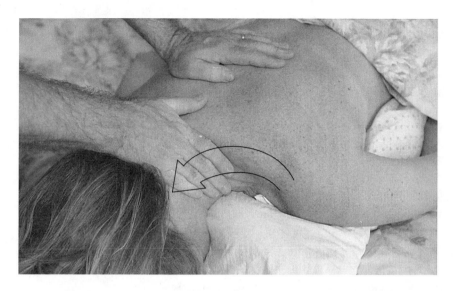

Figure 7-30 The palm and flattened fingers glide together, returning up the neck. As it returns back to its starting position on the shoulder the palm slows for an instant, then begins the cycle again. Repeat several times until this becomes like one continuous, fluid motion.

Finally, the circular effleurage repeated around the upper shoulder provides a sense of wholeness and completion to the area. Remember to apply about the same amount of massage to both shoulders.

THE HANDS

Massaging a client's hands can be a simple act of human to human kindness. For some hospitalized clients, the hands might be the only areas of the body that remain accessible to touch—or for any human contact—especially when a client is in intensive care.

Hand massage can also help nurses, in any context, become better acquainted with their clients. In our personal lives, massaging the hands can be one of the best ways to let somebody who is very special to us know, and feel, how much we care for them and that we wish for them the very best.

Position: For the following demonstration, the client is lying in bed. However, just as easily, she may be sitting up in bed or in a chair. Whether you are sitting or standing, your client's relaxed hand and forearm should be about level with your waist.

1. Squeeze the Palm while Applying Lotion

A. Apply a small amount of lotion to both of your palms.

You want just enough lotion for you hands to "glide, not slide." So start with a "spot" of lotion roughly the size of a dime. (A dime is a small coin, about 17mm in diameter. But there's no need to be so exacting.) Hand massage requires very little lotion but, if the hands are still dry, or rough, you might try another dime, or even "a nickel's worth" of lotion (a spot of lotion slightly larger than a dime).

B. Squeeze and knead the client's hand.

With the client's palm facing down, briefly loosen the hand.

Squeeze, stimulate, and loosen the client's palm and all of the small muscles and joints inside. Use an alternating motion, squeezing first with your right hand, then the left, kneading the hand gingerly (Figure 7-31). Be mindful of your pressure when the client's hands are either frail or particularly small.

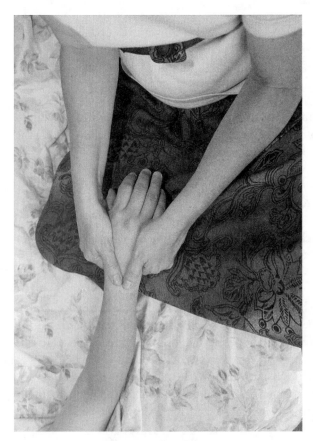

Figure 7-31 With a small amount of lotion on your own palms, begin by squeezing and kneading the client's hand with an alternating motion. Stimulate and loosen any tension and resistance in and around all of the small muscles and delicate joints.

Giving Up "The Grip"

Receiving a simple hand massage, for many of us, may be one of the best exercises in allowing ourselves to let go and receive. Amazingly enough, with a little practice, even the hand of a confirmed "giver" can learn how to let go. If your client lifts up her arm in an attempt to "hand you" her hand, ask her to let the entire arm relax, all the way down from the shoulder joint. Suggest to her, "Can this arm be heavy?" If she tries to "help" you again, touch her shoulder with your one hand and "wiggle" her hand and arm with your other. Demonstrate for her how her hand and arm might just drop, effortlessly, if she were to completely let go of it. Jokingly, tell her, "Think Limp-Noodle, Limp-Noodle," as you wiggle the arm.

How difficult should it be to let somebody else help us feel better? Your client may not be accustomed to receiving so much help and personal attention from others. For that very reason, hand massage might be another good place to begin your entire massage.

2. Rotating Thumbs to the Palm

Turn the client's hand over, with the palm facing up.

A. Apply friction to palm with rotating thumbs.

The motion of your alternating thumb friction is now rotating "backward," toward you. This is in contrast with rotating away from you, as the RTF has been shown in all of the previous examples (Figure 7-32).

B. Cover the entire surface of the palm.

This technique creates a unique, pleasurable sensation in the hand and has a very relaxing effect. Like the soles of the feet, the hands have reflexive areas that, when stimulated, help open up and relax the entire body.

3. Squeeze the Hand Again

Turn the hand back over, palm facing down, and squeeze it again with both of your hands, alternating, just as in step 1.

4. Repeat Steps 1–3 to the Other Hand

THE NECK

Position: The client is lying on her back in a hospital bed. Standing near the client's right shoulder, the nurse reaches across, working on the client's left shoulder.

Helpful Hint: Some clients want no lotion anywhere near their hair. As mentioned, others may not be concerned about the lotion, but just don't want their hair "messed up." The following technique might cause your hands, and a very

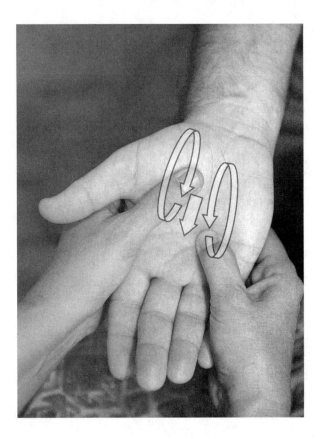

Figure 7-32 Grasp the hand firmly while gently spreading the palm open. In this particular RTF stroke your thumbs' motion is rotating "backward," pulling toward the client's fingers.

small amount of lotion, to touch the occipital area at the base of the skull. In our experience, most clients don't seem to mind having a touch of lotion on their hair, especially on the back of the head near the neck.

If your client voices any concern about lotion on the hair—or if you have a feeling this might be a concern—you can always use the "dry" techniques for the neck (without lotion) as described in the previous chapter.

1. Apply Lotion to the Shoulder and Neck

Ask the client to turn her head slightly toward you, so that she is facing away from the shoulder you are about to massage.

A. Place a small amount of lotion in one palm.

Begin with a drop of lotion about the diameter of a nickel, and spread it evenly on the soft surfaces of your fingers and on both of your palms. This stroke will not need very much lotion.

B. Spread the lotion up the client's shoulder and neck (Figure 7-33).

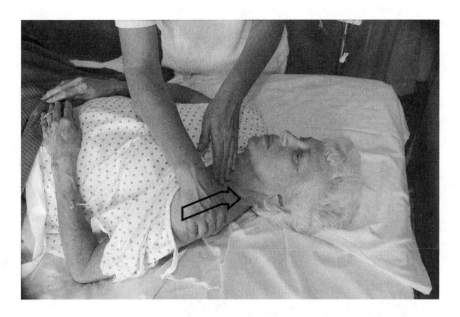

Figure 7-33 Reaching across, apply a small amount of lotion to the client's upper shoulder and the side of her neck with one smooth stroke. Stop just short of the hairline.

With one continuous stroke, using your palm and only a light to moderate pressure, pull the lotion up the fleshy shoulder and neck. Stop just below the hairline.

If the client's skin feels especially dry, you might try using a bit more lotion, possibly just the amount remaining on your other palm. Again, use the lotion sparingly.

This entire technique is intended primarily for the neck. Even though we tend to think of the neck and shoulders as being distinct body parts, the fact is they are inseparable. Relieving stress and tension in any part of this important area helps the whole upper body relax.

    2. Apply an Alternating Friction with the Finger Pads, Up and Across the
        Shoulder and Neck

    A. Place the flattened fingers of both hands on the far shoulder.

Still reaching across the client's body, place the flattened fingers of both your hands on the top of client's left shoulder, slightly above the shoulder joint (Figure 7-34).

    B. Apply alternating friction, pulling across the muscle.

Press into the fleshy muscle slightly with your finger pads as you pull toward you. With alternating hands, work across the soft shoulder muscle. "Finger pads,"

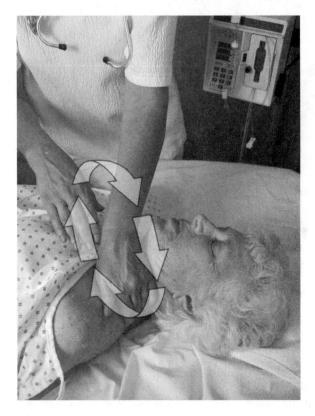

Figure 7-34 Apply alternating friction to the upper shoulder and neck, pulling across with the pads of your flattened fingers.

in this case, includes the fingerprint areas as well as the soft surfaces of all three joints on the first, second, and third fingers of both hands.

The finger pads of each hand work as a unified area of contact and pressure. Both hands begin working together, alternating, onto the skin and into the soft muscle tissue.

This version of the alternating friction technique works much like the RTF, which we have already applied along the back muscles. There are two differences. First, the two rotating areas of contact (all of the finger pads) are now much broader and, therefore, they form a somewhat less specific area of contact than when we worked with the thumbs. Secondly, the continuous rotation is now a pulling motion, working "backward," so to speak, pulling toward you (Figure 7-35).

C. Progress up the shoulder, to the very base of the neck.

Working your way across the upper shoulder, you will gradually come to the very base of the neck (lower cervical area), where the neck and shoulder meet.

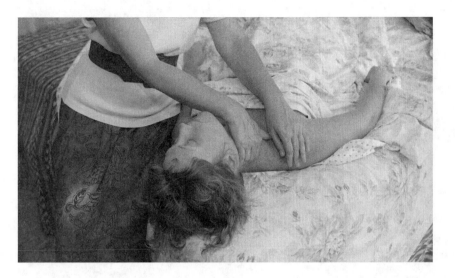

Figure 7-35 With the client lying on a regular bed, work across on the opposite shoulder. Note how the client's positioning, angled out from the corner, provides enough room for you to sit comfortably.

Ask your client for some feedback on how much pressure to apply. With practice, this stroke can create a very pleasant, relaxing sensation for the client's neck.

D. Apply friction up the side of the neck (Figure 7-36).

Continue up the neck, working on the muscles alongside the cervical spine.

E. Apply friction beneath the occipital ridge.

The direction of the stroke shifts slightly as it begins to work its way along under the occipital ridge and out (laterally) toward the ear. Pulling the muscle tension away from the spine, the alternating finger pads rotate along just beneath the bony ridge.

While working so closely near the edge of the scalp, be mindful not to pull the hair.

The client may feel instinctively like moving her head around ever so slightly during this stroke. That's because, with so much tension and soreness having been stored here, the sensation caused by the rotating pressure exploring all the "nooks and crannies" in the muscles of the neck can feel fascinating. The client moving her neck helps your fingers find, and sink into, those particular areas that might feel especially sore. Stimulating these areas helps release the tension in the neck and encourages the whole area to relax.

Try to back off the pressure of your stroke just a bit before you reach the bony protrusion (the Mastoid Process) behind the ear. Avoid any direct pressure to that particular spot because it is often quite tender.

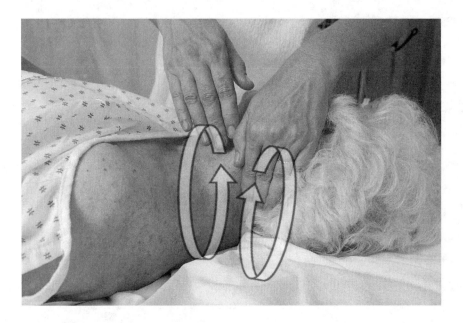

Figure 7-36 The finger pads of each hand apply a continual contact and a gently "pulsating" pressure as they alternate into the soft muscle tissue of the upper neck.

Time permitting, you might repeat this rotating friction pressure up into the occipital ridge. Having someone else perform this stroke on you will illustrate its value, and why it will always be a technique worth repeating.

3. Repeat Steps 1 and 2, to the Other Shoulder and Side of the Neck

The following strokes to the face and head should be considered "Optional." But there may be certain cases where these prove to be some of your most appropriate techniques.

• OPTIONAL: Friction to the Cheeks

A. If the client's skin seems dry, apply a tiny drop of lotion to the soft surfaces of your flattened fingers.

Try not to use much lotion on the face, only what is absolutely needed. Also, avoid any direct contact with the eyelashes or eyelids since even the best lotions can cause irritation.

B. Place the soft surfaces of your flattened fingers together, resting them on the right and left cheeks.

The long, flattened surfaces of the fingers are the only parts of the hands that make contact on the cheeks.

Let the Client Move Her Own Neck

Caution: A very relaxed neck—one whose muscles have just been kneaded and stretched—may like to turn on its own accord to face the other direction, not by being "helped." So allow your client to move his own neck when he feels ready. After you finish applying the strokes to one side of the neck and shoulder, suggest aloud that the client now bring his neck back to a "neutral," or face-up, position. Since those neck muscles have now been elongated, the effort of turning his head should be left up to him alone, by his own internal volition.

Specifically, do not use your own hands to move or "place" the client's head from one extreme position directly into facing the opposite direction. That kind of "positioning" can sometimes seem abrupt, controlled, and even painful for the client, no matter how "carefully" you try to move it. Let the client's muscles do the work from the inside out.

After you have finished working on the remaining side of the neck and shoulder, once again, ask the client to move his own neck back into the neutral, face-up position. Some clients like to stretch their own neck, even rocking it back and forth a few times from side to side after having the muscles stretched so thoroughly.

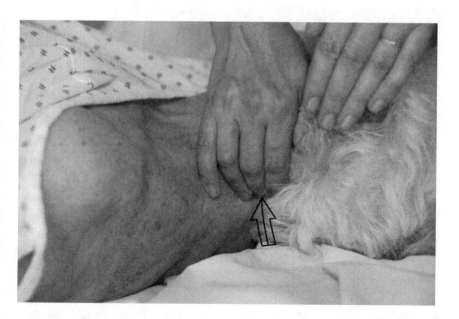

Figure 7-37 Loosen the muscles at the base of the skull by applying a slow, rotating friction to the occipital ridge. This area is often tender, so work gently, yet creating a firm, comfortable sensation for the client.

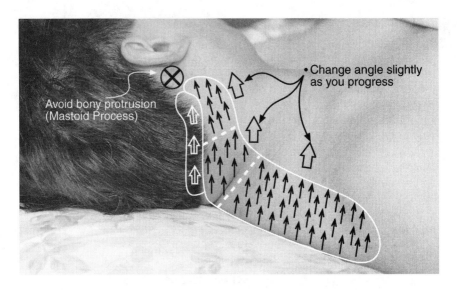

Change angle slightly as you progress

Avoid bony protrusion (Mastoid Process)

Figure 7-38 The arrows indicate the general directions and the progression of your rotating finger pads. The broken lines indicate more specific areas for concentration within the whole, unified region.

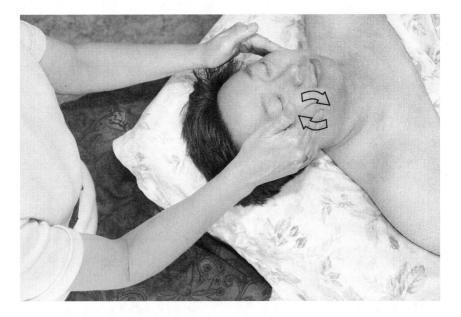

Figure 7-39 We use the jaw muscles, called "masseters," for chewing our food and gritting our teeth. While they are known for being the strongest muscles for their size in the human body, gentle fingers can still encourage them to relax.

C. Apply a light circular friction, simultaneously, to the masseter muscles of both cheeks just beneath the skin.

Since there will be some slight movement of your fingers on the skin, this stroke is, technically, a "friction" stroke. But it should be nowhere near the degree of friction you have applied elsewhere (such as with the RTF stroke).

The majority of the pressure is applied toward moving the muscles around slightly, just beneath the surface of the skin, in small, simultaneous circles. The motion of those circles begins by circling over-and-forward, as indicated (Figure 7-39). The facial features are quite sensitive, so this stroke should only feel pleasant to the client's face.

If the client begins stretching the jaw muscles around in circles in response to this movement's sensation, it is often to help your fingers find those specific areas of tension and soreness. You may, likewise, shift from using the long, inner surfaces of the fingers to applying a slightly more direct pressure with the finger pads (that is, if your fingernails are short) (Figure 7-40).

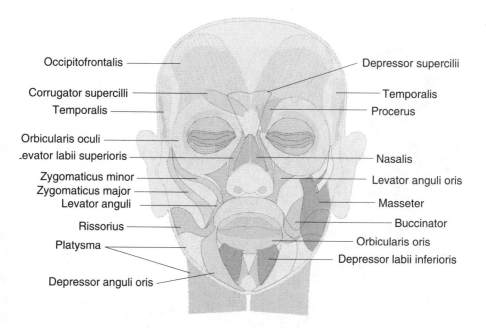

Figure 7-40 The temporalis, frontalis, and masseter muscles are very sensitive, and they provide good indicators for the degree of general mental tension and stress throughout the body. They also respond almost immediately as your massage gently suggests they can relax.

You will not need to be very specific with this movement, though. Just use the slight pressure and hand movement to coax and encourage the jaw muscles to relax. General relaxation is all we are trying to induce.

Unconsciously flexing the masseter muscles in the course of a day can indicate a habit of forceful mental concentration. Occasionally, a client will be made aware that they can't seem to completely let go of their jaw. Ask them to concentrate on the sensation of this stroke and encourage them to relax the muscles of the whole head and neck areas as well. This simple technique can be especially helpful after long hours of study, driving on the highway, or any other activity that requires sustained mental exertion. You can practice it, too, without a partner, by applying it on yourself. See if you don't feel the top of your head and scalp relax as you loosen your jaw.

• OPTIONAL: Friction to the Temples

A. Place the soft surfaces of your flattened fingers together, resting on the right and left temple areas.

The "temple" areas are roughly 1.5 inches in diameter and are located on both sides of the head between the upper edge of the ear and the end of the eyebrow.

B. Apply a light circular friction to the surface muscles of both temples, simultaneously, just beneath the scalp (Figure 7-41).

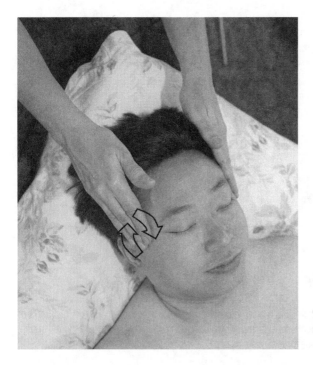

Figure 7-41 A simultaneous, circular friction to the temple areas with your finger pads soothes and relaxes the mind and body.

The temple area may be tender or sensitive to the touch, so be careful not to apply too much pressure here. Rather than the amount of pressure you apply, it will be more about the quality of the sensation your hands create that will have such a relaxing effect. (Just for practice, try this stroke on yourself.)

Technically, this area might be referred to as "where the anterior portion of the temporalis muscle meets the frontal belly of the epicranius muscle, located directly over the sphenoid and anterior temporal bones of the skull." But even more important than knowing their precise anatomical definition, remember *not* to pull the hair. Refer to the illustration for the general location and just massage the entire area. If it is okay to touch the client's hair, you can extend the area of contact to the (temporalis) region of the scalp just above the ears.

• OPTIONAL: Effleurage to the Forehead

A. Place the heels of your palms together on the center of the client's forehead.

Your palms are relatively relaxed, as are your fingers. And the stroke is directed outward (laterally), toward the temples.

B. Effleurage in one smooth, simultaneous motion (as shown in Figure 7-42) off the forehead.

The forehead is also very sensitive, so it doesn't need a lot of pressure to help it relax.

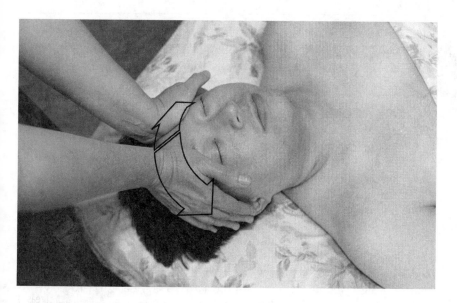

Figure 7-42 Firm but gentle pressure applied laterally across the frontalis muscle on the forehead completes the series for the face and head.

Again, if the skin on your client's forehead happens to be dry, just a hint of lotion (one small drop) spread evenly over the heels of your palms reduces most of the friction to the skin.

Repeat this short stroke at least once or twice.

CAUTION: Once again, in order to avoid getting any lotion on or near the client's eyes, do not touch either the eyelashes or the eyelids with your hands or fingers.

C. After this stroke, rest and relax for at least 5–10 seconds.

This is a good stroke for near the end of a massage. But regardless of where it might take place within a sequence, after applying this soothing stroke to the forehead pause just a few seconds before you begin any other stroke. Let the client savor its effect.

Helpful Hint: Relaxing the face and head can be a nice way to finish a massage. However, you might find that saving the feet for last is also a pleasant way to end. On the one hand, the head and face are very personal, yet the feet hardly ever receive massage. If you have time for only one of these two important areas, we recommend the feet. If you do have time to work on both the head and face areas as well as the feet, be sure to save massaging the hard-working feet for last.

THE FEET

The Journey of a Thousand Miles Begins with a Pair of Feet

Over the span of a lifetime we cover countless journeys and thousands of miles on our feet. Yet we hardly ever give them much thought, unless they happen to tire out or otherwise complain. For many feet, theirs is a destiny of damp darkness confined to a pair of almost airtight shoes. Seldom are they afforded even the simplest of joys, like the warmth of salty sand, luxuriating in the comfort of fresh cool mud, or the soft shuffle of summer grass beneath their smooth, tender soles. In spite of how we treat our feet, or how little recognition they get, they deserve the utmost of care and, at minimum, a measure of respect.

Massage helps us realize how much road tension we're carrying along with us in our feet. Imagine, one day, somebody takes hold of your foot and gives it a good, friendly "wringing out." And if one foot gets massage and the other one thinks it's going to get ignored, you'll hear about it. Who says feet can't talk? How, we think to ourselves, could we have ever let our own feet go so long without

continued

letting them know how much we appreciate them? After all, they have borne our weight through every single step of our lives!

Physically, feet are tender, sensitive, and fascinating. Much more than walking machines, they are living networks of intricate muscle and small, precise bones. Their soft tissue is enlivened by thousands of microscopic nerve endings, especially on their soles. And so it's no wonder that having our feet massaged feels so indescribably good!

One instructor made a point of suggesting that wherever there is a bony joint in the human body there is a corresponding nexus of subtle, bio-electrical current. So by using massage to open up the muscles and joints in our feet we are, in effect, releasing the flow of bio-electrical current throughout the entire body. Adjusting those fine networks of muscles, bones, and joints is like fine-tuning a dozen tiny transducers, similar in comparison to the old-fashioned "crystal set" radio receivers of the early twentieth century. When we rid our feet of all that excess tension and static, the analogy continues, our "reception" is bound to improve. But whatever we may or may not believe about the body's electrical nature—or whether or not we think our feet have feelings, too—nobody will argue with you when you say you feel much better after having a good thorough foot massage.

From a historical perspective, bathing or massaging the feet have long been deemed as tokens of honor. As such, they are powerful and symbolic acts of selfless human service. Going back to ancient times, "anointing" the body with oil signified reverence, and ministering to the feet was considered to be an act of profound humility and respect for another human being. Mentioned specifically in the texts of ancient India and China, improved health was seen as yet another beneficial effect of addressing the feet through massage.

For your clients who may be seriously ill or otherwise incapacitated, a good foot massage can serve to introduce a moment of pleasure and relief into the slow process of recuperation. During almost any illness—or even just after a hard day's work—a foot massage right before bedtime can help make a good night's sleep that much more restful and rejuvenating. Our feet have been kind to us, and now we can return the favor.

Position: The client lies on her back in a hospital bed, while the nurse stands slightly to one side, facing the foot (Figure 7-43). Be sure the bed is adjusted to a comfortable height for the nurse.

1. Apply Lotion to the Foot

Apply just enough lotion to reduce friction on the foot, but not enough for the skin to be slippery. If you do happen to apply too much lotion, just blot the excess off with the sheet.

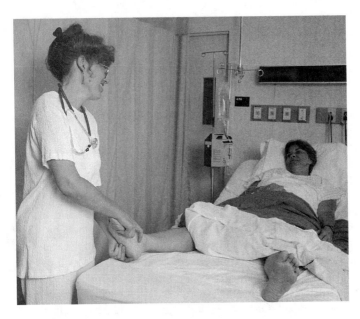

Figure 7-43 In as little as 2–3 minutes you can brighten any client's day with a short, three-step massage for each foot.

Although we won't focus specifically on massaging the ankles, it is important that they always feel included in the general foot massage. So remember to make good contact with the heel, ankle, and achilles tendon areas as you apply the lotion.

Applying lotion leads naturally into the next step, kneading the foot.

2. Knead the Foot Thoroughly

A. Heels of your palms rest on top, finger pads underneath.

Place the heels of your palms side by side on top of the client's foot, your finger pads will work up underneath, into the sole.

B. Knead, alternately, squeezing with each hand in turn (Figure 7-44).

Both hands maintain contact with the foot as you squeeze and knead the "road tension" out of all of the small muscles, tendons, and joints.

Work gradually from back, near the heels, progressing up and forward, toward the toes. Kneading helps the foot regain some of its inherent flexibility.

3. Apply "Stripping" Friction to the Sole

A. Form two parallel lines with your fingers underneath the sole of the client's foot (Figure 7-45).

This initial placement begins on the lower sole of the foot as close to the heel as possible.

B. Strip the tension out of the sole of the foot, heel to toes.

Beginning near the heel and working toward the toes, "strip" the tension out of the sole of the foot.

Figure 7-44 Rest the heels of your palms on top of the foot for stability. Using the alternating finger pads of both hands, apply a squeeze-and-release action up into the sole underneath.

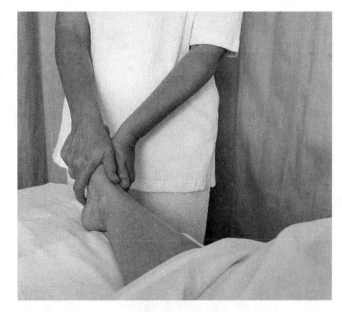

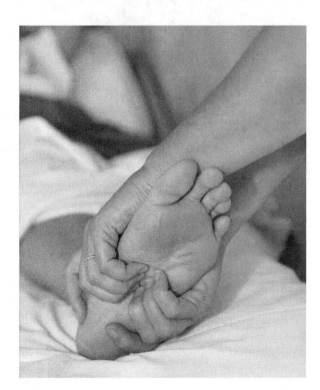

Figure 7-45 Take the foot firmly in both hands, placing your finger pads as shown, and slowly "strip" the tension out of the sole of the foot.

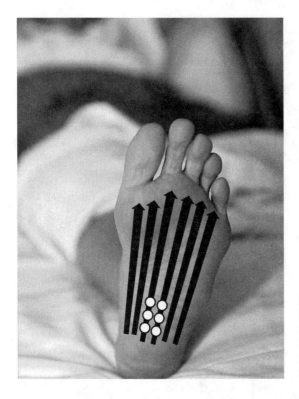

Figure 7-46 Align your finger pads in the lower-center "belly" of the sole, near the heel. Apply a firm, continuous friction—using three long, slow strokes—as you strip the tension out of the foot toward the toes.

Apply a sliding (friction) pressure with the pads of your first, second, and third fingers aligned in parallel (as shown in Figure 7-46).

If your fingernails are suitably short, you can also use the tips of your fingers for this stroke. NOTE: Omit this stroke entirely if you either have long fingernails, or if the client complains about them.

C. Cover the entire sole of the foot systematically.

Apply three straight double lines of friction to the sole. Begin near the heel, and draw the aligned finger pads directly up the sole, toward the toes.

This stroke is intended to draw, squeeze, or "milk," the tension right out of the foot.

4. Apply Rotating Thumbs to the Sole of the Foot

Position: The nurse is now seated in a chair facing the client's foot (Figure 7-47). The foot should be at a relative height anywhere from about level with the nurse's elbows to just below eye level. The nurse's forearms might rest on the bed for support.

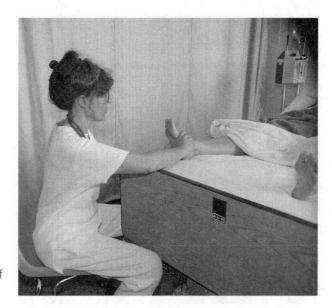

Figure 7-47 Whether at home or working on a client in an adjustable hospital bed, the nurse should be comfortable. Note the positioning of her hands and the general height of the client's foot.

A. Begin near the heel, and work toward the toes.

Focus on the "hollow" (concave) areas of the sole, as well as the mound-like (convex) surfaces. Explore the soft tissue underneath the skin as you stimulate the tissue into relaxation.

Time permitting, you can also reposition you hands and work on the round surface of the heel if you wish.

B. Apply Rotating Thumb Friction systematically to the entire sole of the foot (Figure 7-48).

Progress up and around the contours of the arches, and into the rounded area just beneath the base of the toes.

This RTF stroke may become the heart of your foot massage with lotion, and it can take anywhere from 30 to 90 seconds per foot, or even longer, time permitting. One word of caution: do not overwork your hands and thumbs to the point of tiring them out. And be sure to *relax your own shoulders* as you work.

Allow an equal amount of time for the other foot.

Helpful Hint: The client's rate of breathing is something you might notice. It is a great indicator of whether the sensation of your foot massage is pleasant or, possibly, slightly painful. Ask the client for feedback on the sensation.

Imagine what it must feel like—to these feet—to receive your foot massage. Then try to give exactly the kind of massage you think they might most enjoy.

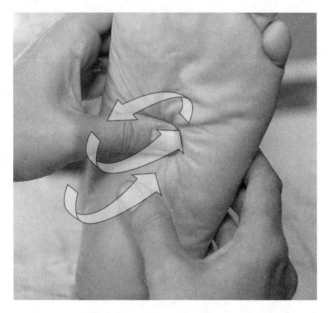

Figure 7-48 With rotating thumbs, thoroughly explore and stimulate the entire sole of the foot.

5. Squeeze and Knead the Foot (once again, as in Step 2)
Position: Stand up again, as before.
Squeeze and knead all of the remaining tension out of the foot, heel to toes.

You won't need any more lotion, since the repetition of this stroke is primarily to create a sense of completion for the client.

6. Repeat Steps 1–5 to the Other Foot

To Give Your Best Massage, Always Remember to . . .

1. Take your time.
2. Stay physically comfortable through every stroke.
3. Put yourself in your client's place.
4. Encourage client feedback, and take it to heart.
5. Get yourself a good massage as often as you can.

GENERAL OUTLINE

The following General outline lists all of the numbered steps and the lettered substeps for the massage routine with lotion. Omitted are all of the detailed instructions and other commentary. Once you have read through all of the detailed steps once or more—and worked through the actual techniques with a practice partner—you may no longer need all of the helpful details. The following General version will save you a lot of time. It is followed by a final Brief outline, which includes the numbered steps only.

BACK MASSAGE

1. Apply Lotion

   A. Place the lotion on the client's upper back.

   B. Now, draw the lotion slowly back and forth, left and right, across the shoulders with your hands.

   C. Draw the lotion down the back with both hands.

2. "Palm Circles" Covering the Back

   A. Begin by placing the hand you are most comfortable using at the top of the client's spine.

   B. Make clockwise circles with your relaxed open palm, progressing down the spine, and into the deep lower back.

   C. Re-position your palm back up near the top of either shoulder.

   D. Repeat this step, now, down the other side of the back.

3. Friction to the Rhomboids

   A. Place both of your hands on the tops of the shoulders as close to the neck as possible.

   B. Apply friction by pulling down, directly across, and over the rhomboids.

   C. Begin the "return" portion of the stroke at about the midpoint of the back, toward the bottom of the rib cage.

   D. Repeat this short stroke 3–4 times.

4. Knead the Shoulders

   A. Rest the heels of your palms on the back side of the client's upper shoulders.

   B. Align your four flattened fingers against the front of the shoulder muscle, positioned so the fingers are opposed the heels of your palms.

    C. Squeeze the muscle mass, then release, alternating, right hand, then left, etc.

    D. Gradually cover the entire upper trapezius area using a slow, steady alternating rhythm.

    E. Begin where the neck joins the shoulders and work out toward the upper bony ridge of the shoulder blades until you run out of muscle mass.

    F. Repeat this sequence to the area a couple of times, remembering to alternate, and keeping a slow, steady pace.

5. Rotating Thumb Friction to Muscles Alongside the Spine

    A. Rest your hands on the client's lower back, and position both of your thumbs on the muscles along one side of the spine.

    B. Start the motion with a small friction stroke, using your right thumb, by moving it forward on the skin.

    C. As the right thumb finishes it's short stroke, lift it up just slightly off the skin, and begin an identical short movement on the skin with the left thumb.

    D. Repeat the movement until the motion of both thumbs becomes rhythmical, cyclical, and continuous.

    E. Guide the whole movement through the muscles, gradually, continually re-positioning your hands (as needed, for support) along the back.

    F. Repeat steps A–E to the muscles up and along the other side of the back.

6. Heels of Both Palms Up the Back

    A. Place the palms of both hands on the sacro-iliac area (the very bottom of the lower back).

    B. Lean some of your upper body weight into the heels of your palms.

    C. Allow your hands to slowly glide, simultaneously, up the long back muscles.

    D. Complete this stroke by kneading the shoulders using the alternating motion.

    E. Repeat the entire stroke at least once.

• OPTIONAL: Petrissage the Neck

    A. Petrissage both sides of the client's neck with your thumbs opposed your fingers.

    B. Apply friction, using your thumbs and fingers underneath the Occipital Ridge at the back of the skull.

• OPTIONAL: Apply Friction to the Scalp

    A. Flex your fingers slightly.

    B. Stimulate the scalp thoroughly.

SHOULDERS

1. Alternating Palm Effleurage Between the Shoulder Blades

    A. Begin at the upper shoulder, next to the spine.

    B. Apply a short, gliding stroke with one palm, down through the rhomboid area.

    C. Follow up with the same stroke, using your other hand.

    D. Repeat continually, allowing a relaxing alternating rhythm to develop between the two gliding palms.

2. Rotating Thumb Friction to the Shoulder Area

    A. Apply Rotating Thumb Friction (RTF) to the Rhomboid and Levator Scapula areas.

    B. Apply RTF to the upper trapezius.

3. Effleurage Around the Shoulder

    A. Begin by resting your hand on the area where the shoulder meets the neck.

    B. Glide your palm out, over the top of the shoulder.

    C. Fingers around the shoulder joint.

    D. Recover up to the neck.

    E. From the original starting position, repeat this stroke at least once or twice.

4. Repeat Steps 1 through 3 to the Other Shoulder

HANDS

1. Squeeze the Palm while Applying Lotion

   A. Apply a small amount of lotion to both of your palms.

   B. Squeeze and knead the client's hand.

2. Rotating Thumbs to the Palm

   A. Apply friction to palm with rotating thumbs.

   B. Cover the entire surface of the palm.

3. Squeeze the Hand Again

4. Repeat Steps 1–3 to the Other Hand

NECK

1. Apply Lotion to the Shoulder and Neck

   A. Place a small amount of lotion in one palm.

   B. Spread the lotion up the client's shoulder and neck.

2. Apply an Alternating Friction with the Finger Pads, Up and Across the Shoulder and Neck

   A. Place the flattened fingers of both hands on the far shoulder.

   B. Apply alternating friction, pulling across the muscle.

   C. Progress up the shoulder, to the very base of the neck.

   D. Apply friction up the side of the neck.

   E. Apply friction beneath the occipital ridge.

3. Repeat Steps 1 and 2, to the Other Shoulder and Side of the Neck

• OPTIONAL: Friction to the Cheeks

   A. If the client's skin seems dry, apply a tiny drop of lotion to the soft surfaces of your flattened fingers.

   B. Place the soft surfaces of your flattened fingers together, resting them on the right and left cheeks.

   C. Apply a light circular friction, simultaneously, to the masseter muscles of both cheeks just beneath the skin.

- OPTIONAL: Friction to the Temples

    A. Place the soft surfaces of your flattened fingers together, resting on the right and left temple areas.

    B. Apply a light circular friction to the surface muscles of both temples, simultaneously, just beneath the scalp.

- OPTIONAL: Effleurage to the Forehead

    A. Place the heels of your palms together on the center of the client's forehead.

    B. Effleurage in one smooth, simultaneous motion off the forehead.

    C. After this stroke, rest and relax for at least 5–10 seconds.

FEET

1. Apply Lotion to the Foot

2. Knead the Foot Thoroughly

    A. Heels of your palms rest on top, finger pads underneath.

    B. Knead, alternately, squeezing with each hand in turn.

3. Apply "Stripping" Friction to the Sole

    A. Form two parallel lines with your fingers underneath the sole of the client's foot.

    B. Strip the tension out of the sole of the foot, heel to toes.

    C. Cover the entire sole of the foot systematically.

4. Apply Rotating Thumbs to the Sole of the Foot

    A. Begin near the heel, and work toward the toes.

    B. Apply Rotating Thumb Friction systematically to the entire sole of the foot.

5. Squeeze and Knead the Foot (once again, as in Step 2)

6. Repeat Steps 1–5 to the Other Foot

With some practice, the flow of this routine's several sequences will become natural and intuitive. Once you have the big picture, and see how all of the details fit into it, the following Brief Outline will be all you need.

BRIEF OUTLINE, "JOB CARD"

This one-page outline is for handy reference. Place it right beside you so you can refer back to it as you work.

THE MASSAGE WITH LOTION

THE BACK

1. Apply Lotion
2. "Palm Circles" Covering the Back
3. Friction to the Rhomboids
4. Knead the Shoulders
5. "Rotating Thumb Friction" to Muscles Alongside the Spine
6. Heels of Both Palms Up the Back
• OPTIONAL: Petrissage the Neck
• OPTIONAL: Apply Friction to the Scalp

THE SHOULDERS

1. Alternating Palm Effleurage Between the Shoulder Blades
2. Rotating Thumb Friction to the Shoulder Area
3. Effleurage Around the Shoulder
4. Repeat Steps 1–3 to the Other Shoulder

THE HANDS

1. Squeeze the Palm While Applying Lotion
2. Rotating Thumbs to the Palm
3. Squeeze the Hand Again
4. Repeat Steps 1–3 to the Other Hand

THE NECK

1. Apply Lotion to the Neck
2. Apply Alternating Friction to the Shoulder and Neck
3. Repeat Steps 1 and 2, to the Other Shoulder and Side of the Neck.
• OPTIONAL: Friction to the Cheeks
• OPTIONAL: Friction to the Temples
• OPTIONAL: Effleurage to the Forehead

THE FEET

1. Apply Lotion to the Foot
2. Knead the Foot Thoroughly
3. Apply "Stripping" Friction to the Sole
4. Apply Rotating Thumbs to the Sole of the Foot
5. Squeeze and Knead the Foot (again, as in Step 2)
6. Repeat Steps 1–5 to the Other Foot

SUMMARY

This concludes the chapter of Massage Techniques with Lotion. If the thought of starting at the beginning of the chapter and working through each stroke in turn seems a little overwhelming, there is another way. Consider skimming over all of the techniques and imagining which among them you would most enjoy receiving. Then, for your earliest practice sessions, learn how to perform only those favorite techniques on your friend. Perform each of those strokes in exactly the way you would want them to feel if your friend were performing them on you. In this simpler approach, by picking and choosing from among your own favorites, your very first forays into massage will be so enjoyable that a desire for learning the rest of the strokes will come naturally. Memorizing the "melodies and scales" of their movements will, indeed, give courage to your imagination and wake up your intuition for giving a great massage.

Your initial learning and early practice are now off to a good start. The following chapter on Practical Considerations covers a number of the things many of us have faced when first learning to practice massage.

PUTTING THESE IDEAS INTO PRACTICE

1. What part of your body do you think would most enjoy receiving a five-minute massage with lotion right now?

2. Which one massage technique from this chapter looks easiest to perform?

3. Write down the page numbers for the three "best" strokes that meet the needs indicated in questions number 1 and 2 (above), and re-read those pages thoroughly.

4. Practice applying those three strokes on your first available friend. Keep this book opened to the General (middle) routine as you walk through the movements for each of those strokes. Read each sub-step aloud, if that is helpful, and then perform it.

5. Ask your friend how each stroke feels, and try to make it feel a little bit better as a result of their suggestions.

CHAPTER 8

Practical Considerations

The happiness of life is made up of minute fractions—the little, soon-forgotten charities of a kiss or smile, a kind look or heartfelt compliment.

—Samuel Taylor Coleridge

OBJECTIVES

1. Demonstrate how to make a quick plan for any client's brief massage.

2. Describe how limitations on time can be positive and constructive.

3. Describe how to use massage to help develop your intuition.

4. List the four aspects of massage as a "practice" from a global perspective.

5. List three characteristics of constructive verbal feedback during massage.

6. Discuss some key advantages for learning massage when working with a personal tutor and organizing a "micro" massage class together with two other nurses.

This chapter covers some of the primary practical considerations that all nurses will deal with throughout their practice of massage. Probably the foremost consideration at this point would be time. That is, "how to fit everything in." We begin with a "1,2,3—Quick Plan," a simple approach for deciding how to choose what body areas to work on, what techniques to apply, and where to begin when you only have a few short minutes to spend with a client. The next most pressing issue will be in accommodating some of the different physical contexts for massage, along with getting relative body positioning figured out well enough so that both you and your client are physically comfortable throughout their massage.

Another more long-term consideration has to do with what form your "practice" of massage will take. Here we offer a more "global" view of practice, illustrating how expanding your perspective on each seemingly separate aspect of practice can enrich the others. In this way, your work with clients can become much more rewarding than simply applying massage technique.

Finally, if you really want to learn more in-depth detail about massage, we suggest two ways to take a decidedly active hand in your learning. First, by working individually with experts and, secondly, learning as a small team with other highly motivated nurses. We begin, then, with making the best use of time, both your own time as well as that of your clients.

TIME: MASSAGE'S BEST FRIEND

Many nurses think they just don't have time for massage. This is a position that is well worth rethinking. For just one moment, then, let's set massage and nursing aside and try to get a very practical and realistic perspective on time, itself. There's really no reason to go any further until we do.

Time is really *all* we have. And since none of us knows for certain how much of it we have remaining, we need to make the most of each moment, each and every day. Time, then, becomes so very valuable, not so much because it is in limited supply, but because it is so de-limiting, to the point that it is liberating, continuously so.

Every day we receive a fresh supply of time, and our main job is how in the world we will ever put it to best use. The greater challenge, then, is not so much a problem of "finding enough" time, because we have little else. Rather it is in sorting through the many wonderful things we can spend our time on and then choosing those that make the most difference according to what we know and believe are the most important and valuable things to do.

This small shift in perspective—from "there's never enough time," to "all time is free time *with choice*"—makes each and every moment of life even more precious and irreplaceable than it already was. Both are equally true if we believe them in our heart, so which will we choose? What if we chose the one that lends us the greater sense of choice and freedom? There is hardly any better way to spend a precious, fleeting moment than by helping another person feel better. For these small but priceless acts of giving, each one of us surely has been given more than an extra moment to spare. That is all massage will ever ask of us, one tiny moment of what we have been given in abundance. Massage takes time, yes, but not that much.

Rather than lamenting over what we are leaving out because of time—out of our client's brief massage, or out of our own lives—it might be more redeeming to accept the hour at hand as a gift and savor everything that we *can* bring to it. If we just don't feel like we have enough time for a two-minute massage right now, we may never feel like we have enough time for anything at all, other than what we have let ourselves grow accustomed to by habit. Because "right now" is, literally, the only time we will ever have. Especially in the midst of "managing busy professional schedules," we can insist on treating each moment as our fleeting gift, and remember that gifts grow with the giving and that we do have much more than a moment to spare. Taking this viewpoint to heart will provide you with time for giving a nice massage. And that is why time is the best friend massage could ever have. It is simply up to us to reintroduce them, to re-acquaint them with each other, again and again. Now that we have some time, at least a moment or two, let's get even more practical about spending it.

Time Enough for Massage

One of the first considerations almost any nurse will have regarding massage is, "How will I ever be able to do all of those massage strokes in just one to five minutes?" The answer is simple, you won't ever have to and you couldn't if you tried. And, anyway, you'll never be expected to do that, unless you want to. The routines you have now begun to practice represent a comprehensive form, a small encyclopedia of skills. When learned as a whole, then used as a reference, your routines will help you feel confident that you have more than enough techniques for giving each of your clients whatever he or she needs. Whatever strokes you do choose to perform, coupled with a little intuition, will always be perfectly suited for your client. And the amount of time you both have available will be "just what the doctor ordered," because it will allow you to accomplish all that can be accomplished for the time being.

Since it is a practical certainty that any amount of massage is better than no massage at all, you will not need to be concerned with leaving out some favorite stroke, or fitting in just one more body area, because you will have included everything you possibly could. Within the focus of your moments with clients, your results will always be far better than if you had given them less massage, or no massage at all.

The key to giving "the perfect massage" is very much like making the most of any other type of quality time: keep things simple, enjoy them for what they are, and make good choices based on the opportunity at hand. All we need, then, is the right perspective and the "know-how" to make a quick plan. Since we have one of the best perspectives possible, which is, "now is a good time for massage," we can make a quick plan in a matter of seconds by answering three simple questions.

The 1-2-3 Quick Plan: Need, Time, First

1. Need: What does this client Need most right now?
2. Time: Realistically, how much Time do we have or want to spend?
3. First: What body area shall we massage First?

The answers to these three simple questions are where your Quick Plan begins and ends. It can be sketched out in a few seconds on a "sticky note," or just drawn out mentally. Ask the client what they think they need, or start where you think they need it. If they have a specific complaint, either address that complaint first, or begin on another body area to help divert their attention momentarily off the primary area of tension or pain. It is almost always a safe bet to start by addressing their area of greatest need.

After you have relaxed into the physical movements of performing that very first massage stroke, you have already established your beginning. Now, think of what one other massage stroke you might want to include. It is always nice to perform at least two strokes, if you can, for variety's sake, even if each of those strokes lasts only 15–30 seconds. Ask yourself, "What stroke or body area would I like to end this massage on?" Then, what you will be left with are any other stroke(s) that might make up the middle of their massage—considering how much time you and your client have, realistically, to spend. This is how to make a Quick Plan, and you can think of every quick plan you make, and each massage you give, as an ongoing experiment in achieving balance within the overlapping framework of time and need. Time and need, then, afford us our creative limits, and those boundaries bring focus to our efforts, making them more effective. Time and need, once again, become our doorway for another opportunity to help.

A two-minute massage can be just as perfectly suited for your client right now as a 10-minute massage might feel at some other time tomorrow or the next day. If you find yourself imagining that you are "leaving so much out," simply remember the client's need along with how much time you have to help them right now. Then address the body area(s) that seem to have the greatest need or want to be massaged the most. The remainder of what to include will occur to you as you listen to the client and the non-verbal information coming to you from their musculature and through your hands. Follow your Quick Plan and stay flexible, and you will end up finishing the perfect massage right on time every time.

The simpler you can make your planning approach the more it will pay off for your clients, not just in the beginning of your practice, but for every massage you give. The following are examples of what you might do within certain time limitations using the Quick Plan approach. This will give you an idea about how a plan might take shape in your practice setting.

A One-Minute Massage

Even one minute—just 60 seconds—if that is all the time you and your client have, can be enough to help them feel much better. In fact, just the first 30 seconds is often more than enough to establish a good personal connection and introduce a physical stimulus into the neuromuscular system that causes that pleasant relaxation response throughout the body. The parasympathetic nervous system (as you may have already noticed from practicing the techniques in the previous chapters with a partner) responds almost instantly to the movement of the hands on and in the muscle tissue.

A one-minute massage, like any other, is aimed primarily toward the client's need, and so it might consist of only one stroke, for example, applied to either the shoulders, neck, or hands. In that case, just that one stroke would have its own beginning, middle, and end: initial contact, induction of a sustained stimulation, and followed by closure. Your goal is simply to induce a feeling of comfort and ease through the medium of that physical stimulation.

You will want to sustain that experience of comfort for a long enough period of time to draw your client's attention fully into an awareness of those physical sensations. This causes the client to shift, mentally, from random thought and perception about their environment into a slightly more subjective awareness. Intentionally stimulating the somatic nervous system brings about a natural parasympathetic response including slower heartbeat and respiration. Sixty seconds of intentionally induced relaxation, in and of itself, can be most worthwhile. If you are still even slightly skeptical, have someone try this on you. Even if you're not skeptical, have someone try it on you anyway, and you will realize that you will always be able to find sixty seconds to spare.

WHERE SHOULD YOU BEGIN?

If you only have a minute to spend with a client, how do you know where to begin? Ask them where they think they might enjoy a couple of minutes of massage. They will almost always offer at least one suggestion, sometimes two. If they suggest four or five areas, ask which of those are the "top two." If they still don't know, just make an educated guess. You can hardly fail to find a body area that wouldn't enjoy 30–60 seconds of massage. Almost any technique you begin with will feel great if you take your time and intentionally relax, yourself, as you work and loosen the soft muscle tissue.

HOW LONG WILL THIS TAKE?

Some clients want to know how long the massage will take. The real question is, How will you know how much time the two of you have, realistically, for a massage? Again, take a guess. What are the reasonable expectations within your immediate environment, or of the people around you? Where are you each going, and when do you each really need to be there? Do you have one minute? Or three? The client's need (pain, soreness, tension, stress, etc.) and the time available for the massage will always be related; pick a modest number of minutes and start. Remember, also, you may be called away, or distracted, even while you are applying the first stroke, so you want to make that very first movement count. Tell your client it will only take "a couple of minutes."

Almost anyone has two minutes, but the difference between planning on a minute versus five minutes, or ten, might be something you should consult with the client about. They may have something pressing on their agenda that you don't know about. Fifteen minutes, for example, might be too long for a client who has never had a massage, or who needs to be somewhere in ten minutes. Three minutes, for them, might sound much better. We can all think up more to do in a day than we will ever be able to accomplish in a month, and many clients just feel hurried sometimes, even though they don't have anywhere urgent to go. Also, many of your clients will not know just how good your massage feels, that is, until you start.

UNDERESTIMATE THE AMOUNT OF TIME AVAILABLE

The main thing about estimating time is to always under-estimate it. For instance, if you think you might have five minutes, count on having four, or three. That way you can leave a little bit at the very end for a moment of conversation, or just letting the client relax a bit before you actually break contact and transition back into your regular activities. In a one-minute massage, this extra time at the end might be as little as 5–10 seconds. That could mean relaxing quietly for a few beats at the end, or having a short verbal exchange before the moment is over. During the slightly longer massage, ten to fifteen minutes in length, for example, you might allow up to 30–60 seconds for that final moment of closure. It is generally better to count on a slightly shorter massage and have a minute or so left over at the end, than to count on the longer time, then let the time slip away on you and have to stop abruptly.

A Two-Minute Massage

If you have two minutes, try picking a couple of body areas, depending on the client's need, and make just those two areas feel absolutely great. A little massage is always much better than none at all and, as mentioned, you can sometimes change a client's whole afternoon with just two minutes. In those opening few seconds, it's not so much about "how much massage you can get in," as it is how much you can both appreciate the sensation and relaxation of that very first stroke. When you feel confident that your first stroke has done its job, just glance at your watch and see how long it took, and about how much time you have remaining. Approaching time with a sense of interest and curiosity helps us to remember to relax as we move, and then decide whether we have time for another stroke or two.

Certainly, you could spend two whole minutes on just one area, such as the back. Two minutes is also enough time to give each foot a whole minute of massage. In one minute, a lot of good can be done for two tired hands! As mentioned above, you might think of the two-minute massage, also, as having its own beginning, middle, and end: making initial contact, inducing a sustained stimulation to the area(s), and completing the (last) area with a sense of closure.

3–5 Minutes

In three minutes you can cover a fair amount of territory, relatively speaking. For instance, spending a whole minute on each of three separate areas, such as the shoulders, hands, and feet (about a half-minute on each hand and foot). This can be made into a very pleasant massage experience. In fact, the 3–5 minute massage might eventually be a good goal to set for yourself and work toward.

While you are spending time on your initial practice and learning, you should allow yourself the luxury of ignoring time altogether and focusing on how satisfying it feels to apply a good technique. Then, after you feel like you have started to master the strokes in one or both routines, try to give as many 3–5 minute massages as possible for as many people as you can. Whether you perform the massage with lotion or without, you can learn to help a client feel better in 3–5 minutes. As a result, your shorter massages will become much easier to give, and the longer ones will be a natural extension and elaboration on your 3–5 minute "gold standard." The organizing principle for all of them, regardless of their length, will be the same Quick Plan: Need, Time, and First—1,2,3.

WATCH THOSE TRANSITIONS

If you spend just 3–5 of your minutes working on several body areas, remember that the time you spend transitioning from one area to the next can mount up quickly, especially if you and the client tend to chat along the way. Thirty seconds spent taking off one shoe and sock, for example, or repositioning the client in the bed, can prove to be significant when three minutes is all the time you have available. At the same time, you should never feel rushed or in a hurry, so don't wait until you have fifteen minutes before giving someone a massage. If the clock is ticking, and the client is moving slowly, remember that whatever massage you manage to give them will still be perfect for that client at that time.

REMEMBER SPONTANEITY

Save some room for a certain amount of spontaneity in your massage. You might discover that your client appreciates just having a couple of minutes to talk with you and, in some cases, maybe about how much he enjoyed having his neck rubbed! On the other hand, his shoulders may need a little more attention than you originally thought, so you spend the whole time on the shoulders instead of finishing with the feet, as you had originally planned. So save a little room for flexibility. You are not "leaving out" the feet if you don't include them; you are including the shoulders, because they turned out, after all, to be the client's primary need.

An Informal Experiment in Intuition

Where is the client's primary area of need, and how can you tell? Try this experiment with a few of your first practice partners. Take a few seconds before you start and make an educated guess about which body area(s) might need to be massaged most. Use your instinctive sense and try to get a feeling for where the most tension, stiffness, or soreness has been stored away in their body. There's no such thing as a "bad guess." Put yourself in their place, take a guess, and be sure to make a mental note.

Then, ask your partner, "What area feels like it could use a massage most right now?" Make a note, also, of their response. Later on, you can compare your initial guess with their first response. You can also compare both of your responses to any other special areas you may have discovered along the way. Over time, your "hunches" are likely to improve because you will gather so much information from guessing, asking, and listening; then finding out "first hand" for yourself where they needed massage. Keep in mind that human bodies already understand each other, and there is a fundamental part of massage that is always instinctive. Developing your intuition is just another way to gather information, and that knowledge can come in handy with clients in the future.

If you are ever called to massage a client who happens to be in a coma, the only thing you will have to go on with respect to what area needs help most and where to begin will be your "best educated guess." Your massage for that client will be based solely on instinct and intuition. By noting and comparing your many experiences across dozens, or even hundreds of clients over time, your "guesswork" becomes much more informed. Make an educated guess on every client— What area could use a good massage the most? Then pay close attention to what you find. The 3–5 minute massage can then become a marvelous classroom for developing your intuition.

Three minutes of massage along the back and spinal muscles with lotion can be very helpful and relaxing. The back is one of those areas where you might be tempted to think it needed much more attention than your three minutes could ever afford. And you may be right. But how many clients would turn down three minutes of massage on their back? Or, how about one long minute or so of concentrated work in the lower back?

If you perform massage on two body areas and still have a minute or so left over, you can always use that minute for address some problem area you might have discovered along the way. You could go back to some particularly sore area in some specific muscle, or maybe addressing some painful area that your client became aware of only after they had finally become more completely relaxed. Also, you could always go back and spend an extra minute on the client's primary area of complaint. When you really slow down and engage the muscles and nerves, one minute of massage on that primary area can be made to feel like a very long time.

A 10-Minute Massage

In a ten-minute massage with lotion, after you have some practice, you should be able to massage the back for 3–4 minutes and still have time for 2–3 minutes on the neck and a minute or so for each foot. This allows plenty of time to help almost any client feel much better. Considering most nursing schedules, a 10-minute massage will probably be viewed as somewhat of a luxury, but you will have occasion to give massage of this length, and longer. The more time you have, of course, the more you can do, but the Quick Plan priorities remain the same.

Sixty to ninety seconds (total) can be enough time, for example, to make both feet feel very, very good. And two or three minutes on the neck is enough for that area to feel like it has been touched thoroughly and loosened up. Of course, double or even triple that amount of time on either one of those areas, when you have that much time to spare, can give you a chance to really explore the area in more detail.

15 Minutes

If you have 15 minutes, try massaging several areas (according to your Quick Plan priorities) for about the first 12 of those minutes. Then spend the last minute or two just sitting quietly with the client. That first 10 minutes is enough to give the back and shoulders a fairly good amount of attention and still have enough time for loosening up the neck, or the hands and feet.

The 15-minute massage is where you really see the importance of one choice that you'll need to make in any massage. You can either cover a smaller number of areas thoroughly, or several more areas somewhat less thoroughly but, still, fairly well. So, that choice is yours to make, but don't dwell too long on the decision-making process. Just start the first area and see where it leads you. As in the earlier 60-second massage, let your client's Need, the Time available and where you Start (1,2,3) help you make those choices from the very beginning and, then, as you move forward.

Sixty seconds of any stroke in either of your routines should be plenty of time for the client to "get the message" of that stroke fully. So in a 15-minute massage you could work on up to 10 body areas for 60 seconds each. Remember that feet, shoulder, and hands, because they are paired, count as two areas each. When you start to think in terms of any one stroke lasting 15, 30, 60, or 90 seconds, there is virtually no end to the number of combinations you can try in a 10–15 minute massage. But arithmetic may be less therapeutic in this case than staying attuned to simple body symmetry and the feeling of need.

Think about time up front in your Quick Plan, then for the most part, forget all about time until you feel you are about halfway through or approaching the end. Regardless of how long a massage takes to perform according to a clock, your human to human connection is what brings the most comfort, relaxation, and relief to each client. That is how you bring such value to even the very first moment.

The Longer Massage

Since most nurses will seldom have a great deal of time for massage in today's typical nursing context, we have focused on the massage lasting anywhere from one to fifteen minutes. Accordingly, most of your massage at work will probably be on the shorter end of that scale, from one to five minutes. But you may have occasion to go a few minutes longer, or even much longer from time to time. If so, you might choose to focus, as mentioned previously, on just a few body areas and work all of the affected soft tissue much more thoroughly. Or you could make a point of performing each step of one of the entire routines presented in this book. Either approach will help your client relax while also helping you become increasingly comfortable with all of the massage strokes as presented. In fact, during your initial period of practice and experimentation we recommend that you do try giving longer massage and apply as many strokes as possible. Perform every stroke, right out of the book, just as described and see how long it takes.

The strokes we have illustrated here, even just those for the back alone (with lotion), might easily take up to 30–60 minutes to perform. If you made an effort to spend time trying to address all of the tension you might find along the way, it could even take longer. But those same strokes will take a lot less time if you perform each one of them just once or twice without stopping to concentrate extensively on any given body area.

The "Rotating Thumb Friction" technique, alone, when applied to the muscles alongside the spine, could take up to 30 minutes, or even longer if you really took your time exploring every square inch of the tissue on both sides. If you ever have that kind of time, and if you determine that this is one of the main areas where your client needs attention most, give it a try. Just be mindful not to place undue stress on your thumbs and wrists, or tire out your back. Let your knees relax too, because standing comfortably always helps your back when you need to stand for a long time.

Keep in mind that professional Massage Therapists typically work for 45- to 90-minutes, or even longer, on practically every client. But in most clinical settings (at this time), especially in the hospital, one minute of massage will be a big help for any client, and five minutes for the client in need can truly be a gift.

Your receiving partner may feel "tired" after having a long massage, but that may be because after having become completely relaxed, the cumulative effects of sleep deficit can finally be felt. A nice nap immediately after a long massage is a very pleasant touch. Their face will appear almost childlike when they awake.

AT HOME WITH A PALLET ON THE FLOOR

If you ever give a massage at home for a friend or family member, you will sooner or later find yourself using a simple pallet on the floor. A pallet consists of several things you probably already have around the house. First, you'll need a couple of blankets folded in half, lengthwise, for cushioning. Then, cover this "base" with a regular sheet and add an additional sheet for your partner or, "client," to use as a cover. You might also need another blanket if the room happens to be even slightly cool down at floor level. Add a small squeeze bottle of lotion and a couple of regular pillows and you're ready for a massage.

Note: Regarding the pallet, we'll assume that you are massaging a personal friend or family member, but we'll still use the word "client" to indicate the person receiving your massage.

The positive side of using the pallet is that it's easy, informal, and a lot of fun. The relaxed setting can be a good experience for both yourself and your client. For many, it brings back pleasant memories of our childhood "camp-outs" and "sleep-overs," evenings spent in sleeping bags either on a friend's floor or out in the backyard. Just because we're big kids now doesn't mean we can't still have a little fun.

The negative side of working on the pallet may be all the getting up and sitting down, and scooting yourself around down at floor level. Using a pallet means you'll need to either kneel or sit on the floor for most of the strokes, which is something you may not be accustomed to. Try using a nice, thick pillow to sit on throughout the entire massage. If you decide to kneel on some of the strokes, place that pillow between your heels/calves and your buttocks. This kind of physical activity might be something entirely new, so it can take a little practice getting used to it. Just make sure you're aware of your knees and don't cause them undue physical stress or strain.

If you are physically capable of the floor work, but just not as limber as you used to be, all of the ups and downs can be a little cumbersome at first because you'll probably need to reposition with almost every stroke. If you haven't been exercising much, you might even be sore the next day. Either way, the floor activity will loosen you up. And if you are in good physical shape, the soreness the next day will remind you of the effects of a good round of exercise.

Even if you're into regular exercise, that activity might take more exertion and repetition than either agility or flexibility. Repositioning continually at floor level can help you become much more comfortable with using your body in new ways. Since so many of us spend too much time sitting in chairs working at a desk, driving in cars, and just relaxing back on the couch, the incidental benefits of performing a massage on the floor might be something a lot of us could benefit from.

If you're not accustomed to it, don't try to pretend that you are; it won't be very convincing to your "client," and you'll probably give yourself away by grunting a lot because you'll need to breathe freely as you move around. Go ahead and breathe, even grunting is ok! For the first few times on a floor, though, make sure your practice partner is someone who appreciates the effort you're making for "science," and who's willing to laugh along with you. Remember, too, that your client won't care a bit if you need to move around, as long as you don't step on them!

Another good reason for practicing on the pallet at least two or three times is because, sooner or later, you will find yourself giving someone a much-needed massage, and the only place available will be down on the floor. And it's always better to have had some rehearsal before having to give a "real" performance.

The Floor is Cooler Than the Room

As mentioned in the chapter on creating the healing environment, room temperature becomes more important than ever when you're receiving a massage. And nothing will help you realize this more than receiving a massage down at floor level. Since hot air rises, cool air sinks, so the floor is always a few degrees cooler. And everyone likes to be warm enough when they receive massage. Seventy-eight to eighty degrees is usually comfortable, and even warmer won't be unpleasant for your client. If the room is 80° at "thermostat level," it may feel "hot" to you while you're doing all the physical work of giving the massage. But you can be sure it won't feel overly warm at floor level, in fact, it might still feel slightly cool. Therefore, the room needs to be warm enough so that, if you were lying down on the pallet with lotion covering your back, you would still feel warm and comfy. Your lotion, even if you warm it up, will cool off very quickly as you spread it on the skin, and so it will draw off some of the body's heat, too. So, in short, make it—the lotion and the room—a little warmer than usual.

A nice massage on the floor, in front of the fireplace—maybe with candlelight and some relaxing music—can be one of life's most exquisite pleasures; an experience you might not want to miss. If the idea appeals to you and, after

---

Assemble Your At-Home "Massage Kit"

A massage kit is made up of several common things you probably already have. If possible, before you ever give your first massage on the floor, gather up all the things you'll need and store them in a closet rolled up in a bundle

1. BLANKETS: Two *soft*, thick blankets, one to fold double for the base of the pallet and another for your client to cover with (or to use as extra padding for the base).

2. SHEETS: Two sheets, one to lie on, and one for covering.
Cotton sheets are nice, but any material you like is fine. Flannel sheets can feel especially nice in the winter.

3. PILLOWS: A couple of regular pillows, with pillow cases that can survive having a little lotion on them.

4. LOTION AND BOTTLE: One small plastic bottle about 2/3 full of your favorite massage lotion. Those little fold-down plastic spout tops are ideal. Also, you might have a spare bottle of lotion handy, just in case you ever need it.

• BUNDLE AND TIE: Wrap up all these items neatly inside one of the blankets. Tie everything together with a long piece of thin rope or heavy cord, and store the whole thing in one corner of a closet.

• OPTIONAL—FOAM PAD: a narrow foam pad provides some extra cushioning for the floor. You can buy one (or two) pads at almost any discount store.

Now you'll have your own handy "Massage Kit" whenever you feel like giving (or receiving) a massage at home with a pallet on the floor.

giving it a try, you do enjoy the experience, we make the following recommenda-tion. Don't pass up the chance for a massage just because you forgot to plan ahead. The best way to be prepared for a good massage is by putting together your very own Massage Kit.

THE PRACTICE OF MASSAGE: A GLOBAL VIEW

The practice of massage includes much more than just "giving massage." Many of us have heard of, or have known, someone who "maintains a massage practice." We think of a "massage practice" as someone scheduling regular appointments and applying massage technique for the benefit of their "clientele." With respect to the purely vocational or professional aspect of practice, this image is fairly accurate. However, if you are not interested in considering a career change right now, but you are interested in massage from the perspective of integrating it into your nursing practice, entertaining a slightly different viewpoint of practice might be helpful.

Like the practice of meditation, martial arts, or prayer, allowing massage to become a regular part of your life can turn out to be a much richer experience for you than just taking on another nursing specialty. It might, eventually, emerge as a new aspect of your vocation or turn out to be just a very pleasant lifelong hobby. But you will find that regardless of whether it takes on a vocational role or stays a leisure-time activity, massage is an excellent practice for continual self-develop-ment. In short, like music, martial arts, or gourmet Zen cooking, approaching massage as a practice for developing awareness can truly enrich your life.

A greater appreciation of the depth and value of massage can be gained with no extra labor by viewing its practice in terms of *learning* about it and *giving* it paired equally with *teaching*, or sharing it with others and making sure you *receive* enough massage, yourself. At first glance, giving, teaching, receiving, and learning massage might sound like a big job, a much greater commitment of time than you originally bargained for. But this larger, more global, perspective is primarily just that—a greatly expanded point of view. And the sum is much greater than its parts combined.

There is a good chance that your life will change—or, perhaps more accu-rately, your life will start to change you for the better—as a result of learning and practicing massage. One of the best ways to get an idea about how potentially enriching the practice of massage can be is by considering it from the view of what you are already starting to do with it, right now. Let's start with learning and then look at how our four major facets of massage practice are intimately tied together and consider what that could mean for you.

Learning Massage

First of all, every time you give a client a massage, you will learn more about massage. It would be practically impossible not to learn more about the human body, physical performance, and even some interpersonal psychology. You will learn specifics, too, such as what a particularly painful muscle can feel like to the touch, or how much pressure is "too much," for either a general type of body or during the early recovery stage after some specific injury. Learning is "built in" to every massage you perform, and you won't have to try very hard to learn a great deal, even if you never take a formal massage class.

Over time, depending on your approach to practice, you may gain insights into subtleties of human behavior, such as how long-held attitudes can, over time, help reshape our habits of posture (both physical and emotional) and the liveliness we bring to our carriage. These same attitudes and habits can then begin to reflect themselves in the consistency of muscle tissue as you ply your way through them and encourage them to loosen and relax in response to your touch. Long-held muscle tension releases itself sometimes in the form of life stories recollected and traumatic events that we have been holding onto, adhering themselves to our bodies and psyches for years, even decades.

We could tell you some about what happens when you give massage every day for five years, or ten, and we could speculate on the meaning of that experience—and you could read about it in a book. But wouldn't you much rather learn about it from a client's muscles telling your hands how it all works, what it means, and how it all fits together? What if a hundred muscles told you almost exactly the same thing about some emotional attitude and its relationship to the general resiliency of soft tissue? For example, what do "generous" people feel like? How about people who seem "driven?" If you have an inclination to learn, performing massage will provide you with more than the equivalent of thousands of hours and hundreds of volumes of somebody else attempting to connect all those dots for you.

Thus your giving of massage will continuously improve as a result of the kind of deeper learning it naturally brings about. How, then, could we ever actually separate the two, giving and learning, except arbitrarily? Sooner or later, the sum of all your learning will become more than you can manage to keep to yourself, and you will feel impelled to share it with others.

Teaching Massage

There may be clients, and other nurses, who want to know why you performed certain strokes and not others, or how you performed them exactly the way you did. "How did you learn to find those sore spots?" they will ask. Among the more curious people, someone will inevitably ask you how they, too, could learn some massage. The more we learn, the more we see there is to learn, and this old axiom is especially true for massage. And one of the best ways to learn something is by teaching it.

Massage, then, is a good "practice" for making new friends from a position of humility and helping. Because, as you can see, our friends have a lifetime of knowledge that we don't have, and a curiosity and wisdom all their own. They are asking us to help show them something we could never know all about. In fact, we can never learn all of anything. Yet we have been asked to share. But we should share it, even if we think we know very little. Teaching is learning, too.

The more you explain and demonstrate any part of your massage—even the two simplest strokes—the better you'll understand all the rest of them, yourself. And the better you understand your massage, the better your performance of it will become. So teaching comes directly out of giving because they reinforce and improve each other directly and, in essence, they are really one in the same. Teaching is sharing what you know with someone who wants to learn. But it is a certain fact that some of the most instructive experiences you will ever have in massage will be while you are playing the role of its recipient.

Receiving Massage

One of the very best ways to learn the innermost secrets of massage, and any other mode of therapeutic touching, is through receiving it. Therefore, we should each make a point of receiving massage, ourselves, as often as we can. Many nurses, as well as massage therapists, give dozens and dozens of massages for each one massage they receive. You will need to find a balance in this giving-and-receiving equation that works best for you. But if you must err in achieving that balance, please do it on the side of receiving more than your share of massage (if there could possibly be such a thing) rather than too little of it.

Feeling what each stroke is intended to feel like, by putting ourselves on the receiving end of it, builds a "cognitive model" of that stroke inside our "muscle memory." Your neurons will record and be able to recall that peculiar subjective sensation. Through allowing ourselves to receive massage, we assemble, inside ourselves, the most complete picture possible of its deeper, lasting effect. And this is what we're aiming for, with respect to improving our client's subjective experience: to know massage, and feel it, from the inside out. This is how we convey its healing through the motion of our touch.

Even when the person giving us our massage has had little or no training, or maybe they are just learning, we can still feel the potential in each stroke they perform. Sometimes we feel it because it is not yet fully realized, but by sensing its absence we realize its potential presence through our subjective experience. Every motion of their hand, when it is motivated by an intention to help release our inner resistance, will become a part of our own process of thinking, feeling, and unfolding as a human being. Not only will we enjoy the pleasant sensation and its attendant physiological benefits, unique insights will occur to us regarding the healing nature of touch according to our willingness to see. By receiving massage, we'll be able to imagine—viscerally—what that very same stroke might feel like if it were performed just a little more slowly, or with just a little bit more pressure, on the soft pliable muscle tissue of our next new client. Receiving massage, then, is learning. And simply by receiving our massage in our own personal way, we offer the opportunity for insights, likewise, to the friend giving us our massage. The better we are at receiving, the more clearly our friends will learn what it is like to receive their own massage through our responses to it. In becoming better at receiving, then, we teach effortlessly, without even trying.

In receiving, we'll also see first-hand why it is so important to be relaxed as we perform our massage. We will sense in our own body the overall feeling state of our good friend as they apply their best slow strokes on us. How could we ever hope to learn such practical lessons about giving by any means other than putting ourselves—literally—"in the place of the client"? Receiving is learning, especially when we are of a mind to learn.

Receiving is an integral part of giving, because the best receivers of massage are usually those who seem to know how to open us up so we, ourselves, can receive the most from their massage. People who truly love massage, and know how to bring the most benefit to us through their giving of it, almost always have the knack for getting the most from it when it comes their turn to receive. Therefore, if we want to learn through giving, those nurses and friends who know how to give a good massage will probably become some of the most appreciative receivers we'll ever have. "Givers" make some of the best practice partners, too, once we take time to share with them some hint of what they might be able to expect.

As you become better and better at receiving, when it does come time to perform massage for your own clients, you'll be able to apply all that you've learned from having received those and similar strokes, yourself. It won't matter whether or not you can remember "all of the strokes" you have learned, because your body will have learned what it needs to do. Through receiving, we have learned to teach touch from the inside out. And if a client, or colleague (or student) ever happens to show an interest in learning massage, it may be that through your hands will be the very best way to share with them what you, yourself, have really learned.

Giving Massage

Giving massage is allowing oneself to play a very special role in the life of another. It is offering ourselves to become an instrument of our client's self-appreciation. Giving is offering one's time and breath in service to another's desire to become more whole again. The more we give through ourselves, the more we open ourselves up as a doorway, or portal, of more life and its giving. In giving, we receive so much. Through giving wholeheartedly, we learn that this is a central part of what we have come here to do. Massage is a gift for teaching us all of these things, in vibrant, living color. And the best way we can learn to teach the joy of giving is through modeling it: *letting ourselves be seen learning how to receive.*

In summary, the practice of massage is like the practice of gardening. There is much, much more to gardening than just planting seeds. Yet, as the garden bears fruit only after the seeds have been planted, this instinctual urge to give—to extend oneself, to touch, and to share our life with others—is where this deeper practice of massage almost always begins. Being able to appreciate and tap into all the information flowing back and forth among the many aspects of every massage experience—giving, receiving, learning, and teaching—is what we mean by entertaining a more global view of its practice.

GIVING AND RECEIVING QUALITY FEEDBACK

Simply by trading with partners—without benefit of any additional learning support, such as books, or workshops, etc.—it is conceivable that you could learn to give a very good massage. However, since there are so many excellent books, videos, and classroom workshops available, making the most of someone else's years of expertise distilled down into a well-crafted learning format is bound to be helpful. Nevertheless, trading massage will become a valuable part of your learning, and all of the input you receive from your partners and clients will be extremely helpful.

It is practically impossible to receive your own massage, especially a back massage, so a partner is essential for practice. Working with several partners is even better, because the character of the massage you'll experience from each of them will vary, as will your opportunities for working on different body types. But most of all, practicing with partners will bring you some of your most valuable lessons through what kind of feedback they can give you. And one of the best ways of fully developing your style and technique is by learning how to elicit, receive—and how to give—good, constructive, verbal feedback. In fact, aside from receiving massage, receiving detailed verbal feedback in the form of intentionally helpful critique might be the most important source available for learning more about, and improving, all the massage you give.

Some Suggested Criteria for a "Good" Massage

Each of us can choose our own criteria for what makes a "good" massage "great." But we would suggest considering the following standards when deciding on your own criteria for a "good" massage:

- Creates a pleasurable physical sensation for the client

- Conveys an ease of rhythm and a comfortable rate of movement through each stroke

- Proceeds at a steady, unhurried pace from one stroke to the next

- Works an area thoroughly and gives a sense of completion

- Has a relaxing effect, especially in the case of massage for nursing

- The client perceives the nurse's personal presence as positive and helpful

- The client feels cared for both during and after the massage

You may think of even more defining characteristics of a good massage or, perhaps, even fewer. But regardless of your criteria, the relative success of a massage might be based on how well these, or other characteristic traits, were met on an ascending scale from "Poor" to "Excellent." We might critique our own massage for improvement, of course, but the client's viewpoint is what we should be concerned with most.

Good Feedback is Voluntary

Most of your professional clients will not want to give you much, if any, detailed verbal feedback. First of all, they probably won't know exactly what "detailed feedback" is regarding massage. Secondly, they probably agreed to receive a massage expecting to relax, not talk. Feedback should never seen be like chore, it should come forth because the receiver feels motivated to offer it. It is a special skill when you consider what it entails.

Giving detailed feedback during a massage means intentionally staying in a "left-brained" state of mind. You need to be awake, mentally active, analytical, and verbal, all at the same time while receiving a massage. That's not easy for everybody, and it could become a little tedious (and distracting) if your client or partner isn't accustomed to it, or simply doesn't care to give it a try. Put yourself in their place. If they're not talking, they either don't know that you want them to, don't know what to say, or they need to relax more than you need the feedback. So you can just give them a great massage and accept their silence as a compliment.

Always be on the lookout for partners who can give you at least 10–15 minutes of great verbal feedback before they become quiet and fall off to sleep. Occasionally, a partner might stick with you throughout their whole massage. If so, let them know how much you appreciate it. So return the favor—if they ask—when you receive a massage from them. If you do this several times you will both help refine each other's massage to such a degree that very little feedback (from either of you) will be necessary. Then you can just listen to the rhythm of their breathing, which provides some of the most vivid positive feedback of all.

Some Topics for Detailed Feedback

If both you and your receiver are committed to learning massage, and you both want to improve your work as effectively as possible, try to offer each other feedback on some of the following:

- The most comfortable amount of pressure. Too light? Too deep? Or just right?

- Relative degree of soreness in an area.

- Particularly "good" spots: parts of a body area that are sore to the touch but the soreness feels good and beneficial. "That hurts good."

- Particularly "bad" spots: areas that are very sore to the touch and could use a few extra seconds of attention. These may *almost* "hurt bad," but, as the receiver, you feel like it needs it, so you breathe through it and let them keep going. "Go easy right there."

- Speed of technique: For example, the rate of motion for the Rotating Thumb Friction. Or how fast/slow an effleurage stroke should feel in order to be most effective as it glides up the back.

- Rate of movement: "Pacing" from one technique to the next, or from one area of the body to another.

- "Too Much": Note how the tissue felt just before the receiver said it was too much. Practice breaking contact immediately when your partner says, "those Magic Words," and then proceed more lightly.

Examples of Detailed Feedback

Some of the most helpful and effective feedback might go something like this:

- "That spot you just passed over—go back there—that feels especially sore."
- "Go to the right an inch . . . Yeah, right there . . . Ooh, that's really tender!"
- "The place where you started that stroke was kind of sore, but then the next couple of inches felt kind of numb. It was almost like I couldn't even feel the sensation of your hands as much. Then, just above it, it started to be sore again."

Clear, detailed feedback will improve your massage and deepen your own appreciation for every massage you receive. But in order to participate in that rich conversation you will need to find others from among your friends and colleagues whose interest in that kind of dialogue is as keen as your own.

LEARNING MORE WITH A PERSONAL TUTOR

There will always be so much more to learn about massage, and there are any number of good ways to learn about it. In addition to the many excellent books, instructional videotapes, and workshops now available, one of the most effective learning experiences available might be in finding and hiring your own personal tutor. A tutor is a massage teacher who provides instruction for individual students, or who is willing to work with very small groups by special arrangement.

One of the greatest advantages of a tutor is that, unlike in a classroom, you will have your teacher's full attention and guidance through each step of the instruction. His or her only objective will be to explain and demonstrate massage technique, then monitor your personal performance on each stroke. This helps to make you almost certain that you can perform each technique comfortably and effectively. Also, establishing a personal relationship like this with a private teacher signifies—both to your teacher and to yourself—that you are ready and willing to learn a great deal more about massage.

Motivated teachers can help kindle a student's natural enthusiasm, but the reverse is true as well. Your active interest and receptivity to hearing and understanding everything your instructor demonstrates and explains can become like a dynamo, bringing out the best of everything your teacher has to offer. Quality instructors and motivated learners help draw out the very best in each other.

One seeming disadvantage of tutoring, for some students, might be in receiving almost a little too much personal attention during practice. Occasionally a student might even feel a little uncomfortable having their instructor watching so closely over their shoulder. But because your tutor's close attention is wholeheartedly supportive it will only help improve your massage.

Three Students and One Teacher

Another innovative way to learn massage—that is, if you have two friends with equally high levels of interest and intention—is in what we call a "Micro-Class." In other words, hiring a tutor/instructor to teach just you and two other nurses. This requires a certain level of intention and dedication because, first of all, you and your two colleagues will need to take initiative in order to make it happen. Secondly, interest level and commitment are essential because you'll need to be able to count on each other to make every meeting and practice between every session if at all possible.

Patience is also a factor, because one partner will, at times, only watch and learn. That partner will observe a round of demonstration and practice in detail while you perform a short series of massage techniques on the third. Learning to observe closely—without actively doing—is one of the best ways to enhance learning any new manual skill, especially massage. You need to allow yourself to relax and observe. As baseball legend Yogi Berra once said, "You can observe a lot just by watching." Your observation in this case will be deliberate and intentional, it's purpose being to improve your immediate upcoming performance. Here is how it works.

ROUND ROBIN

Very briefly, the three students practice in "Round Robin" style. First, the instructor demonstrates anywhere from two to four new massage techniques on one of the students. To illustrate, let's suppose you are the first student to perform the new strokes on one of your partners. Your third partner watches the instructor's demonstration, then watches your hands as you move through performing the short series of strokes for the first time. Your instructor guides you through the nuances along the way. You also receive verbal feedback from your partner as they are lying on the table receiving your massage. The third, or observing partner can, of course, ask questions or offer suggestions any time along the way but, for the most part, it's their turn to watch, and allow the visual and verbal elements to all soak in. The urge to do is re-directed into a heightened perception, like carefully watching a demonstration on a big-screen TV, but this time the action is live and in-person.

After you have completed your turn performing the short series of strokes, the three of you will rotate places. For example, since you have just completed performing the strokes, you might take your turn lying on the massage table and receive those same strokes from the partner who just observed. The student who just finished receiving the massage becomes the observer. Each of your experiences of the second massage will be unique, having just experienced those same strokes from a slightly different point of view.

Finally, after you have received your partner's massage, the three of you will rotate, changing places once again, and work through the same techniques a third time. Now, you are the observer, and the first partner, who originally received the massage from you, then watched, has a turn to perform those, now, very familiar strokes. When this third and last round is complete, and after a short break, your instructor demonstrates another three or four techniques and the process begins anew.

"Do one, receive one, and watch one" may be one of the very best ways to learn massage, one small handful of massage strokes at a time. Then follows a very rich "de-briefing" conversation between the three of you and your instructor, another unique benefit of this "micro-class" format.

The only time any one of the three students actually needs to spend a whole set strictly observing is when the group is learning strokes for a part of the body that is singular, such as the (one) back or the (one) neck. During those "singular" segments, one student needs to observe while the other performs on the third. On the hands, however, two students can work on the third partner at the same time, that is, with one student on each of the two hands. The same would be the case for the legs, or the feet, etc. While learning techniques for these "dual" areas, each of the three students will get ample opportunity to practice while, at the same time, being able to observe the exact procedure while it is being performed by another student. The experience is like a "mirror-image" effect, again, like watching yourself practice on big-screen TV but with real sensation and rich feedback, both verbal and tactile.

Needless to say, during your role as the receiver, having two students perform the same strokes on you simultaneously can be very relaxing. Try as you might, you may not be able to mentally keep up with all four of those hands and what they are doing. So it's not uncommon for the receiver to doze off after a few minutes of this "dual massage." When the receiving partner does finally get up off the table—and it's now her turn to participate—she may be so relaxed that following along by observing the techniques is about all she can manage to do. For other students, the best thing might be to move right into performing the next physical activity in order to help them stay awake. You will sleep well at night after each session like this.

RICHER ENVIRONMENT, RICHER RESULTS

A great deal of material can be learned quickly when three students team up with one instructor. For example, suppose (conservatively) that each learning session covers only six to eight new strokes. Then, in just four to six sessions, each of three nurses would be able to learn somewhere between 24 and 48 massage strokes! More importantly than learning how to perform "x" number of strokes, all would know exactly what each of those movements were intended to feel like from having felt and heard them described several times apiece. In addition, each partner would have taken part in a rich, ongoing conversation of verbal feedback between and among the other two nurses and their instructor as well. Perhaps most importantly, each of the three partners would now know someone personally whom they could rely on to give (and receive) a very good massage, and they could also count on to receive excellent quality feedback for furthering their own massage practice in the future.

Instructors generally tend to use their own short, descriptive phrases when describing and directing the hand movements for each technique. These phrases can become shortened in a class into phrases with rhythm, which become like the words to a rhyme or song. With all the repetition, those phrases become easy to recall as you start to give massage to your clients. The physical sensations of having received, observed, and performed each of one of those movements several dozen times—along with those key phrases—will, in effect, become imprinted on each student's muscle memory as well as in their thinking. Overall, after having participated with two other nurses in four to six tutoring sessions like the one described above, each of you will have a considerable amount of in-depth training and a good, solid foundation for providing simple and very effective massage for all of your clients.

The social bonds formed between yourself and your two friends will support your own commitment to massage, and motivate you to continue your practice. After completing the initial series of sessions, getting all three of you back together from time to time for an evening of practice will be beneficial for, even if nothing more than, the personal rewards of friendship and fun. For these reasons and others, we believe this three-student approach to learning massage with a tutor/instructor may have the greatest number of advantages, and the least number of disadvantages, of all the different avenues for learning massage. Certainly, when compared to books, videos, and workshops—all of which can be outstanding and extremely rewarding—this is the most people-intensive, conversation-rich approach of all. Learning with friends will enable you to experience, first hand, the many aspects of "global practice" taking place all at the same time.

Three Rules of Thumb

- General, Specific, and General Again

   General strokes help us get acquainted with a body area, and also help the area become acquainted with the sensations of receiving the massage. Specific strokes explore and loosen the area, showing us where the greatest needs may be, such as tension and soreness. Closing with another general stroke gives the body area a sense of completion and finality, so it feels much better about our having to move on.

- "Too Much"

   Reminding our client is, also, reminding ourselves that every massage we perform should feel good. So if some particular stroke "hurts good," we encourage the client to breathe into the physical sensation of soreness and let that sensation "fall right out" with the exhalation. What you want every client to come away with is the clear, simple insight that, "Massage feels good, and I feel better." Some practitioners sincerely believe that a massage isn't really helping a client unless it hurts a little. But for our nursing clients, we wouldn't want to cause any more pain in their lives if we can possibly help it. The client's massage should feel very good—from the client's point of view.

- A Graceful Close

   Some clients drop off into a very deep sleep near the end of even a short three-minute massage. It's as if they were just waiting for permission to let go. Toward the end of another client's massage, they may open their eyes with a story to tell. A number of clients will "come back" as if nothing out of the ordinary has taken place at all. And for those occasional clients who never fully relax or, perhaps, even talk throughout their entire massage, a friendly, matter-of-fact finish on your part is perfectly fine and appropriate. In offering our massage, we honor our client's expectations and the way they see their world. That includes whatever they might reasonably expect from the closing moment of their massage experience.

   Occasionally a client will be surprised, even amazed, at how wonderful they feel. It is up to us to hold open the possibility, then, for that one extended moment of *deeper rest* at the very end of the massage. This is our way of honoring that client's potential for being delighted and surprised—even speechless. For that reason, it can be a nice courtesy to just "sit and be with" your client, just for a moment or so, if possible, when their massage is over.

SUMMARY

From the perspective of the "global" view of *Practice*, your own personal practice of massage has now begun. You have already learned and considered a great deal about massage. The giving of massage, if it hasn't already started, can't be far behind. Whatever your experience so far, either in nursing or with massage, you are now much more fully engaged in the process of your practice of *Service* in the same global sense. Now you can plant the seeds of teaching by showing one person—someone you already know—that one simple massage stroke, the one you like most. Then, ask him or her how it feels. The answer will be your feedback and, as you have probably noticed, feedback from clients is the cohesive element that activates the several aspects of "practice" and infuses their interaction. Feedback is the essence of every learning process, and learning to teach effectively through the simple act of giving and receiving will become the path to your success in the practice of massage.

Success in healing is less about the quantity of the help we bring—or what personal outcomes we, ourselves, should expect or derive from our helping. Success is in the quality of feeling we are willing to generate into the world around us out of own impulse to share of ourselves. This chapter, then, has attempted to bring to light some of the most practical things we could consider with respect to massage. Now we can begin to embrace a deeper understanding of what it means to practice the massage *with heart*.

PUTTING THESE IDEAS INTO PRACTICE

1. Imagine you are about to massage your "Friendliest Client of the Day." Sketch out your "1-2-3 Quick Plan" for that massage on a sticky note. Remember: the client's need, plus the amount of time available, indicates what body area and stroke to begin with first.

2. Give what you think is a "short" massage to your closest friend and see how long it actually takes.

3. With a pencil and piece of paper, write out the following headings down the left side, 1 minute, 2–3 minutes, 3–5 minutes, 10 minutes, 15 minutes. Be sure to leave a couple of lines between them. Now write down what body areas you would like to have included for each length of time if a friend were to perform their massage techniques right now *on you*. For example, if a friend were to spend the next 3–5 minutes massaging you right now, which body areas would you most like having massaged in that amount of time? Do the same exercise for the remaining time categories. Remember to follow the Quick Plan strategy.

4. List two friends or colleagues who might like to form a "micro"-massage class with you. Sketch out a Quick Plan for each of them on separate sticky notes. Then give them each a three to five minute dry massage.

5. Write down the names of three people, or the names of three businesses, that you could call to find the name of your first potential tutor. Call and ask this person how much they charge for a 60-minute massage.

Massage as a Bridge
for Connecting

INTRODUCTION TO PART III

In this section we introduce HeartTouch, an *internal maneuver* that helps us give a massage that is more than technique—a massage with heart. To do this, we must first explore the power of what we think and feel. On the one hand, this internal maneuver takes a minute or less and is very easy to do. It is intentionally choosing and focusing on a thought. On the other hand, it may take a lifetime to be able to intentionally choose our thoughts and focus our awareness, no matter what the situation.

In step one of HeartTouch, we use our thoughts and feelings to create an inner connection with our own heart energy. Providing foundational material for this step, Chapter 9 helps us realize the effects that different thoughts and feelings have on the body. Chapter 10 suggests techniques for intentionally choosing what we think and feel, especially in stressful situations. Both of these chapters are helpful because it is not always easy to adopt new habits of thought. A variety of techniques and an understanding of the myriad benefits of conscious thinking encourage us to try.

In steps two and three of HeartTouch, we use our thoughts and feelings to connect with others, creating a pathway for healing. To address the question of how this might occur, Chapter 11 discusses energy, energy fields, and energy-based healing. As we explore energy-based healing, we find that we must consider spirituality in the massage/healing experience if we are to provide a thorough foundation for practicing HeartTouch.

With this underlying knowledge base, in Chapter 12 we discuss the steps of HeartTouch in detail, with supporting research, and in the final chapter we use it to give a *massage with heart*. HeartTouch is a technique that can be used not only as you give a massage, but in many situations in your professional and personal life when a return to the heart makes a difference.

Psychoneuroimmunology, the Bodymind Connection, and Massage

We are what we think.
All that we are arises with our thoughts.
With our thoughts, we make the world.

—Buddha (563–483 B.C.)

OBJECTIVES

1. List the players in the psychoneuroimmunology network, describe how they communicate with each other, and discuss the role our thoughts and feelings play in the network.

2. List three specific thoughts/feelings and describe their effects on the health of the bodymind.

3. Explain the difference between a stressor and stress, and list two internal and two external potential stressors.

4. Explain how prolonged perceived stress can lead to chronic disease.

5. Discuss ways in which massage affects our thoughts and feelings, and our thoughts and feelings affect the massage we give.

Can you remember a time when you were feeling depressed about something going on in your life? You may have noticed a headache or a knot in your stomach. All of a sudden, a friend calls, and you talk about your situation. You receive kind words and suggestions. You get off the phone, your head feels better, and the knot is gone. There is a smile on your face, and your world looks very different. Nothing physical in your world has changed. You still have the same amount of money, your job is the same, your family has not changed.

What happened? This is the power of your thoughts and feelings to affect your body.

·

Can you remember a time when you didn't get enough sleep for several days in a row? Have you ever experienced pain for a few days, maybe a sore muscle? You may have found yourself feeling angry or irritated with almost anyone who came near you.

What happened? This is the power of your body to affect your thoughts and feelings.

These scenarios illustrate the connection between the body and mind, and psychoneuroimmunology (PNI) is the science that studies this connection. PNI looks at how specific thoughts and feelings (TF) affect the chemistry of the body, and how what is going on in the body affects what we think and feel. Do our TF impact our health? Can we consciously choose TF? What role do our TF have in the stress we experience in our lives? If we experience stress every day, does it cause illness? These are questions that research in PNI is finding answers for, and questions we will address in this chapter.

Why is PNI included in a massage book? Thoughts, feelings, and the giving and receiving of massage are intricately interwoven. When we give or receive a massage, our TF change. When we more fully understand how TF change physiology, we gain a deeper appreciation of the benefts of receiving, and giving, massage. Secondly, stress greatly affects the healing process of our clients, and our own lives at work and home. Understanding the power of our TF gives us a full picture of what stress is, how we can change our experience of it, and how massage helps to relieve it. And finally, your TF while giving a massage affect the one you are massaging. What you think and feel determines whether your body and mind are relaxed or stressed, which has a dramatic effect on the way you perform the actual massage techniques. And choosing your TF is necessary to practice HeartTouch (Chapter 12) which helps you bring heart and meaningful connection to massage and other interactions as well.

Becoming aware of and choosing your thoughts is one of the most difficult challenges you will ever undertake. It is necessary, however, if you want to live a life of happiness and health. We are all more likely to undertake difficult challenges if we fully understand why they are important. This chapter discusses the *why*. We discuss the communication network within your body, ways in which different TF affect different areas of the body for health and illness, and how TF affect stress. Chapter 10 offers some techniques for the *how*, how to recognize and change unwanted TF.

Throughout this chapter you will notice that we talk about thoughts and feelings individually because they are different. Thoughts observe, analyze, and consider, and usually precede, and instigate, feelings. Feelings carry e-motion, the movement of energy. This energy has the power to create changes in the bodymind and create communication between individuals. To change our feelings, we usually must become aware of the thoughts that caused them.

People from all walks of life including nurses, doctors, physicists, neuroscientists, and religious leaders are realizing that the body, mind, and spirit are not separate. Harvard Medical School sponsors five workshops on different aspects of mind/body medicine and a conference on Spirituality and Healing in Medicine. The research in PNI has shown us that we are not a body and a mind, but more a bodymind, and really, a Spiritmindbody. We are entering an era of fundamental change in healthcare. Understanding the power of our TF to affect the mind and body is on the leading edge.

It is, and always has been, the very nature of nurses to address the whole person. Nurses have the opportunity to be leaders in this new exploration of what creates health, and who we are as individuals.

PSYCHONEUROIMMUNOLOGY: THE BODYMIND CONNECTION

The greatest discovery of my generation is that human beings, by changing the inner attitudes of their minds, can change the outer aspects of their lives.

—William James (1842–1910)

Nightingale in her *Notes on Nursing*, first published in 1860, discusses the healing relationship between the body and mind. She says,

In the hospital it is the relief from all anxiety which has often such a beneficial effect upon the patient. A patient can just as much move his leg when it is fractured as change his thoughts when no external help from variety is given him. It is an ever recurring wonder to see educated people, who call themselves nurses varying their own objects many times a day, and while nursing some bedridden sufferer, they let him lie there staring at a dead wall, without any change of object to enable him to vary his thoughts . . . I think it is a very common error among the well to think that "with a little more self-control the sick might, if they choose, "dismiss painful thoughts" which "aggravate their disease."

Nightingale knew that the TF of the clients played a large role in their health, and she realized how difficult it sometimes is to change TF. She believed that people need help to change their thoughts, especially if they are sick. It was a nurse's responsibility to keenly observe the patient, notice if he was anxious or depressed, and help him vary his thoughts.

As early as 1926, Walter Cannon discussed the fight and flight response where the adrenal glands of the endocrine system were stimulated in response to feelings of fear or threat. So we knew that feelings could affect the endocrine system. In the 1970s, two startling discoveries were made. In 1973, Candace Pert and Soloman Snyder discovered endorphins, chemicals secreted by the body that create feelings of euphoria (Pert, Pasternak, and Snyder, 1973). It was the first realization that the chemistry of the body affects our TF. In 1975, Robert Ader and Nicholas Cohen (1981) found that the brain communicates with the immune system. Previously, science believed that the immune system functioned independently, protecting our body from invading organisms and disease, not influenced by anything else. In 1976, Pellitier and Peper demonstrated that meditators could control pain, bleeding, and infection from wounds. These were the early beginnings of PNI. It took quite a while for the scientific community to believe, and begin to research, the fact that the body and mind were intimately connected. The question soon arose wondering if people could consciously affect the immune system, which would have far reaching implications for healing.

In the 1990s, we saw the first studies suggesting that we can use our thoughts to consciously direct specific functions and movement of the cells of the immune system. Highly motivated college students with simple training could use mental imagery to bring about significant changes in their white blood cell (WBC) count, the movement of the WBCs, and so the potential area of their activity (Schneider, Smith, et al., 1990). Hall demonstrated that conscious thought could improve the functioning of the WBCs. He used a variety of self-regulation techniques, including biofeedback, relaxation, meditation, and imagery. In 18 of 22 studies that were reviewed, the subjects were able to voluntarily alter their immune function (Hall, Minnes, and Olness, 1993).

Before we go any further, it is time to address the subject of "guilt and blame." What if you try many healing techniques using your thoughts to heal your body, and the body doesn't heal? What if a family member or client is ill, you teach them these techniques, they try them, and the body doesn't heal? People often say, "I am still sick because I couldn't be loving enough," or "Why can't you let go of your anger? You would get well." If physical healing does not occur, there is no place for guilt or blame. No one did anything "wrong." Remember our discussion of healing in Chapter 1? There is much more to life than meets the eye. We are much more than physical bodies. We may not be totally aware of all the reasons we are living our life the way we are with the people we are. Some parts of life are mysteries. There may be a reason we do not know of why the body doesn't heal. Perhaps people are drawn closer. Perhaps healing of the spirit occurs, and that is the real purpose. Becoming aware of thoughts and feelings brings about healing on many levels. The physical may not be one of them. As we become more aware of what we are thinking and feeling, we can look deeper into the heart. Here we find our real purpose, and true healing.

We are entering an exciting age in healing and human development. In the near future, healthcare will include learning how to use the power of our TF to connect with the cells of our bodies for the prevention of illness and the promotion of health.

Methods of Communication within the Bodymind

How do the mind and body communicate with each other?

ELECTRICAL: NEUROTRANSMISSION

For a long time science has known that messages are sent throughout the body via the nerves, or neurotransmission. Electrical impulses are stimulated by input received through our five senses and activities going on inside the body. These impulses pass from nerve cell to nerve cell until they reach their destination. This process occurs in milliseconds. When you touch a table, you instantly know it is a table; it is hard, flat, and made of wood. The impulses travel along a nerve until they come to a tiny space between the nerves called a synapse. At the synapse, these impulses stimulate the release of chemicals, called neurotransmitters, from the end of the cell. They flow across the synapse and connect to the next nerve cell, or tissue cell, by connecting to receptors attached to the wall of the cell—it is somewhat like a lock and key. The neurotransmitter changes the structure of the receptors. This change stimulates changes in the receptor's cell. In this way, the electrical signal continues on. Depending on the type of electrical signal, the activities of the cell can be stimulated or depressed (Rossi and Cheek, 1988).

CHEMICAL: NEUROMODULATION

The other method of communication, neuromodulation, is the principal method involved in PNI. Chemicals are secreted from an area, travel through the body, and connect to cells in other areas of the body. Neuromodulation takes from one minute to days, but is longer lasting.

These chemicals are called information substances. Some are neurotransmitters that convey messages within the brain. Some are hormones from the endocrine system, and some are steroids, like cortisol, from the adrenal glands. The remaining overwhelming majority, 95%, are peptides. Peptides are proteins that play a part in the regulation of almost all life processes. The information substances travel through the blood, cerebrospinal fluid, lymph, and intercellular spaces to their receptors throughout the body. They then affect the functioning of the receptor's cell. If it happens to be a heart cell, it affects heart function, or a kidney cell, it affects kidney function. The information substances can also affect the electrical transmission of information along nerves. They float into the synapses and connect to the receptors, occupying the receptor so that the neuro-transmitter from the nerve cell cannot connect (See Figure 9-1). For example, when your toe touches a freezing mountain stream, your electrical system imme-diately says: NO, pull the toe out! You can override it with conscious thought (chemical system), and jump in for the thrill of it.

Information substances trigger changes in all cells. They affect pain, hunger, and reproduction. Information substances play a role in how motivated we are, how we learn, and how we feel. They affect the replication of new proteins, which are the building blocks of all cells. These proteins also make possible communica-tion within the cell, as well as between all cells of the body. Some of the informa-tion substances are transported directly into the nucleus of the cell and affect

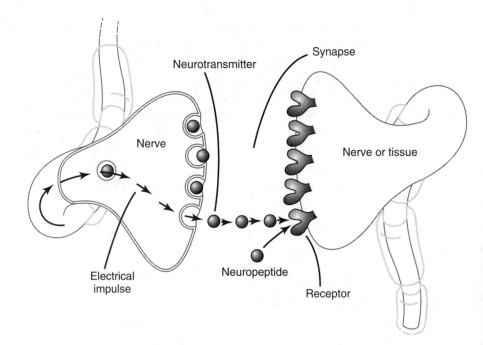

Figure 9-1 Electrical impulses stimulate the secretion of neurotransmitters into the synapse (neurotrans-mission). Information substances float into the space between cells and connect to the receptors on cell walls, increasing or decreasing activity within the cell depending on the function of the information substance (neuromodulation).

DNA expression (Rossi, 1986). DNA is the blueprint, the control tower, of each cell. In July of 2000, scientists finished mapping the DNA molecule. There are many "junk" genes whose function is unknown. What if we can use our TF to direct information substances to affect our DNA via "junk" genes?

Initially, PNI focused on the interaction between the immune, endocrine, and nervous systems. Researchers found that the communication in the body does not only come from the brain to the body, but the body sends messages to the brain through these traveling information substances. In addition, the endocrine and immune systems communicate back and forth with each other. The immune system makes hormones just like the endocrine system, and so is able to communicate with all glands of the endocrine system. The immune system can begin the stress response because it also makes adrenocorticotropic hormone (ACTH), like that made in the endocrine system. The immune system makes and secretes endorphins that travel to the brain and alter mood (Blalock, 1983). The immune system may function as a "sensory organ" signaling the central nervous system that bacteria, viruses, toxins, or tumors exist in the body (Rossi, 1986). The endocrine system makes chemicals that travel to the brain and immune system, sending messages to them.

The PNI Communication Network

During these last 25 years, Candace Pert has continued to lead research in the area of PNI, describing this adventure in her excellent book, *Molecules of Emotion*. She discovered that there is a body-wide network including all major systems continually communicating with each other via information substances. By the early 1980s, Pert, Francis Schmitt, and others were finding that the messages exchanged between systems of the PNI network appeared to be carried primarily by peptides. Peptides were not only in the brain and spinal cord but found in organs all over the body. Receptors for the peptides were found to be great distances from where the information substance was made.

Peptides released into the bloodstream can be received within a minute by all peptide receptors throughout the body. They affect many functions, including consciousness, memory, digestion, and immunity, almost simultaneously. The peptides and their receptors form a communication network through which the different areas of the body communicate with each other, coordinating bodymind function, including fighting disease and maintaining health (Pert, Ruff, Weber, and Herkenham, 1985; Pert, 1997).

In the mid-1980s, Pert analyzed the mapping of peptide receptors in the limbic system of the brain using a technique called positron emission tomography (PET). PET provides a "window" into the actual functioning of the live brain, showing in living color how the brain works (Pert, Ruff, Weber, and Herkenham, 1985; Pert, 1986). Neuroscientists believe that the limbic system is the area of the brain that deals with emotion. The fact that 85–95% of the peptides Pert studied had receptors in the limbic area of the brain strongly suggested that the peptides may be the molecules of emotion. In other words, the traveling peptides may cause us to feel emotion, and emotions we have may be able to direct the movement of peptides!

There are nodes, or areas where the concentration of receptors for peptides is very high, in several areas of the body. Receptors for opiate peptides (endorphin family), are especially high in these areas. Because peptides and emotions so greatly influence each other, what we feel especially affects these areas. These areas also make and release peptides into the body. These nodes seem to exist in the largest numbers in the areas of the brain and body associated with pain, emotion, and processing of information from the five senses. However, there are receptors for the peptides on all cell membranes.

We want to give you a brief description of these peptide nodes (Figure 9-2) to help you see where your TF have the great influence. The following information supplements Figure 9-3.

CEREBRAL CORTEX IN THE BRAIN

Our TF may be designed to determine how we interpret what comes in to our brain from our five senses. Even what the brain *permits us to see* in the first place is greatly affected by what we are feeling and what we believe. The part of the brain that controls the eyeball, and what images are permitted to fall on the retina, has a high concentration of peptide receptors. Have you ever watched an emotional scene in a movie with someone else and later, you each have two different memories of what happened?

LIMBIC SYSTEM AND HYPOTHALAMUS AREAS OF THE BRAIN

The amygdala of the limbic system and the hypothalamus have a higher concentration of opiate peptide receptors than any other area of the brain. The cortex has many connections to the amygdala. These connections may enable people to consciously control their emotions and affect the automatic functions of the body, including healing.

Since the entire cortex, limbic system, and hypothalamus are changed and affected by the constant flow of new peptides, our memory, learning, and our interpretation of reality are being constantly affected by the peptide flow. The peptide flow is influenced by our feelings. "The stability of memory and learning that is necessary for daily living is a precarious illusion dependent upon how well our body is able to maintain a certain level of homeostasis, or constant, balanced functioning" (Rossi and Cheek, 1988). This homeostasis, controlled by the hypo-thalamus, is greatly affected by the emotions we feel. So, what we are feeling affects everything we have remembered and learned in the past, all new experi-ences in the present, and what we will learn in the future.

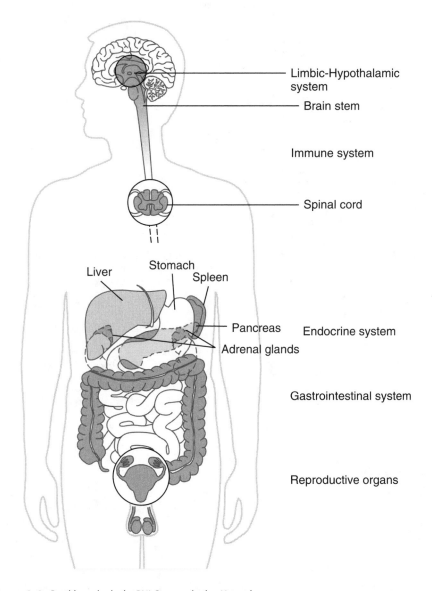

Figure 9-2 Peptide nodes in the PNI Communication Network.

Area	Function	Peptides influence
cortex (brain)	conscious awareness, receives and processes information from five senses	personality, creativity, abstract thought, filtering of incoming sensory data and so affects what we pay attention to
limbic system (brain) amygdala hippocampus	creates emotional states, coordinates emotion, motivation, memory, and learning, interprets sensory data	how we remember the past, how we interpret the events in our world, how we feel in daily situations
hypothalamus (brain)	controls homeostasis and all autonomic functions, release of chemicals that create body response to sensory input	blood pressure, healing, metabolism, breathing, all automatic functions
periaquaductal gray area (brain)	pain perception, expectation (placebo effect)	pain control, healing of all body systems according to what we expect
dorsal horn of the spinal cord	nerves from body make first contact with the brain	prioritize what signals get attention first,
gastrointestonal tract	digestion, metabolism, sugar balance, elimination, detoxification	weight control, eating disorders, nutritional intake, constipation
endocrine system		
pineal gland	regulates biocycles	sleep/wake, etc.
pituitary gland	growth, reproduction, stress, stimulates other glands to action	fertility, all aspects of the stress response, proper function of entire endocrine system
thyroid gland	metabolism, calcium balance	weight control, energy levels
parathyroid glands	calcium balance	muscle tension, nerve function, bone function
thymus gland	growth in children, matures T-cells (immune system)	proper T-cell function (decreases contribute to cancer and HIV)
pancreas	blood sugar balance	diabetes, hypoglycemia
adrenal glands	stress response	cardiovascular function, blood pressure, immune function
gonads ovaries, testes	reproduction, sexual characteristics	fertility, pregnancy and lactation, appearance
immune system tonsils, adnoids, thymus gland, bone marrow, spleen, lymph system (nodes, vessels, lymphocytes), white blood cells	identify and destroy harmful, invading cells, filters blood, destroys mutated cells within the body, regulates immune response	healing, infection, tumor growth (cancer), autoimmune diseases (lupus, etc.), skin problems (psoriasis, etc.), allergies

Figure 9-3 Areas greatly affected by thoughts and feelings due to high concentrations of peptide receptors.

PERIAQUADUCTAL GRAY REGION IN THE BRAIN STEM

One way we are able to intentionally tune into this area is by focusing on the breath. Yogi's and women in labor, through focused breathing, are able to consciously raise pain thresholds so that incoming pain stimuli are lessened. We may be able to intentionally plug into the network at any point in similar ways and affect any other point (Pert, 1987). What we expect, or the placebo effect, plays a large role in healing in the body. It can be 60–90% effective in relieving a wide variety of ailments, including chest pain and asthma (Benson, 1996).

GASTROINTESTINAL TRACT

The entire gastrointestinal tract from mouth to anus is rich in peptide receptors. Feelings can cause a knot in the stomach or diarrhea. Eating if rushed or emotionally upset disrupts the peptide regulated process of digestion. Observing the patterns of our digestion and elimination can alert us to emotional upset we may not be aware of. Conversely, as the stomach and intestines digest food, the mental state often changes. Many people feel comforted when they eat ice cream or chocolate.

ENDOCRINE SYSTEM

Each gland of the endocrine system secretes chemicals called hormones (information substances) that are picked up by the body and initiate vast numbers of activities. What we think and feel affects all of these activities. Feelings of stress can influence the pituitary gland and the ovaries, affecting fertility. And what is happening in these glands affects how women think and feel. Before the menstrual cycle, some women have pre-menstrual syndrome, with hormones traveling to the brain making it difficult for many women to think as clearly as usual.

IMMUNE SYSTEM

Our first line of defense against outside invaders includes the acid pH of the skin, the mucus membranes of the body, and the acidity of the stomach. The second line of defense consists of the traveling white blood cells that engulf and digest invaders or malfunctioning cells. The next line of defense involves the lymph system, including the lymph nodes and T and B lymphocytes.

A white blood cell travels through the bloodstream and decides where to go by following chemical cues. It has receptors for every peptide that has been discovered on its cell surface. When it "scents" a peptide, because it has receptors for it, the WBC travels to the peptide. When it reaches the peptide, the WBC binds with it, and the WBC's internal activities begin to be increased or decreased depending on what kind of peptide it is. Some of these WBC activities are recognizing and digesting foreign invaders, wound healing, tissue repair, and communicating with B and T lymphocytes. Thoughts and emotions can trigger and direct peptide travel. WBCs are then attracted to the peptides in these areas to perform the above functions. Peptides, then, appear to control the movement of WBCs. We may be able, in this way, to consciously use thought and feeling to aid in the healing of disease. It is important to also realize that our TF may contribute to the creating or prolonging of illness as well.

What is happening in the immune system affects our thoughts. When you are sick and the immune system is working hard to help you, doesn't your brain seem to shut down, making it hard to think, so you will go to bed? And our TF affect all of the functions of the immune system. Looking at Figure 9-3, you can see that we could not live long without our immune system. It is important to be aware of situations that adversely affect it.

What are some of the things that can cause decreased immune system function?

1. Being in a situation we don't like, and feeling we can't change it
2. *Unresolved* emotion—including anger, guilt, resentment, fear, depression
3. When someone close to us dies
4. Not enough sleep
5. Eating poorly
6. Pollution of our environment
7. Changing residence or job status
8. Watching violent or scary movies
9. Prolonged periods of stress

Because emotions influence the travel of peptides, and peptides affect all of the above systems in the PNI network, our TF affect the functioning of these areas. When we maintain rigid control over our lives, believe we cannot change bad situations, will not try new things, and believe we do not deserve happiness, the functions of all these areas are decreased. The body is more susceptible to illness, the mind is confused and dull, the emotions are either held in or out of control, and our spirit has a difficult time getting our attention. Conversely, when we have hope, look at life as a challenge, and choose to enjoy our moments, the functions of all these areas are enhanced. They work together easily to keep the body healthy, the mind thinking creatively, the emotions felt and expressed, and the spirit able to intervene, allowing us to realize our potential.

THE PEPTIDES AND THEIR RECEPTORS

Let's look a little more closely at how peptides work in the body so that we have a better idea how we can influence them. Recall that peptides are cells made largely of protein. A receptor is a molecule that is a long string of proteins. Part of the receptor extends out beyond the cell wall into the space around the cell, and part of the receptor extends deeply into the cell. There may be millions of receptors on one cell, with at least 70 different types. Each receptor will only accept a few kinds of visiting cells (information substances, chemicals, etc.), so a peptide flows through the body until it finds its receptor.

A fascinating characteristic of peptides and their receptors is that they dance together. A receptor is a single molecule, very flexible, able to change its shape easily. **Receptors respond to visiting cells by vibrating.** The vibration produces waves of sound and energy. The receptor changes shape, switching back and forth between several possible arrangements, vibrating and "humming," moving to music that we do not yet hear. As the potential dance partner, or peptide, approaches, the two begin to interact, adjusting their vibrations to see if there is a fit. The receptor only accepts a peptide if the peptide can match its vibration. The peptide repeatedly touches the receptor, encouraging it to change its shape to see if the two can vibrate in synch. If this match occurs, the two bind. The information the peptide is carrying is transferred by the receptor into the interior of the cell. Depending on the type of peptide, the information might stimulate, depress, heal, or harm the cell. Even antibodies produced by the B lymphocytes in the immune system begin to vibrate as they approach a virus, bacteria, or tumor cell, changing shape to try to gain entry to the cell and destroy it (Pert, 1997).

In static terms it could be looked at as a lock and key, but they are not static. The receptor and the visiting cell dance and sing. They are much like two people singing in unison who must produce sounds (vibrations) of exactly the same frequency or tone. We are discovering that there is magic and mystery in the way we are put together. Perhaps we are vibrating energy more than we realize. Many of our internal functions may be regulated by vibration, or energy. These receptors that are so sensitive to vibration are likely to be affected by other types of vibration, such as microwaves, televisions, computers, or electric blankets. Energy in the form of colored light, music, feelings, or energy from the hands may affect the cells by affecting the receptors.

The Opiate Peptides

The opiate peptides, or the endorphin family, are a large and interesting group of peptides chemically similar to morphine. Opiate peptides are produced by immune cells, cells in the gastrointestinal tract, testes, the brain, and many other areas of the body. Receptors for them are on cells all over the body, meaning they can attach to these cells and affect their function. Some opiate peptides released in response to chronic stress have harmful effects, like decreasing immune system functioning.

Others have very positive effects in the body, such as increasing immune function by improving natural killer cell activity and the function of lymphocytes (Kaye, Morton, Bowcutt, and Maupin, 2000). Some researchers believe that they are necessary to maintain a normal emotional and physiological state. Certain types of opiate peptides cause an increase in the brain waves associated with relaxation. Some create feelings of happiness and are associated with expanded consciousness.

These "positive" endorphins are released when the body or mind is stressed, whether a "good" stress (challenge) or a "bad" stress (threat). They are also released regularly in response to natural daily circadian (24-hour) biorhythms. It is almost as if the body is programmed to give us continual opportunities for happiness. Many experiences have been shown to cause the release of endorphins, including exercise, orgasm, and breathing. Women in labor who practice breathing exercises release endorphins. When we are moved by art, beauty, and nature, endorphins are released. Laughter and smiling cause the release of endorphins.

According to Charles Darwin, facial expressions for anger, fear, sadness, enjoyment, and disgust are identical among all people. When a wolf bares his fangs he uses the same facial muscles as a person does when angry. Based on these commonalities, Darwin believed that emotions must be crucial to survival. He said that when the molecules of emotion were found, they would appear over and over through evolutionary changes in many species, because they were so important. The opiate peptides fit this criteria. They are found in the brains of fish, reptiles, birds, mammals, and insects. They are even found in one of the most primitive, one-celled organisms, the tetrahymena (Pert, 1997).

It seems that most creatures have the opiate peptide receptor in common, perhaps enabling us all to communicate with, and understand, each other in ways we have yet to discover.

Receptors and drugs

All drugs, prescription and illegal, have potentially harmful effects on the body because of what they do to the myriad receptors all over the body. When drugs bind with the receptors that produce anti-anxiety and euphoria, the body sends a signal not to produce any more of the natural peptides that create these states. This sets up a dependence on the artificial substance. Once the drug is withdrawn, the receptors can return to normal sensitivity, but it often takes a long time. Our bodies are millions upon millions of peptide and receptor interactions all depending on each other, occurring continually, to keep us healthy and happy.

When we introduce outside substances that attach to these receptors, we have no idea what cascade of events we are initiating all over the body and mind. For example, antidepressant drugs prevent serotonin from being reabsorbed. There are also receptors for serotonin in the intestines and on immune cells. We may not be sure of all of the effects.

Sometimes drugs are necessary under certain circumstances, but they should be taken with caution and awareness. Under the supervision of a doctor, it might be possible to stop taking a drug to see if it is still needed, or try taking the lowest possible doses.

Cancer, AIDS and peptides

We are going to take a moment to discuss cancer and AIDS because they affect so many of our clients and our personal lives. Decreases in immune system functioning occur as a result of unresolved emotions, stress, and lack of social support. Because of this, these feelings may be linked to the cause and progression of cancer, infectious illness, and HIV (Kiecolt-Glaser and Glaser, 1995). We are seeing that emotions influence the movement of peptides. There seems to be a relationship between peptides, cancer, and AIDS.

Pert and Ruff demonstrated that the cells so rapidly dividing and doing damage in small cell lung carcinoma were mutated macrophage cells from the immune system sent there to clean up toxic materials (Ruff and Pert, 1984). Many different kinds of cancer cells have receptors for peptides on their cell walls. Peptides, the chemicals that are affected by our emotions, are able to affect the growth and movement of cancer cells. Could our emotions play a part in creating peptide behavior that can increase or decrease cancer?

By 1986, Pert had focused her work with peptides and receptors on the AIDS virus. She found that the AIDS virus entered the cell through the T4 receptor site. From her work with the opiate receptor, she knew that if there is a receptor, the body must make a peptide to fit it. If she could find the natural peptide, make an artificial copy, and inject it into the body, it might occupy all the T4 receptor sites. The AIDS virus could not get into the cell and do its damage. They found the naturally occurring peptide, VIP (vasoactiveintestinal peptide) that blocks the T4 receptor and created a copy that could be produced in a lab. They named it Peptide T.

Other researchers found that Peptide T was 80–90% effective at inhibiting the virus from growing in human cells in a test tube. The immune cells of people infected with the virus for a long time who show no symptoms, secrete a substance that blocks the virus from entering the cells. Since peptides are released in response to emotions, it might also be possible to discover which emotions cause the release of VIP in the body, and which emotions might inhibit its release. Long term survivors of AIDS typically have hope for the future, high self-esteem, a happy outlook on life, and the will to change to survive. Peptide T is in the opiate family. Perhaps emotions can direct this blocking substance.

As of 1997, Pert's discoveries of Peptide T for AIDS, and receptor-related possibilities for a cure for cancer were finally being funded for research and human trials.

HOW DOES PNI WORK IN DAILY LIFE?

We now have an idea of what happens as we think and feel on a cellular level. Let's see how these cellular dances manifest in daily life. We will look at how TF affect the way we interact with people in our world, the power of what we expect or believe, and the effects of specific TF on the bodymind.

Who is Thinking?

We begin our exploration of this topic here, and discuss it further in the remaining chapters in the book. To intervene in the scenario of thought and effect, we must first separate the thought from the one having the thought. We often live our entire lives completely immersed in the river of TF, to the point of allowing it to control our destiny. Sometimes we have a pleasant float down the river, and sometimes we are terrified, wildly thrown around in the rapids. It never occurs to us that we can leave the river at any time we want to. Suddenly one day, we crash upon a rock and crawl out onto the land. As we sit on the grass and look around, we see the world from an entirely different perspective. The river flows by in front of us, but we are not part of it. We can choose to re-enter and take a ride whenever we want to, or we can choose to observe it from the shore.

Our TF continually flow through us, but they are only part of who we are. As we learn to pull ourselves out of the river of our thoughts, we see the world in a completely different way, from a new point of viewing.

Interacting with Our World

Interaction with another begins with the process of input. When we see something, hear something, touch, taste, or smell something, that input enters the body and creates an electrical impulse that travels to the brain. These electrical impulses travel to the limbic system. Here, the impulse is changed, or interpreted, based on learning, emotions, and memories that are stored there. This modified information is sent to the hypothalamus in the brain, which sends the corresponding cascade of chemicals throughout the body. Many of these chemicals are peptides influenced by our emotions. These chemical substances transmit information by traveling to all parts of the body and binding with receptors on cell walls, affecting all of the functions that go on in the body.

Here is an example of the above process. If as a small child I was bitten by a dog, the memories of dog in my limbic system are especially connected to feelings of fear. As I get older, when I see a dog, that electrical visual input goes to my limbic system and is colored with fear. The interpreted input goes to the hypothalamus. My hypothalamus will then cause the secretion of chemicals necessary to initiate the stress response. On the other hand, if I had loving dog experiences as a child, when I see the *same set of visual cues* as the first child, they are interpreted completely differently. Because of the memories stored in my limbic system, my hypothalamus will get a different chemical array. It will release a whole different set of information substances that create relaxation, joy, and love.

When trying to understand and improve our interactions with other people, we must realize that tones of voice and body postures are stored as memories and associated with certain TF. For example, imagine a family where parents never argue. When there is disagreement, it is never talked about or resolved. After a few hours, everyone acts like the conflict never happened. But not really. There are subtle tones of voice and facial expressions. The little children watch this mode of dealing with conflict, and learn it as the way people treat each other when they disagree. In another family imagine a lot of loud raising of voices in response to conflict. The children in that family learn that yelling words that cause pain is the way to disagree.

What do you think will happen if the children from these two families marry? If they have not taken intentional steps to change their childhood programming, they have completely different sets of learning and memories in the limbic system of what to do when conflict arises. One is silent, the other yells. They "go unconscious" in the midst of arguments because the other person's response is so unfamiliar and so painful. They do not physically lose consciousness, but begin to experience an extreme stress response. The higher centers of the brain are turned off, and the instinctual part is activated. The two begin reacting based on old habits learned in childhood. The interaction they are experiencing is so incongruous with what they thought reality was "supposed to be," the brain will not acknowledge what the senses are picking up. After a certain point, they each literally may not be hearing what the other is saying. Under these circumstances, it is very difficult to choose a response that is different from their programming. They may not even remember what they said or did later on. Have you ever found yourself in a situation where you were being yelled at, and you were staring at the person's face but thinking about something else, not hearing a thing they were saying?

This phenomenon can happen with any situation in life because we are only physically able to view the world through our own unique set of memories. It is a miracle that any two people ever communicate effectively because we are all experiencing different worlds.

There is good news!

The limbic system is not cement. The memories laid down in the past can be changed with conscious intention. We can teach ourselves to interpret our world in new ways. We can look at the memories and thoughts that are stored in our limbic system and reinterpret them. New patterns in the brain are then created. We can learn to detect early warning signals that we are entering old, familiar situations that cause us to "go unconscious." (See Chapter 10.) When we notice these signals, we can choose to respond with different thoughts, emotions, and actions. For example, say as a teenager my aunt gave me shoulder massages for headaches. Although she meant well, she talked constantly in a loud voice as she brusquely squeezed my shoulders like she was washing overalls on a washboard. She insisted on doing this every week, and you can imagine the headaches were especially bad just before she came over. I decide early on that I never want a massage again and avoid people who talk incessantly. Years later, when I become a nurse, I learn that massage really helps clients, and find that many of my clients seem to need to talk. I decide I want to change my feelings about massage and the value of listening. I start by reading books about the benefits of massage and simple techniques I can do. After receiving a few private massages from an experienced massage therapist, I realize that I feel wonderful. I even notice that as I relax, I talk more than usual, and the therapist listens. The learning and memories in my limbic system begin to change. After a time of practicing new thinking, when a loud talkative client can't sleep, I ask, "Would you like a massage?" and enjoy every minute of it.

A similar procedure can be used to change habits of thinking and feeling that are no longer serving us in many areas of our lives.

As children, we learn about ourselves and the world from our parents and those we spend a lot of time with. We imitate how they think, feel, and handle situations in life. We have a great responsibility to the children in our lives to be conscious of what we say to them, and to each other in their presence. For example, from the very beginning of our nephew Eli's life, we all repeatedly told him, "Eli you are so smart, you are a good boy." As he turned two and was chattering all the time, he would run around the house saying, "Eli cute boy, Eli smart boy, Eli good boy." Eli is nine now and still teaches us many things, including how much our view of who we are is formed by the people around us.

What if we learned behaviors and ways of viewing ourselves and the world that make us sad or angry, and are not serving us? If we want to live a healthy and happy life, we must know that our parents did the best they could with who they were at the time, based on what they learned from their parents.

This is some refrigerator wisdom that continues to change my life.

"Every human being alive, at every moment of their life, did the only thing they were capable of doing with the prevailing awareness that they had at that moment.

There is no one to blame."

The past is gone. It is now a memory. The only life it has is what we continue to give it, with our energy. We often think that to forgive an action means we are approving of it, and so we cannot forgive. When we continue to relive a situation over and over, past the point of exploring it to learn from it, we create physical states that decrease immune function. Eventually our health deteriorates.

Another way to view forgiveness that might make it easier is that releasing the emotions allows the flow of information, in the form of peptides, that is necessary for a new perspective. Intentionally engaging in activities that create a movement of peptides helps hurt to move out, and we sever the hold that the memory has on us. We become free, and healing begins. (See chapter 10 for activities that create peptide movement.)

The Power of Belief

A belief is a special combination of thought and feeling. A key to turning on self-healing may be a belief that it can be done. In the last few years there has been a renewed interest in what has been called "the placebo effect." When we hear "placebo," we have learned to think that it is something that really has no benefit. Yet, doctors used to give people placebos, or sugar pills, and they worked. We know that the sugar pill itself had no healing power. But then why did people get well? People didn't know it was sugar, and they believed it would work. Our beliefs are more powerful healers than we ever imagined. Placebos are 60% as effective as most medications. "Placebos" have been shown to have significant effects 70% of the time when treating angina pectoris (chest pain), bronchial asthma, herpes simplex, duodenal ulcer, and coronary artery disease (Benson and Friedman, 1996). Congestive heart failure (Archer and Leier, 1992), pain (Turner, et al., 1994), and rheumatoid arthritis (Tilley, et al., 1995) show significant improvement with the use of placebos. These findings indicate that when we expect that a healing technique, drug, herb, or surgical procedure will work, we engage our internal healing system. Our body has the ability to manufacture the exact amounts of the right chemicals and send them to the right places for our healing. We can intentionally enlist its aid by choosing what we expect. Some techniques are suggested in the next chapter. It is important to mention that we can also create the nocebo effect, which is when we have poor expectations, and decreases in health often occur. Since 60–90% of the illnesses that take people to healthcare providers are poorly treated by drugs and surgery, it is time to learn how to turn on the healer within (Benson, 1996).

The Power of What We Expect, or Believe

Two Japanese physicians, Ikemi and Nakagawa, asked 13 high school students who were very sensitive to a Japanese plant similar to poison ivy to participate in a study. The students closed their eyes. They were told that their arm was being touched by the leaves of the poisonous plant. All of them had skin changes of redness, itching, and raised swollen areas. In reality, they were touched by leaves of a harmless plant. Next, they were told they were being touched by a harmless plant on the other arm. Eleven students showed no skin changes. In reality they were touched by the poisonous plant. This study suggests the power of our beliefs to alter the immune system and affect the body (Barber, 1978).

Herbert Benson (1996) suggests using the term "remembered wellness" to refer to the placebo response because bringing about the placebo effect in the body is dependent upon remembering or expecting feelings of well-being. If we expect that something is about to happen, the brain often begins making necessary changes in the body 20–30 seconds before the event actually occurs, suggesting the ability of expectation alone to change the body.

Effects of Specific Thoughts and Feelings

The effects of specific thoughts and feelings are becoming a topic of much research. A study in the *Journal of the American Medical Association* reported that common emotions such as tension, frustration, and sadness can cause a drop in the blood supply to the heart (Gullette, et al., 1997). See Figure 9-4 for the effects of different feelings on the body.

Three specific feelings seem to be emerging in research literature as having profound effects on the body: anger and hostility, perceived control (belief that we have the ability to change what we don't like), and social support (support, caring, and love gained from positive relationships).

ANGER AND HOSTILITY

Our thoughts and feelings greatly affect the cardiovascular system (heart and blood vessels). How many times have you seen a client's blood pressure reading

Feeling	Effect on Body
Depression	70% increase for chance of heart attack than those not depressed (Barefoot and Schroll, 1996)
Anxiety	Creates as significant a risk for sudden death from heart disease as cigarette smoking and lack of exercise (Frasure-Smith, Lesperance, and Talajic, 1993)
Marital conflict including hostile, negative behavior during problem solving	Decrease in immune and endocrine function, and increased blood pressure (Malarkey, et al., 1993, 1994)
Chronic stress of Alzheimer caregivers	Slower wound healing (Kiecolt-Glaser, Marucha, et al., 1995)
Pride, excitement, enthusiasm	Increased immune function (Stone, et al., 1994)

Figure 9-4 Effects of specific feelings on the body.

unusually high because he was anxious about coming to the doctor's office? High blood pressure is a major risk factor for heart disease, and is the most important risk factor for stroke. According to the American Heart Association, between a quarter and a third of adults in the United States have high blood pressure, and nearly half of these people do not know they have it. In response to our emotions, cells of the immune system secrete peptides that can increase or decrease the buildup of plaque in the coronary blood vessels. Blood flow is closely regulated by emotion peptides by signaling receptors on blood vessel walls to constrict or dilate. If emotions are felt and expressed, peptides are released that help blood flow more easily. If they are blocked, blood flow can become chronically constricted (Pert, 1997).

Heart disease is America's number one cause of death. Heart attacks account for almost half of all deaths in the United States (Williams, 1993). A study of 12,986 white and black men and women, age 45–64 years old, suggests that proneness to anger predicts coronary heart disease in middle-aged people independent of the established risk factors, including cholesterol level, smoking, diabetes, age, or alcohol (Williams, et al., 2000).

One study examined the relationship between hostility and coronary artery calcification in 374 black and white men and women, aged 18–30 (Iribarren, et al., 2000). Hostility is defined as the tendency to behave antagonistically, think cynically, and frequently feel anger. There was a significant relationship between hostility scores and calcification of the coronary arteries in the heart, after adjusting for demographics, lifestyle, risk factors, and physiological variables. Notice that these changes are seen even in very young adults.

It almost seems as if we are designed so that the body functions better when we are not constantly angry or hostile.

Anger is a normal response in life designed to get our attention that change needs to occur. Noticing it, constructively expressing it, and letting it go contributes to health. The problems in the above studies occur when anger and hostility are frequent responses to situations in life, are expressed in a destructive manner, or are held in and never dealt with.

BELIEVING WE HAVE CONTROL, OR CHOICE

Control in this context means the power to choose and make changes. You are the only one who has the power to change the way you perceive your world and how you want to respond to it. We are often taught that others can make us feel certain things. In the past we may have learned that when another person does or says something in a particular way, there is only one way to respond. In reality, people can't make us feel things any more than they can make us answer the phone if we don't want to. We choose to feel a certain way, just as we choose to pick up the receiver. Part of having conscious choice is choosing which people to spend our time with.

Perceived control benefits us in several ways. Since 1964, Martin Seligman has researched the phenomenon of learned helplessness (See Chapter 10 for more information). If a person, dog, roach, or goldfish learns that he has no control over his environment, or that nothing he does matters, he will become helpless. He won't even try to move away from a shock. Helplessness is very similar to depression. Feeling helpless can lead to decreased immune function, low self-esteem, poor performance at school and work, and hopelessness (Seligman, 1990). Having a hardy personality (sense of personal control over life events, views change as a challenge, and is committed to the people and activities in his or her life) contributes to improved immune function (Dolbier, et al., 2001) and a 60% lower risk of early death (Pennix, et al., 1997).

Secondly, in a study of 10,000 British civil servants, those who felt they had control, regardless of job status, had significantly less heart disease. This was true even after accounting for the risk factors of smoking, cholesterol, high blood pressure, physical activity, and obesity. Perceived control included input into job tasks, decisions about who they worked with, and flexible time. The intensity of job demands and social support did not contribute to the difference in heart disease (Marmot, et al., 1997).

A third reason to look at the control we feel we have in our lives is because it is perhaps the greatest determinant in the amount of stress we experience in a situation. In situations of high demand and little control, stress levels are very high and can be predictive of the development of heart disease. Lansbergis (1988)

This example is given to illustrate how much happens in the bodymind in response to one particular consistent thought or belief.

A belief that we have no control, or no power to affect change leads to . . .

1. Decreased norepinephrine which leads to:
   Decreased arousal, activity, motivation
   Lack of proper focus on the environment
   See self as the cause of all negative events
   Think a single setback is a never-ending pattern
   Worst is assumed unnecessarily
   Decreased coping abilities
   Decreased ability of muscles to function

2. Decreased dopamine leads to:
   Decreased sense of reward or pleasure
   Decreased cognitive function that affects bodily movements

3. Decreased serotonin leads to:
   Decreased mood regulation
   Decreased ability to relieve pain
   Decreased ability to raise and lower endorphins and enkelphalins
   Increased impulsive and violent acts

4. Increased cortisol leads to:
   Decreased WBC
   Decreased function of thymus, lymph nodes
   Decreased number of lymphocytes and plasma cells
   Decreased antibody formation
   Progressive loss of nerve cells in hippocampus area of brain
   Speeds aging
   Decreased bone density

5. Decreased connection between brain cells
   If we have hope and self-efficacy (believing we have the ability to perform the task), we have:
   Increased serotonin and endorphins (regulate mood and relieve pain)
   Decreased cortisol
   Decreased epinephrine and norepinephrine (stress hormones)
   If we view life as a challenge, and feel we have some control, we have:
   Increased immune function
   Decreased cortisol
   Increased motivation
   Active learning
   Broader range of coping skills

found that feelings of a lack of control led to arousal of the sympathetic nervous system and increased cortisol (stress response), as well as withdrawal. Chronic increased cortisol leads to decreased immune function and decreased cognitive functions, such as memory and learning. People who felt they had little control in their environment also had decreased coping abilities, decreased motivation to improve the environment, and increased feelings of helplessness. However, *people in the same situation who felt they had some kind of control* and viewed it as challenging, had sympathetic arousal, but their cortisol levels were not elevated. Situations of high demands and high control led to high motivation, creativity, and job satisfaction. They were stimulated, but their immune systems were not compromised. Chronic high levels of cortisol are found in persons who are depressed or feel hopeless (Lazarus and Folkman, 1984; Kiecolt-Glaser and Glaser, 1997).

Robert Karasek (1979), originator of the demand-control theory of work stress, suggests that we have basic needs for activity, freedom, competence, and control. When the demands made upon us and our ability to make decisions about how to solve the problems match, more active learning occurs. We have greater belief that we can solve problems, which enables us to develop a broader range of coping strategies. When we experience lack of control for a long time, we begin to experience a loss in our ability to solve problems, make judgments, and tackle challenges (learned helplessness). Increasing a person's control in a situation counters the effects of learned helplessness.

It almost seems that we are designed so that to be healthy and happy, we must feel that we have choice in the events in our world.

A sense of increased control can come from a number of sources. Perhaps the most important is taking responsibility for discovering what our unmet needs are and being sure they are met in a life-giving way. It is important to start by taking small steps that can be easily achieved. People also begin to feel they have more choices in life when they learn new coping skills, adopt a more positive outlook, and seek needed information to be better prepared for upcoming events. Building a support system and placing faith in a Higher Power or someone who is deeply trusted can increase a sense of control. A nurse might use the above suggestions to help clients feel a greater sense of control over their environments. Control can come in small ways such as being able to choose when to eat and get a bath. Some techniques for meeting needs and gaining control are mentioned in the next chapter. Buchanan, Gardenswartz, and Seligman (1999) offer various techniques for changing thoughts and feelings of learned helplessness into learned optimism.

SOCIAL SUPPORT

Social support means that you feel supported, cared about, and/or loved. For some it may come from feeling part of a group—such as a church, bridge club, or

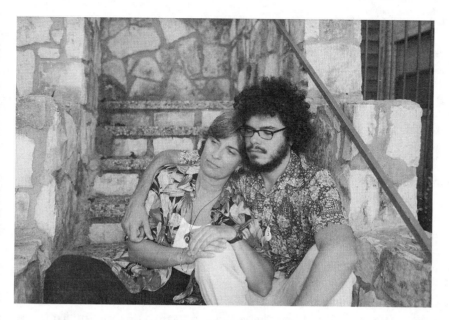

Figure 9-5

playing sports on a team. For others it is a caring relationship with a pet, friend, family member, or Higher Power. It is knowing you have someone you can call on, during the good and the bad times (Figure 9-5).

In a groundbreaking study of 4,725 men and women spanning nine years, those who were socially isolated were twice as likely to die during the study compared to those who had close social contacts, including being married, having contact with friends and relatives, and/or having church and group memberships (Berkman and Syme, 1979).

It almost seems that the body is designed so that to be healthy, we must interact with others in supportive ways.

In a review of 81 studies, social support was very beneficial to the cardiovascular, endocrine, and immune systems (Uchino, et al., 1996). When people with heart disease, including those who had a heart attack, had supportive relationships, their life expectancy was three to five times greater than those who did not feel like they had someone they could count on (Woloshin, et al., 1997).

Social support increases feelings of self-esteem, self-identity, and control over one's environment, which tend to result in enhanced immune function. In one study, people who said they had one to three supportive relationships had four times the risk of getting a cold when exposed to the cold virus than those who had six or more supportive relationships (Cohen, et al., 1997). Women with metastatic breast cancer who participated in a support group lived twice as long as those not in a group (Spiegel, et al., 1989). One group of people with malignant melanoma participated in a support group intervention, and one did not. Those who replaced depression with hope, determination, and a will to live had increased immune function. After six years, 10 of the 34 in the group with no intervention had died, while only 3 of 34 in the support group died, and they had less recurrence (Fawzy, et al., 1993).

Research also shows that when we help others, we benefit physically and emotionally. In a study of 3,000 men and women for 9–12 years, those who volunteered to help others at least once a week lived longer than those who did not (House, Landis, Umberson, 1988). Recall in the massage study where Elders massaged infants that the Elders benefited more by giving massage to the babies than by receiving one (Field, Hernandez-Reif, Quintino, et al, 1997). Giving and receiving love and kind interaction helps us realize our optimum potential for health.

In eight community-based studies between 1979–1994 the relationship between social isolation, and death and disease from all causes, was studied. These studies were conducted all over the world, and they found that if we are socially isolated we have two to five times the risk of premature death than those with a strong sense of community and connection (Ornish, 1998).

It almost seems that the bodymind is programmed to self-destruct when we feel consistently angry, helpless with no power to choose, and are isolated without love and support.

THE BOTTOM LINE OF PNI

We are designed so that every day, for our entire lives, our mind-stream can run our lives with very little conscious attention. When we are not happy or healthy, it is a signal that it is time for us to intervene. Our thoughts and feelings are our tools for this task.

When we choose to view ourselves, our lives, and the people in them as irritations or distractions, keeping us from having what we want, we send peptides flooding all cells of the body, creating sadness, isolation, and disease.

When we choose to view ourselves and the events and people in our lives as challenging teachers, offering an opportunity to learn what works and what doesn't, we send peptides flooding all cells in the body, creating happiness and healing.

As we learn more and more about how the body works, we find that vibration, or energy, plays a huge role in whether interactions occur in ways that contribute to health or disease. Receptors on cell walls vibrate and so are affected by vibrations, or energy. Energy comes in many forms, including feelings, energy from the hands, microwaves, and even the electromagnetic field of the Earth. We are a fascinating miracle of energy and chemistry working to create our experience of life, and who we are.

STRESS AND PNI

We now discuss stress in detail for several reasons. First, the phenomenon of stress is a perfect example of PNI, with our TF playing a major role in the stress response. Secondly, most of the people who will want you to give them a massage have tension due to stress. Because massage interrupts the stress response, learning more about stress adds to your knowledge of the benefits of massage. Third, nursing is one of the most stressful occupations, and our clients are usually in one of the most stressful situations in their lives. Finally, in our world today, 90% of the problems of the bodymind are believed to be stress-related.

Increasing numbers of nursing studies are using PNI as a framework to discover new links between our TF, stress, and the health of the body (Zeller and McCain, 1996). Wells-Federman, et al. (1995) suggest that PNI provides a psychophysiologic explanation for the therapeutic properties of traditional nursing interventions such as empathy, social support, massage, Therapeutic Touch, meditation, imagery, prayer, and listening. Schrader (1996) presents evidence that clients with traumatic injury have multiple stressors leading to decreased perception of control which leads to a subjective stress response. This perception of stress contributes to excessive increased cortisol which leads to decreased immune function. Interventions for the bodymind are suggested. Kaye, Morton, Bowcutt, and Maupin (2000) use PNI to look at the relationship between stress and depression in neurological clients. They report that high stress is significantly related to high depression. With prolonged stress, norepinephrine levels in the brain become depleted, resulting in depressed mood and distorted thinking. Perceptions of lack of control can also lead to depression. They suggest that nurses "need to assess and recognize the PNI response involving stress, depression, and immune dysfunction."

What is Stress?

A stressor is an event that occurs. Stress is our response to the event. Some events like constant noise, not enough sleep, and unhealthy food, water, and air create a stress response in almost everyone. With many events, however, the degree of stress we feel is determined by the thoughts we think and feelings we have about the event. Have you ever been sitting safely on the couch in your home in the evening, thinking about work that day, and suddenly you're feeling anxious and your heart is pounding? The original event is past. Your TF created the stress response.

What we think and feel plays as big a role in coloring the events occurring in present time. The TF we choose as an event is occurring, begins, or prevents, a stress response. Standing in line at Disneyland in the summer is an example. The first thing many adults talk about is how long the lines are, how hot it is, and how many people there are. Their children are standing right beside them in the same line, and their story is usually very different. They tell about the exciting rides they have been on or the rides they want to go on next. They don't mention the lines and weather. The parent appears to be stressed, and the child is having a great time. They are very likely thinking and feeling very different things as they wait for the rides.

Feeling stressed is a signal that change needs to happen. Stressful situations present an opportunity for learning and growth.

Potential Causes of Stress

In 1926, Hans Selye began observing the way people responded to certain situations, and began noticing a pattern. In 1936, after observing this pattern in rats, he described the biological stress response, or General Adaptation Syndrome. He discovered that a variety of "noxious agents" introduced into the body over time produced the same syndrome of gastric ulcers, shrinkage of the thymus gland, lymph nodes, and spleen, and over-activity of the adrenal glands (Selye, 1974).

In Selye's later work of 1976, he differentiates between stress that causes illness (distress), and stress that enhances health (eustress). The crucial element seems to be whether the individual believes he has control over his situation. Our TF come into play again. To feel continually frightened or hurt with no control over the situation are examples of distress. We experience eustress when we are running a marathon, teaching a workshop, creatively solving problems, or going out on a first date. We view this event as a challenge, and it can be stopped when desired.

When the demand in the environment exceeds our control over it, eustress changes to distress (Landsbergis, 1988). As mentioned previously, one of the greatest causes of stress in the body and mind is feeling a lack of control, feeling that we cannot change a situation that we don't like. One of the best ways to dance with stress is to remember that there is **always a way** we can change our situation if we don't like what is happening, **even if the only thing we can change is how we think and feel about it.**

There are many other potential causes of stress. Hippocrates, 2,400 years ago, diagnosed all human ills as being the consequence of change. Any extreme, whether too much or too little, is potentially stressful. Multiple stressors are another source of stress. Most of us can handle one or two stressors fairly well, but problems come when we have several stressors happening all at once. For example, if the car breaks down, we can usually handle it. If we have a bad shift at work, we can usually handle it. However, what happens when we are late for work, we go out to the car, and we remember we have left the dog in the house. As we get out of the car, we spill coffee on our clothes. We get to the door, and realize we have locked the keys in the car. One child falls down and starts crying, and the other child is scattering the transparencies for our presentation in the flower bed. We just might sit down in the yard and cry. For many of us, these scenarios happen more often than we would like to remember. The body is not made to handle it.

Have you had the feeling that life is speeding up? Constantly feeling rushed, or "on" also creates a stress response. Before you know it, a month is gone. We wear beepers, have car phones, are expected to check e-mail every hour, and have personal fax machines. The expectations on us all are too great and create new sources of stress.

We can't avoid stress. It's everywhere. To be healthy and happy in today's world we must learn to dance with it.

When we want to discover where our stress lies so we can do something about it, we must do a thorough search of our lives. We look at sleep, food, childhood, relationships, environment, daily, repeated activities, and feelings. Sometimes we have been experiencing a particular stressor for so long we have forgotten when it started and what caused it. For example, when a client wonders, "Why does my neck hurt?" we ask, "What activities do you do every day? Do you carry a briefcase, purse, or child on one side? Does your computer arrangement fit your body? Do you read in bed at an odd angle? Is your pillow the right thickness? Is there someone or something in your life that is a pain in the neck? Is there something you're not saying?"

Dr. Barbara Howard, a pediatrician, says that 25% of the children that come to see her have stress-related problems (headaches, abdominal pain, urinary frequency), and the numbers are rising. Frank Treiber of the Medical College of Georgia, says that if a child comes from a family that is chaotic, unstable, and harbors grudges, there is greater blood pressure reactivity to stress as an adult. Cortisol levels are elevated, and they tend to get very angry quickly in response to conflict. If the early home is secure and loving, children can experience discomfort without a stress response (Adler, 1999).

We often are not aware of some of the things that produce stress in the bodymind.

Potential External Stressors
　　Lack of supportive relationships
　　Change in family relations, divorce, and death
　　Change in where you live
　　Unsatisfying communication with others
　　Job competition
　　Prolonged exposure to low-frequency electromagnetic fields (Becker and Selden, 1985)
　　Constant noise
　　Air and water pollution
　　Unhealthy food
　　Not enough sleep
　　Overcrowding
　　Victory in sports
　　Speaking in public
　　A passionate kiss
　　A raise in pay
　　Getting married
　　Temperature or altitude change
Potential Internal Stressors
　　Feeling a lack of control, helplessness, hopelessness
　　Poor self-esteem
　　Boredom, feeling that what we do has little value
　　Depression
　　Fear of failure
　　Frustration due to unmet needs
　　Unexpressed feelings, such as anger, resentment, hostility, grief
　　Not living up to expectations
　　Extreme joy

Even though we may not be conscious of it, an underlying element of many causes of stress is a feeling of separation. Think about a situation in your life right now in which you feel particularly stressed. I know that I often feel most stressed when I feel separate from things I love. The stress we feel in this separation is beckoning us to examine our lives. Why does this separation occur? In my own life, I get caught up with the details of life that seem to come faster and faster. I forget to keep the main thing, the main thing. Feelings of separation from loved ones can be caused by unresolved feelings. Feelings of separation from my own inner self happen when I don't make time for activities that bring me peace and pleasure. Many feel alone, separate from everything. From one point of view, stress of any kind occurs only when we mistakenly believe we are separate from the Divine, forgetting that we are all, always, connected.

Stress-related Disease

As early as 1975, Dr. Herbert Benson wrote about stress-related illnesses. In America, stress is now considered to be an epidemic with 70–80% of all visits to physicians being for stress-related problems (Scofield, 1990). Eighty percent of all diseases including chronic diseases are considered to be stress-related (Goldberg Group, 1993). According to the Anxiety Disorders Association of America the cost of stress-related illness is $44–$65 billion per year.

Conditions Affected by Stress

Heart disease, high blood pressure	Infertility and impotence
Immune system problems such as allergies, rheumatoid arthritis, infectious disease, and cancer	Diabetes
	Over active thyroid
	Obesity
Asthma	Grinding of teeth
Pain	Tension headaches
Skin conditions such as herpes, psoriasis, acne, warts, eczema	Insomnia
	Arthritis
Anxiety disorders such as panic attacks	Ulcerative colitis
	Diarrhea, constipation
Depression	Stomach ulcers
Menstrual problems	

Early Warning Signs of Ineffective Coping with Stress

Has anyone ever said, "You sure look stressed out." And you said, "I'm not stressed. I'm perfectly fine." Very often we don't even realize we are stressed. If stressors increase slowly, the body learns to function with greater and greater demands placed upon it. We begin to think the stressed state is normal. This can be dangerous because harmful levels of stress can be reached, and we are not aware that it is building up. The bodymind cannot handle large amounts of stress forever. Before we know it, a crisis occurs.

There are early warning signals that tell us it is time to make some changes in our lives (Mast, Meyers, and Urbansky, 1987).

Early Warning Signals

Physical signs	Emotional signals	Behavioral signs
Dilated pupils	Feeling inadequate	Sleep disturbance
Pounding of the heart	Depression	Being accident prone
Cold hands and feet	Negativity	Forgetfulness
Shortness of breath	Not caring what	Urinary urgency
Frequent sighing	happens	Unnecessary motor
Unusually large amounts	Being unaware of	movements (hair
of gas and belching	feelings or events	twirling or fingernail
Abdominal cramping	Feeling panicky and out	biting)
Dry mouth	of control	Eating disorders
Change in bowel habits	Feeling "keyed-up"	Substance abuse
A lump in the throat	Irritated emotional	Being overly-
Muscle tension	reactions and a	competitive
Weakness	quick temper	Speaking difficulty
Grinding of teeth	Suspicious attitude	Sexual promiscuity
Increased perspiration	Blaming others	Problem solving
Hot and cold flashes	Inappropriate laughter	difficulty

If you, or anyone you know, is having several of the early warning signals, it is time to stop and review life. If current levels of stress continue, the symptoms will increase, eventually leading to disease. If someone you care about has become very difficult to be around, it might be that they are extremely stressed, don't realize it, and need your help. Does this sound like a teenager? This is a particularly stressful time of life. They need to know they are loved and supported even if they act like they don't need it, or care. If you notice clients in the hospital having these behaviors, it is very likely due to the extreme stress they are under. Your help in reducing their stress, and your compassion, is what they need most.

The Stress Response

Examining what happens in the body during a stress response is helpful because often you, a client, or family member may notice symptoms that appear to be unrelated. However, if you know what stress does to the different systems of the body, you can see that these apparently unrelated symptoms point to a chronic stress response. Understanding the stress response lends insight into how stress can lead to the chronic diseases on the rise today.

Since the beginning of humankind, the stress response was designed to help us freeze, run away, or fight in threatening situations. These situations typically only lasted for a short time, and did not occur very often. The physical effects of the stress response are beneficial in the short run. However, when stress happens for days and months and years, continuously, with many different stressors at once, the once beneficial responses cause disease.

Learning what stress does to the body helps us understand why it is so important to be aware of what we think and feel when we are in a potentially stressful situation. Learning what stress does to the body also helps us realize the need for massage. An event occurs. Our five senses direct the information to the brain. Due to the memories in our brain, a judgment is immediately made whether the situation is threatening or not. If the situation is determined to be threatening, the stress response begins. The adrenal glands are stimulated, and the heart starts beating faster. **This is where we usually first notice the response and have the opportunity to change our thoughts.** If we do, we can stop the stress response. If we don't notice it, the response continues.

The stress response has two parts. The first part is electrical, and happens in milliseconds. Hydrochloric acid secretion to the stomach and small intestine is increased. Epinephrine is secreted from the adrenal glands which increases mental acuity, sweating, heart rate, and respiratory rate. We have increased blood sugar, blood clotting, and general metabolism. In the short run, we want more blood clotting in case we get cut, we want to breath faster and have a high heart rate to run and fight. We want increased blood sugar for more energy. In the long run, if stress continues day after day, increased heart rate and blood clotting can lead to strokes and heart attacks. Increased blood sugar can lead to diabetes. Increased acid in the stomach and intestines may contribute to ulcers and digestive problems.

Norepinephrine is secreted and increases blood pressure, blood flow to the skeletal muscles, and constriction of the blood vessels in the arms and legs. In the short run, we want extra blood to our arms and legs for running and fighting. In the long run, the internal organs such as the kidneys, intestines, liver, pancreas, and spleen are not getting the blood supply they need. Digestion, sugar metabolism, and detoxifying the body are impaired. With constriction of vessels in the peripheral muscles, cramping, pain, blood clots, and nerve disorders may result. In the short run, high blood pressure ensures that the brain and body have all the blood they need to run. In the long run, strokes and heart problems develop.

In the second part of the stress response a different part of the adrenal glands secretes cortisol (a steroid). In the short term, cortisol is designed to aid in adapting and coping. It increases sugar (glucose) and fat (cholesterol) in the blood. In the short term, increased fat and sugar in the blood gives us extra energy to run and fight. In the long run, we might develop high cholesterol, narrowing of the blood vessels, or diabetes. Prolonged cortisol decreases bone density. Aldosterone is also secreted that causes water retention. In the short term, increased water protects us if we start loosing blood. In the long term, this can lead to high blood pressure and heart problems. If we then start taking diuretics and blood pressure pills, we may be headed for kidney problems.

If the stress continues, continual cortisol production causes increased stress, yet increased stress causes increased cortisol. A vicious cycle can develop. Cortisol decreases protein stores needed for healing and building all cells, including information substances. Continual high levels of cortisol circulating in the blood stream change the activities of other peptides in the body. These peptide changes affect our thoughts and emotions, making it difficult for us to choose new ways to respond to situations. We get stuck in habitual, negative responses that are very limited, and see no way out. Chronic depression can result. Depressed people typically have high levels of cortisol in their bloodstreams.

In a meta-analysis of the literature on the effects of stress on the immune system, Herbert and Cohen (1993) found a strong relationship between stress and decreased immune function. One reason seems to be that prolonged cortisol production decreases the function of the thymus gland, spleen, and lymph nodes of the immune system. It decreases the white blood cell count, number of lymphocytes, number and function of natural killer cells, and antibody formation, all crucial for the immune system to destroy invaders to the body such as viruses, bacteria, and malfunctioning cells such as cancer cells. In the short term, the body is not concerned with immune function when we are running from a bear. In the long term, diseases such as increased infection, cancer, and AIDS can result.

A survey of research on stress and memory loss concluded that in animals and humans, memory loss and even partial amnesia is caused by cortisol secreted in response to stress, affecting the hippocampus of the brain. These effects are most pronounced in elderly people, people with previous emotional trauma, and those experiencing a high level of stress at the time of the event (Joseph, 1999; Markowitsch, 1999). Some elderly people are less able to adapt to stress, and so have prolonged levels of high cortisol after a stressful experience and so decreased immune function. Prolonged stress even in young animals causes changes in the hippocampus that mimic the effects of aging (McEwen, 1990). Can it be that experiencing chronic stress could play a part in Alzheimer's Disease? Perhaps learning to effectively handle stress at young ages may prevent problems with learning and memory as we age.

So, when we continue in situations that we view as stressful, over the long haul we begin to suffer from the chronic diseases we see in the world today, including the number one and two causes of death in America, heart disease and cancer. When we have increased blood pressure, water retention, heart rate, and fat in the blood, we set ourselves up for heart disease, stroke, and heart attack. When we have decreased immune function, decreased protein stores for healing, decreased ability to detoxify the body, and decreased digestion and assimilation of food and water, we set ourselves up for cancer. People are dying at younger and younger ages from heart disease and cancer.

It almost seems like the design of the body is such that it begins to self-destruct when we view life as stressful for prolonged periods. This is perhaps an indicator that we are designed for happiness and health.

After the stressor is gone, the body returns to homeostasis and all is well if the damage is not too great. However, if the stressor continues, such as continual noise and polluted air, living with someone we are not compatible with, or working at jobs we hate, the adaptation phase of the stress response begins. Outwardly, most functions return to normal if the stress is compatible with life; however, large amounts of energy are required to maintain homeostasis if events are persistently perceived as stressors. A return to a non-stressed state does not occur (even though it appears to) as long as the perception of stress continues. This can be very dangerous because we think all is well when it is not. Immune function continues to diminish over time (Kiecolt-Glaser and Glaser, 1993).

If the stressor, or how we look at it, is not changed, the body eventually experiences the exhaustion phase. Physical and mental coping mechanisms begin to fail. Have you ever had your back go out from bending over and picking up a piece of paper? Have you known anyone who burst into tears because someone ate the last cookie? In chronic stress, endorphins decrease, which can lead to depression. Conditions begins to occur such as migraines, infertility, ulcerative colitis, arthritis, heart disease, cancer, early aging, and death (Gherman, 1981). When stress begins to cause disease, there is an information overload. The mind-body network is so overloaded by trauma or emotions not dealt with, that it has become clogged and cannot flow freely, in terms of circulation, peptides, or energy. The largely automatic processes that are regulated by peptide flow, such as digestion, elimination, blood flow, breathing, and immunity do not function in a healthy way (Pert, 1997).

Luckily *we do not have to suffer this fate*. In some situations we can get rid of the stressor. When we can't, we must change our internal environment, considering flexible ways of viewing the inner and outer world. Life can become a classroom full of amazing lessons to be learned.

PNI AND MASSAGE

PNI helps us realize the power of thoughts and feelings. We now return to the question, why is this important in massage? First, learning about PNI and the bodymind connection allows us to understand the magnitude of the benefits that receiving a massage can bring to a client, or ourselves. We have learned that when TF change, physical changes occur in all parts of the body. Conversely, when changes occur in the body, we begin to think and feel differently. For example, the stress response can begin with mental/emotional responses that create physical changes. If we experience situations in our lives as threatening, we may feel worried, angry, resentful, or sad. We may begin to think that we are worthless and have no power to change the situation. As we feel more and more stressed, muscles tighten, intestines become upset, and immune function decreases.

Or the stress response can begin with a physical condition that leads to mental/emotional changes. Blood pressure goes up, blood vessels constrict, and muscles tighten. When we have tension and pain in the muscles, we become mentally distracted. It is hard to think, and it is certainly difficult to have creative thoughts. As we become more distracted, we begin to feel irritated, which often progresses to anger and hostility. Our thoughts become skewed causing us to have incorrect perceptions. We often begin to feel anxious or afraid. And so the stress cycle continues indefinitely, mind affecting body and body affecting mind.

To stop the stress, we must interrupt the cycle. Massage interrupts the stress response by changing thoughts, feelings, and physiology. When the body gets massaged, muscles soften, and the mind is changed. Our thoughts turn to how wonderful we feel, and how great the world is. We feel cared for. We begin to contemplate things we enjoy. When we have these kinds of feelings, peptides are released that enhance the flow of information in the body, creating healthy functioning of the systems in the body. Blood flows more freely, immune function is enhanced, and muscles become more relaxed. The stress response ends.

Massage benefits the bodymind in many other ways. The part of the nervous system (parasympathetic) that initiates the relaxation response is activated by massage (Field, 1998). Massage causes the release of serotonin (Ironson, et al., 1996) which helps with mood regulation, the ability of the body to relieve pain, and the ability to raise and lower endorphins. Massage also directly causes the body to be flooded with endorphins, contributing to feelings of well-being (Pert, 1997).

The spinal cord and the skin and muscles along the spine are areas of high concentrations of peptide receptors (nodes). The nerves in the spinal cord, and the nerves leaving the spine for the body are affected by peptides coming to these centers. Stressful feelings can send peptides that create tension in back muscles. On the other hand, as we begin to have feelings of relaxation during a massage, different peptides are sent to the nodes along the spine that relax back muscles and enhance nerve flow.

Massage can also help heal childhood experiences. When infants and children perceive events as stressful over and over, stress hormones increase. The receptors for these hormones on the cells are constantly flooded. The memory of the trauma is stored by these changes in the receptors. With constant stress, these emotions are stored all over the body, not just in the brain. These memories can be retrieved by touch therapies. Massaging the body firmly creates a peptide flow that can release emotional patterns held at the receptor level. Touch causes just the right amount of peptides to be released at just the right times so that our mind, body, emotions, and spirit grow and heal in the best way possible (Pert, 1997).

Second, what we think and feel as we give a massage affects our own body. As you perform the slow, gliding massage strokes, your body relaxes along with the receiver's. As your body relaxes, peptides are released that encourage all body functions to work at their greatest potential. The natural movement of the peptides encourages any stress in the body and mind to be released.

Third, perhaps the most important reason to include information about PNI in this massage book is because what you think and feel as you massage affects the quality of the massage you give, and so the bodymind of the receiver. See Chapters 12 and 13 for more information. As a giver of care and massage, it is our responsibility to learn to notice and choose our thoughts and feelings. In massage we intently focus on what we are doing with our hands, bringing our awareness to the present. It is an opportunity to become aware of what we are thinking and feeling. We can tune in to the ongoing internal dialogue of the mind. When we notice, we can choose. If we don't like something we hear the mind saying, we can substitute a thought that creates the feelings that we want. Massage is a very effective technique for noticing and directing our thoughts and feelings. What we think and feel as we are giving a massage creates relaxation, or tension, in our body. This is felt by the receiver and contributes greatly to the benefit gained from the massage.

SUMMARY

Learning about PNI and stress shows us that what we think and feel about an event determines to a great degree how much stress we experience, and how well the entire bodymind functions. Clients often have muscle pain and feel overwhelmed, are chronically tired, mentally cloudy, and emotionally on the edge of crying or screaming at someone. Nurses and other healthcare providers often have these same feelings. We can use what we've learned about PNI to create the lives we want. As teachers and healers, we have a unique opportunity to teach the principles and techniques of PNI to help our clients handle stress and heal to their greatest potential.

We are here to have fun, to love, and to serve. PNI in a nutshell. All of the information and research we have discussed about PNI is telling us that when we do these things our bodies are healthy and live for a long time. Our minds are creative and happy. Our spirits are free.

We now realize the importance of what we think and feel, but how do we go about changing our point of view, especially in situations that really push our buttons? The tools that have helped us the most make up the next chapter.

PUTTING THESE IDEAS INTO PRACTICE

1. Take five minutes to do a personal stress assessment. Pick a physical stressor (a physical pain) or an emotional one (worry, anger, sadness, etc.). You can do both. Make a list off the top of your head of one or two word phrases that might explain the cause of these stressors.

2. Is there a client or colleague that you have trouble getting along with? For the next week, every time you see that person, notice the thoughts running through your mind. Intentionally substitute kind, life-giving thoughts.

CHAPTER 10

Techniques for Choosing Thoughts and Feelings

Thoughts tremble, they are unsteady, they wander at their will. It is good to control them, and to master them brings happiness.

Your worst enemy cannot harm you as much as your own thoughts, unguarded. But once mastered, no one can help you as much.

—Buddha

OBJECTIVES

1. Describe three ways in which what we think and feel creates the reality we experience each day.

2. Discuss four reasons suggesting that techniques for changing thoughts and feelings are beneficial to health.

3. Discuss four ways of noticing what we are thinking, especially in stressful situations.

4. List two internal and two external activities that change what we are thinking and feeling.

5. Describe the process by which we can create our Quality World.

Many of us have taken numerous workshops and read countless books on how to manage stress and be happy in our lives. We feel great during and right after the workshop. After a few days, life is the same as ever. What happened?

For most of us, those wonderful comprehensive plans involving many changes are truly what we want to do. Unless we make the effort to learn to become aware of what we are thinking and feeling, even in the bad times, we go back to our familiar old ruts. Unless we get to the bottom of those thought habits, the best laid plans are forgotten in a few days or weeks. The part of us that is comfortable in those ruts becomes afraid and overwhelmed.

So what can we do? Take baby steps. A dear friend of mine was contemplating the journey to greater health and happiness. She said, "Tell me everything I can do to feel better." I suggested, "Drink a quart of water a day." She said, "That doesn't seem like much." She agreed to try it for a week, and just that simple action began a cascade of change in her body, mind, and spirit.

The previous chapter discussed the effects of what we think and feel on our health and well-being, and the value of being aware of our thoughts and feelings (TF) while giving a massage. This chapter suggests many techniques for changing our TF, creating the life experience we want. These techniques seem deceptively simple upon first glance, yet often the unseen, most simple things are the most powerful. We are also more likely to actually try tools that are easy to use wherever we are. You may be wondering, "How hard can it be to change a thought?" You may find it more difficult than you think. That's why there are lots of tools to choose from. We are all different. Hopefully, you will find one, or a combo, that works for you. Some of these tools help you begin to notice what you are thinking in both the easy and difficult times. Others suggest ways to change thoughts that are not creating the feelings and behaviors you want, to those that help you be the person you know you are on the inside. No matter how much time we spend debating foreign affairs, in the long run, if we don't have clean air to breathe and water to drink, nothing else matters. In the same way, no matter what we try to do to improve our individual lives, in the long run, if we don't notice and choose what we think and feel, nothing else matters. This awareness and choice is a step in our growth as we realize our full potential as the spiritual beings that we are.

WHO IS THINKING?

As we continue on our journey, we again ask, "Who is thinking? What is the conscious aspect of who we are that feels and thinks?" If we are going to notice our thoughts, there must be someone there to do the noticing and changing. We often think of ourselves as the body. Take a moment and ask yourself, "Am I my foot? Am I my stomach? Am I my brain? Am I my thoughts? Am I my feelings?" Then who are you?

When we learn to make a regular habit of experiencing the Self directly, both in our quiet moments as well as in our daily movements, we come to know ourselves in a very deep and profound way. When we try to describe it to another, words often fall short. This growing sense of understanding and inner knowing never ends. Self-knowledge is as boundless as the canopy of the heavens and as deep as the capacity of our hearts for love. In this inner knowing, we flourish perpetually and have our connection with the Divine. This is the Self that we bring with us as we begin each massage.

The Self has a body full of moving parts, a mind full of TF, and a field of energy surrounding and permeating it. Yet, it is more than the sum of its parts. As we learn to separate the Self from our TF, we experience more and more deeply who we are in our heart of hearts.

CREATING YOUR REALITY

Now, why is it crucial that you learn how to notice and choose your TF? They create your reality, what you experience on the inside as well as what you experience in the outside world.

In 1979, Ellen Langer at Harvard conducted an amazing study showing the power that our TF have in creating our reality. A group of 75-year-old men became physiologically younger by shifting their awareness. For one week they went to a retreat center that took them back to 1959, when they were 55. The newspapers, furniture, radio programs, clothing, everything was from 1959. A control group went to a retreat center and was in present time. At the end of the week, biological markers for aging were measured, as they had been at the beginning of the week. The faces of the experimental group looked younger, their fingers were longer, stiff joints were more flexible, and their postures had straightened. Muscle strength, intelligence, vision, and hearing had improved as well. This was only one week! **When the men thought that a certain reality existed, their bodies and minds changed to fit that reality.** The control group decreased in several measures. Langer believed the results were found because: (1) The men were asked to behave as if they were younger. (2) They were treated as if they were younger. (3) They were asked to follow complex instructions about their daily routine (Chopra, 1993).

What we think and feel creates the reality we experience in at least three ways:

1. Influences our bodymind, our vehicle for experiencing this world.
2. Allows us to reinterpret past memories, and form new memories that we use to guide our future.
3. Affects our reception and interpretation of input from the five senses, creating our present reality.

Emotions and Peptides Influence the Bodymind

If you've ever been sick and gone to work anyway, you know that the state of your body colors your experience of reality. If you've ever been worried about a loved one in the hospital in another state, you know your mind also colors the world you experience. When the body and mind are functioning at their greatest potential, we have the best chance of creating and experiencing the kind of reality we want.

As you recall from the previous chapter, the activities of the peptides in the body influence what emotions or feelings we have. When peptides are not flowing through the body as designed, emotions become blocked, and it is more difficult to express our feelings. Conversely, our emotions affect the activities of the peptides. When we do not freely experience and express our emotions, peptides do not move in optimal ways. Imbalance and disease of the bodymind occur.

If we continue to have the same TF over and over, the same peptides are released over and over, sending the same messages to organs, muscles, and nerves, creating the same body and mind, over and over. Prolonged or repeated emotions like anger, guilt, resentment, hatred, sadness, and depression continually create a body that functions less and less efficiently, contributing to disease.

By influencing the flow of peptides in the body, TF are designed to be our tools for entering the ongoing activities of the bodymind to create healing. When we change our TF, we release different peptides, and this creates a new body. When you feel happy, take note. Be sure your life includes many moments like these. Feeling love, happiness, joy, compassion, and appreciation causes the release of their corresponding peptides, creating a healthy body with increased immune functioning, efficient heart functioning, and relaxed muscles. The constant, harmonious movement of emotions and peptides creates health.

Recognizing, expressing, and letting go allows emotions to move through and out of the body. Some people express emotions by talking to others, some by writing in a journal. When we do anything that reduces our experience of stress, including exercising, getting massage, eating properly, and sleeping well, our peptides move as designed. When we engage in activities that cause the peptides to move freely, it is also easier for our thought processes and emotions to be flexible and change. With a flexible body and mind, we can best create the world we want.

Emotions and Peptides Influence Memories

The smooth functioning of our world, and our enjoyment of it, is dependent on our memories from yesterday, and since we were born. We can affect these memories, and our interpretations of them, with the TF we have today. How much of your time do you spend thinking about something that happened a few minutes, days, or years ago? These memories can still cause you to feel emotions as strong as you did when the event occurred. If the memories are unpleasant, they can ruin your day. If the memories bring a smile, your day is brightened.

Emotions, by the release of peptides, create memory at the cellular level, all over the body. When receptors on a cell are frequently flooded with a particular peptide, they change the cell membrane. Information pathways are created. The next time information comes to the cell, it will most easily follow the pathways created by the peptide flood. This flooding of receptors, and changes in cell membranes, creates lasting changes in what pathways information takes into cells. Strong feelings create these floods of peptides. So, when an event is accompanied by emotion, it is easier to recall (Pert, 1997). When an opinion is accompanied by emotion, it takes more work to change it.

For example, you go to a Caribbean restaurant. The service is lousy, and the food makes you sick. You are angry, and tell everyone you know. Floods of peptides are secreted in response to your emotions that attach to receptors causing changes and creating memory. In the future, if someone suggests getting Caribbean food, you will immediately remember the name of the restaurant, what you ate, that you don't want to eat there again, and you might get mad all over again.

On the other hand, if you feel very loved when you are with a particular person, large amounts of different peptides are secreted. In the future, when you need to be comforted, you remember that person, and seek them out. Thinking about certain people and places recreates the feelings we have when there. Whenever I go into a basement, I remember my grandmother, her basement, and the cookies she lovingly and secretly left in a bottom drawer in the kitchen so we could find them when we were little.

Because quantities of peptides create pathways, when we frequently think the same thoughts and have the same feelings, good or bad, there is a greater likelihood we will continue to think and feel them in the future. For example, the more we choose to have negative thoughts about someone, the greater is the likelihood that we only notice the things they do that we don't like. The good deeds don't catch our attention. Conversely, when we fill our minds with thoughts that are curious and accepting, we are more likely to give a person the benefit of the doubt, and expect a rewarding future. An open mind with flexible opinions enables us to easily change, have more options for behavior, and enjoy a richer life experience.

Memories created in the past by certain peptide floods can be reinterpreted by intentionally having new feelings about the event, as we think about it in the present. New peptides will be released that create new "pathways." When we remember the situation in the future, we will feel differently about it. For example, as a child your parent walked away instead of talking about upset feelings. One day, your parent tells you about what his childhood was like, and you discovered that anger was dealt with in a violent way. You realized your parent's behavior in your childhood was an amazing behavior change, considering his past programming. It ended the chain of violence and protected you. Now when you look at how your parent behaved in your childhood, you see it in a new way. The walking away and not talking was indeed a very loving and courageous act.

When we feel emotions in a situation, that situation will be remembered most easily in the future. If we find ourselves in a situation that we want to remember in the future, either to create more of, or avoid, allowing ourselves to strongly feel the emotions attached to the situation will help to secure the memory in the bodymind. Just as childhood emotions contribute to how we experience the present, what we choose to feel today creates memories that will influence our future reality.

Emotions and Peptides Determine the World We Allow Ourselves to See

I have always disliked bluejays. They make a terrible racket and are bullies in bird world. One day I saw a hurt bluejay in the road and picked it up so it could die in peace. It didn't die. It fought for life and survived. I began to notice bluejays. One day I heard a most beautiful melody, very lilting, that I had heard several times before. I looked into a tree and saw a bluejay. I had heard the sound before, seen bluejays in the tree, but still thought it was another bird I couldn't see. Because I disliked bluejays, it had never occurred to me that they could sing such a beautiful song. I thought they only made screeching noises. Because of my increased appreciation of bluejays, my mind (peptide array) allowed me to connect the melody and the bluejay for the first time. My view was forever changed. To receive new information we must allow ourselves to entertain new thoughts. New thoughts can change our views, the chemistry of the body, and our lives.

We have learned that the thoughts we have and the emotions we feel cause the release of peptides that travel to the brain and connect to receptors in the cortex and limbic system. Recall that these areas govern our personality, input from the five senses, memory, and learning. So, these peptides affect how we interpret sensory input, and what we learn and remember. Peptides connected to cells in these areas play a role in what images from the five senses we are given the opportunity to pay attention to. Recall that peptides affect the movement of our eyeballs, and what they are allowed to look at. If we have strong, rigid feelings about the way things are in the world, these corresponding peptides will only allow input from the senses to reach consciousness that vibrates with, or is in harmony with, what we already believe. The brain can only bring to our conscious awareness the information it is prepared to find, based on its internal patterns and past experiences. Perhaps we can only experience what we are open to, what we are willing to believe is possible.

We know that concepts can radically affect precepts. Thus the native islanders could not see the first white man's ship anchored in the bay because they did not have the concept for such a thing The limited conceptual frame-work that came with the use of their language made them unable to see a sailing ship.

Similarly, the limited conceptual framework that comes with our modern use of language may make us unable to "see" . . .

—John Heron

Our external reality, or what we *literally* see, hear, taste, touch, and smell, is greatly determined by what we think and feel.

The brain cannot process and have in conscious awareness all the input from all the senses and internal workings of the body all the time. We could not focus effectively on anything. If you focus on the details of your visual input alone for one minute, it is so much information you could never listen to what someone was telling you at the same time. What makes it to consciousness is only a speck of what is actually there.

We Create the Reality We Experience

Jim, a lawyer, told us this story.

One day I was standing at an intersection waiting for the light to turn so I could cross the street. The light turned red. A car was coming that was clearly going to run the red light. Another car had the green light and was coming at about 40 miles per hour through the intersection. I saw that a wreck was about to occur. Knowing this, I paid special attention realizing I would be the only witness. I am used to paying close attention to detail and realize the weight that is placed on the story of an eye-witness.

The collision occurred, and no one was seriously injured. The policeman arrived and asked if I had seen the whole thing. I gave him a detailed account of exactly what I had seen. He looked at me strangely for a moment and asked if I was sure that my account was correct. I said, "Definitely. I knew this was about to happen so I paid special attention."

He led me over to where the crumpled cars were. They had not been moved at all. He pointed out that from the skid marks and the positions of the cars, the event could not have happened the way I described it.

I was shocked. He was right. After I thought back over the incident, I realized I had expected that one car would hit the other in a certain way. I saw what I expected to see. I would have sworn in a court of law that my account was what happened.

The reality Jim expected to see was exactly what he saw. According to him, he saw what was really true, or reality. If two people had seen the wreck, most likely there would have been two different stories, and two different realities. No doubt, what we choose, and expect to happen, creates the details of the world we experience each day, in many ways. We make decisions that create our futures based on what we believe reality to be today.

How can we possibly talk about an objective reality, or one experience that is real for everyone? All people have different memories within their bodies and brains, creating different filtering mechanisms going on all the time. Some cultures teach their children that wise Elders go to mountain-tops and commune with spirits and bring back wisdom that the entire community follows. Other cultures teach children that old people who isolate themselves and hear voices are crazy. Those two groups of children have different realities concerning the elderly, being alone, and attuning to spirit. Each is convinced that their world, their thoughts and feelings, are real.

What if we are told all our lives that it is bad to get dirty. Can we experience the thrill of swimming in a spring-fed creek with the ducks and turtles floating by? What if we are told that all that exists is the three-dimensional world of the senses. Can we feel or see the energy that flows around all things? What if we are told that we are separate from God? Can we ever allow ourselves to feel oneness with the Divine?

If the view of reality we have always had does not serve us for health and happiness, we can change our thoughts, and so change the peptides coming to the receptors, and so change the receptors and the cell function. If we are willing to believe that there are many explanations for events, and that the answer may be something we have not yet thought of, the corresponding peptides may allow us realities we have not yet imagined. The more expansive our willingness to entertain the unknown, the more of the uni-verse we will be able to be conscious of. We can create a new reality.

The techniques in the following sections are intended to help break old patterns of thought, feeling, and behavior, allowing us to experience a new world.

SUPPORT FOR THOUGHT-CHANGING TECHNIQUES

A 20-year study conducted by the University of London School of Medicine determined that *unmanaged mental and emotional* reactions to stress present a more dangerous risk factor for cancer and heart disease than either cigarette smoking or eating high cholesterol foods (Grossarth-Maticek, et. al., 1988). "Unmanaged mental and emotional reactions" means TF we are not intentionally choosing. Techniques to address TF are becoming more and more popular due to research indicating their effectiveness and their need. Recall that roughly 42% (a 10% increase in five years) of the American public is searching, and paying, for complementary healthcare techniques to maintain health and prevent and treat illness, indicating clear public demand (Eisenberg, et al., 1998). Most of these techniques involve a change of our perspective, or how we view a situation. Sometimes we engage in an activity that changes our thinking, like massage or exercise, and sometimes we intentionally direct our thoughts in a new direction, as with imagery.

Many of the techniques that help us become aware of and change our thoughts can also create relaxation and stress reduction. They affect the autonomic nervous system which controls the stress response, breathing, healing, pain, digestion, heart rate, and all of the other automatic or "unconscious" functions of the body. These techniques have been shown to reduce blood pressure, respiration, heart rate, and to enhance immune function (Benson, 1996; Blumenthal, et al, 1997; Hall, Minnes, and Olness, 1993). They have also been credited with improving chronic anger, headaches, acute and chronic pain, psoriasis, asthma, cancer, and heart disease.

As you recall from PNI, the more we feel stressed, the more our immune function decreases. Many of these techniques that help us change TF also improve immune function.

Research suggests that immune function increases when we:

1. Laugh
2. Watch funny or caring movies
3. Have close support system: friends, family, colleagues
4. Have pets and plants to care for
5. Eat balanced meals with enough protein
6. Get enough sleep
7. Recognize and express feelings and needs
8. Recognize our choices for changing our situation
9. Use guided imagery and visualization
10. Talk and write about traumas

In 1992, healthcare costs in the United States exceeded $800 billion. By the year 2000, that figure was projected to double, making up roughly 20% of the projected gross national product (Goleman and Gurin, 1993). This is a large

Condition	Technique	Results
Surgery	Imagery	Shorter hospital stay, need less pain medication (Kiecolt-Glaser, et al., 1998)
Inpatient psychiatric	Relaxation exercises (progressive muscle relaxation, focus on breathing, guided imagery, soft music)	Significant reduction in anxiety after exercises (Weber, 1996)
Coronary artery disease	Quit smoking, exercised three times/week, support group, vegetarian diet, stress management one hour/day (choose from yoga, focused breathing, progressive muscle relaxation, meditation, imagery). Some improvement even if they didn't do all of the above.	After one year, no chest pain, less hostile, angry, depressed, anxious. Significant decrease in cholesterol **without drugs**, 82% had regression of narrowing of coronary vessels. Control group had increased chest pain and progression of vessel narrowing (Ornish, et al., 1990)
Heart disease	Group 1–standard care, 2–standard care and exercise, 3–standard care and relaxation, reducing hostility, looking at events as challenges, monitoring and changing thought patterns	In five years, Group 1–30% further problems, 2–21% further problems, 3–10% further problems, reducing risk of further problems by 75% (Blumen-thal, 1997)
Depression in women (ages 18–24)	Reduce negative thinking (thought-stopping and positive self-talk and affirmations), increase self-esteem, reduce depressive symptoms	Over six months, significantly lower depression scores, significantly less negative thinking (Peden, et al., 2000)

Figure 10-1 Research Support for Thought-Changing Techniques.

incentive to find cost effective, preventive techniques. Techniques for reducing stress that involve changing thoughts, such as meditation, imagery, and relaxation skills, have been shown to be as, and often more, cost effective than current medical treatment, with greater health outcomes (Herron, et al., 1996; Caudill, et al., 1991; Friedman, et al., 1995). In 1984, the NIH recommended meditation over prescription drugs for treating mild hypertension because of its effectiveness in reducing stress and tension (Goldberg Group, 1993). Massage very effectively relaxes the bodymind. Thoughts of worry and hurry change to peaceful contentment. By so doing, the stress response is interrupted, immune function improves, and pain is relieved (Field, 1998). See Figure 10-1 for research supporting thought-changing techniques.

Have you ever noticed that the more stressed you are, the harder it is to figure out how to get back to your self that is relaxed and enjoys life? Remember the cortisol cycle? Stress causes cortisol secretion, and cortisol continues the stress response. Cortisol affects our thinking process. The more stressed we get, the harder it is to think of new ways to change the situation. This is why it is so important to create a plan ahead of time, before a stressful event occurs, that includes techniques for interrupting the stress response. The first step is to remember to look in on the thought train, to notice **that** we are thinking.

NOTICING THAT WE ARE THINKING, BECOMING CONSCIOUS

We must notice *that* we are thinking before we can change *what* we are thinking.

The Buddhist master, Luangpor Teean Jittasubho says that when we are not aware of our thoughts as they arise, there is the opening for suffering. Thought itself is not suffering. When a thought arises, if we do not see, know, and understand it simultaneously, greed, anger, or delusion arises, and brings us suffering. Suffering also is one way to begin the process of self-awareness. Pain has the ability to bring our thoughts to the present moment. It can help us become more aware of what we want to change in our lives. Jittasubho says that doing activities that help us be aware are like raindrops filling a bucket. They continue to accumulate until one day we are awake.

Most of the time there is a constant flow of thoughts through our minds, and peptides through our bodies, that help us live our daily lives. We are not consciously intervening very much at all. As we discussed in the PNI section, we frequently react, especially in stressful situations, based on old habit patterns. Our brains have an interesting function designed to ensure our physical survival. When we are stressed, endorphins and ACTH act together to block out the function of the cortex, the area where conscious, rational thought resides. Our behaviors are then governed by the instinctual part of the brain. This may be helpful when we need to move very quickly. It may not be so helpful in the mental/emotional stresses we usually experience. This may explain why in stressful conversations we may "go unconscious" or find it very hard to react in new ways that are different from old patterns.

According to Deepak Chopra, M.D. (1993), we form "premature cognitive cognitions." For example, a group of goldfish are put in an aquarium and a divider is placed in the middle so that the fish can only swim in one half of the aquarium. After some time the divider is removed. The fish continue to swim only on that one side. Once habits are formed, they are hard to break, for fish or humans. If you have ever tried to stop smoking you know how hard it is because smoking is interwoven into so many parts of the body and of life. It is just as hard to learn to respond to someone who is yelling at you by speaking softly and kindly. Most of us have learned to withdraw or get angry.

Remember how repeated floods of peptides form pathways that direct incoming information. These pathways can become "thought ruts" that are often deep. Have you ever been driving on a dirt road and found yourself in a hardened rut made by cars in drying mud? It is easy to move if you stay in the rut. To move in a different direction, it takes much force to turn the wheel out of the rut. Often wheels spin and cars swerve. With enough gas and focused attention you can escape the rut. In the same way we can learn to be conscious.

You may be saying, "But I am conscious! My eyes are open, I am walking around." Have you ever been driving down the freeway and noticed you missed your exit? Where were you? You were not conscious in the moment because you didn't intend to miss your exit. We all have done this. When our TF are not focused in the present moment that we are living right now, we are effectively unconscious, unable to choose our responses. When the Self is not engaged, the body and mind run on auto pilot, reacting, not responding. If this can happen while we are hurling ourselves down the road at 70 mph, it can surely happen in a situation when we feel fear or other uncomfortable emotions.

So, the first step in waking up is becoming aware in the present moment. Thoughts precede feelings, even if the thought is very fleeting. A thought can be a belief, or a way we have learned to explain a certain situation. We must first realize *that* we are thinking, and then notice *what* that thought is.

> ### Refrigerator wisdom:
> When patterns are broken, new worlds emerge.

The Breath as a Cue

The breath is an invaluable ally for noticing that we are thinking. About every five seconds, all day long, we take a breath. At any moment, no matter where we are, we can use our breathing as a tool to bring us to the present. When we focus on the inhale and exhale for a breath or two, our stream of thought is momentarily interrupted. We can then notice what has just passed through our minds and the accompanying feelings we are having.

To get into the habit of noticing your breath, once every hour for a week take a few deep sighs. When I do this I find I am transported from wherever else I am, back to the present. It gives me a chance to ask, "Is this what I want to be thinking? Is this how I want to be feeling? Is this what I want to be doing?" I become aware of areas of tension that I need to let go of. My body relaxes. Remembering to take a breath during a stressful situation brings you to a point of power from which you can intentionally choose a response.

Thought Checks

Thought checks also get us in the habit of noticing that we are thinking. Once per hour notice what you are thinking. Set a timer if you have to. Tune in to the usually unconscious thoughts that are running the flow of peptides, and health, of your mind and body. If you don't like what you notice, replace the thought with what you really want to think. It is our responsibility to direct the mind when it wanders astray just as it is our responsibility to direct our feet in the direction we want to walk. If you find your mind repeating something over and over, you must take charge. Your mind may say, "But that would not be real. That's fake." **We can fill our minds with whatever thoughts we want to.** Sometimes the mind must be reminded that we run the show. If we allow it to control the inner workings of the body and how we feel, we get into trouble. What we put our conscious attention on grows in our experience. This occurs whether it is positive, "This is a great day," or negative, "I will never lose weight." You will soon create a new habit and catch yourself thinking all kinds of things.

Feelings as Wake-Up Calls

Most of the body functions are designed to maintain homeostasis, a balanced healthy functioning. For the body and mind to survive, our temperature must stay somewhere between 96 and 104 degrees. That is only eight degrees. Only five minutes of feeling anger or appreciation begins to affect heart function and immune system. We are finely-tuned machines. Do you think the efficient functioning of such a finely-tuned machine would be left to chance? Internal controls are built in. We have just not been taught how to use them. The controls are the emotions.

We may not notice our thoughts because they disappear so quickly, but we are designed so that it is very difficult to ignore our feelings. **Feelings are red flags.** Feeling peaceful, having plenty of energy, and being happy are signals to keep doing just what you are doing. Upsetting feelings are trying to tell us that we must change the situation we are in because it is not contributing to growth, health, or happiness. We can use our feelings as wake-up calls. Sadness and grief get our attention. Anger and resentment fill our entire experience. Feeling thrilled, peaceful, or in love also make us stop and take notice. Emotions tell us to check our thoughts. What were we thinking immediately prior to the feeling? Does that thought lead to feelings and behaviors that we like? What do we want to change? Emotions alert us to check the world around us and be sure it is really what we want, and what is healthy for us.

When I notice myself feeling confused and frustrated, that is my cue to sit down, set my alarm for five minutes, and begin taking slow, deep breaths. I let my mind float to the beach. The chemical stress circle is broken, and I can think more clearly.

Physical Cues

If we ignore the feelings, we often begin to get physical cues. Emotions make the body feel relaxed or give us "butterflies" of excitement. Emotions can create a lump in the throat or a knot in the stomach. They cause the face to flush and the body to sweat. If we still don't listen and look at our situation, our heart will pound, and we get diarrhea. The body is made to function pain free and have plenty of energy. Headaches, constipation, pain, low energy, depression, and anger are all warning signs from the bodymind. If we heed them and make changes, homeostasis is maintained, and we are healthy and happy. If we ignore these signs, we get more and more severe signals until we get an illness. Constipation or diarrhea can become ulcerative colitis that can become colon cancer. We are just trying to get our own attention so we will change the things in our lives that are not fun. Emotions cause physical sensations, so we can use these physical cues to notice emotions we may be unaware of. If we have a chronically tight neck, we can ask ourselves, "What in my life is a pain in the neck?" A physical cue can be your signal to stop and notice what is happening around you and within you. Frequent illness, allergies, or persistent physical symptoms are trying desperately to wake us up to the world we are creating.

With practice we can learn to become aware of physical cues to bring us back to the present moment so we can choose our responses. When I am in one of those "difficult situations," I often notice that my heart starts pounding, my face feels flushed, my throat begins to constrict, and I feel like I have a knot in my solar plexus. I have learned that these are my cues that I am feeling fear in some form. There is danger of my "going unconscious" and saying things I don't really want to say. I stop, take a breath, or four, and move my focus of awareness away from the situation for a moment. Then I at least have a chance of choosing my feelings and responses. If you notice a physical cue, there is most likely a feeling and a thought behind it.

Even though you have every intention to choose a new response the next time that familiar, uncomfortable situation occurs, you may still go unconscious the next ten times.

Be patient with yourself.

Keep having the intention to notice the feelings and physical cues.

Eventually you will notice, after the fact, that you went unconscious. Then you start noticing that the situation is beginning to occur, and you are conscious. You are noticing the cues. You are able at last to choose a response instead of reacting in old ways that have never worked, and never will.

The Fork in the Road

Let's say that as you drive out of your driveway, you back into a tree and dent your car, spill your cereal on your shirt, have an argument with your son, are late dropping the kids off, and have a headache. You come to work hungry, angry, in pain, and thinking about how you will repair your car.

There is potential here for catastrophe, or great healing.

Scenario One

Yesterday, your friend asked you to give her a short massage this morning because her back has been killing her, and she has a very important afternoon meeting. You run into her office, out of breath, with your feelings and your stomach churning. She gruffly asks you why you are late, reminding you she is on a tight schedule. You begin defending yourself, in heated tones, telling her you are, after all, doing her a favor. She begins to yell at you, telling you she certainly doesn't need extra stress, and that her back is beginning to hurt worse. You storm out, slamming the door behind you. Neither person was able to pull out of the drama of the mind and choose heartfelt responses.

Scenario Two

You are a nurse working in a clinic. It is your job to see each client for 15 minutes before the doctor does and assist them with stress management. On the way to the clinic, after the above experience, you feel your heart pounding. You know this is a cue to stop and tune in to what you are thinking. You decide to consciously change your TF by taking a few deep breaths and thinking about your favorite vacation spot. When you arrive at the clinic you are relaxed. The first client has been waiting for you and is irritated because you're late, has forgotten the papers he needs for an important meeting after his appointment, has back pain, and has had nothing but coffee the entire morning. He gruffly asks you why you're late. You are able to slowly and calmly apologize for being late, and for the cereal on your shirt, and tell him you had a close encounter with a tree. The frown in his forehead softens. You both laugh. You ask him where his pain is, and you begin to slowly massage his back. Within five minutes he is telling you how much better he feels. Because you were able to stay aware, he was also able to let go of his irritation.

We have all had both of these kinds of experiences between nurse and client, parent and child, with friends and spouses. How we choose to respond creates what we experience on the inside and in the outside world. How do we begin to become aware so we can choose? We start with the intention to do so.

Once we are able to be conscious with some regularity, we notice our perspectives on life. If the ways we are looking at life and the behaviors we are doing are not working, it is time to change.

You say, "Well of course." But how many times have you noticed yourself wanting someone else to change this or that instead of you? You keep acting and talking the same as ever, expecting something to change. Chances are very slim. When two people are engaged in a pattern of responding, the pattern continues until one changes. As soon as one changes, the other must change. It's like a row of dominoes. The only person in this world we can change is ourselves.

> **Refrigerator wisdom:**
> If we continue to do what we've always done,
> we get the results we've always gotten.

CHANGING AND DIRECTING THOUGHTS

After we consistently notice what we are thinking and feeling, we can begin to make changes. The TF that usually give most of us trouble include fear, anger, guilt, and resentment. Yoda in the *Stars Wars* movies said, "Fear leads to anger. Anger leads to hatred." The Dalai Lama (1995) said that a negative thought or emotion is a state which causes disturbance within our mind. Anger causes such a disturbance. The ultimate source of happiness is peace of mind. Nothing can destroy this except our own anger. Most of us feel anger from time to time. If we don't try to reduce it, it stays with us and may even increase. We will immediately get angry, even with small incidents. Once we begin to notice anger, understand it, and change it, even big events will no longer cause anger. Dissatisfaction, frustration, and hurt lead to anger. Anger leads to hatred. To change anger, we can look at it from a new view. Those events or people that upset us are precious teachers. They give us the opportunity to practice tolerance and patience. When we feel anger or hatred, it can be a cue, a signal that this is one of those valuable opportunities.

Gary Zukav, author of *Seat of the Soul,* says that our darkest and most frustrating times are really our greatest opportunities for learning and growth. They are our **holy moments.** In these moments we have the chance to develop the gifts we were born to develop.

If you practice one or several of the following techniques, you will begin to notice that you are using your TF to create your inner- and outer-world.

However many holy words you read, however many you speak, what good will they do you if you do not act upon them.

—Buddha

External Activities That Change Our Thoughts and Feelings

We will discuss several of the above external activities. They change the chemistry of the body, which changes what we are thinking and feeling (See Figure 10-2).

Tools for Changing Thoughts and Feelings

External Activities
Food
Exercise
Sleep
Looking at art and beauty
Laughter and humor
Being in nature
Massage
Yoga, Tai Chi
Social support
Sound, music, light, color
Energy based therapies such as
    Therapeutic Touch and Healing
    Touch
Meeting needs—both external and
    internal

Internal Activities
Changing breathing patterns
Progressive muscle relaxation
Imagery
Meditation (Relaxation Response,
    Mindfulness Meditation)
Freeze Frame
Changing to optimistic point of view
Stepping out of the box, seeing with
    new eyes
HeartTouch (Chapter 12)

Activity	Effects
Food	
sugar	stimulates, then depresses
carbohydrates (bread, rice)	calm, peacefulness, sustained energy
protein	mental clarity
Exercise	releases endorphins (happiness)
Adequate sleep	reduces cortisol (feelings of control, personal power, high self-esteem)
Looking at art and beauty	releases endorphins (happiness)
Massage	balanced peptide flow (peacefulness), see world in new way, (See chapter 3)
Smiling and laughter	releases endorphins (happiness), pain decreases, immune function increases, stress hormone blocked, heart arrhythmias decrease

Figure 10-2 External Activities and Their Effects on TF.

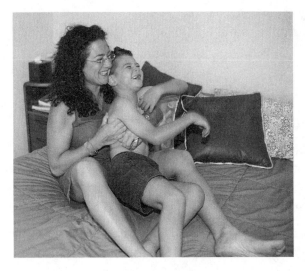

Figure 10-3

Regarding **food,** you are what you eat. Twenty minutes of mild **exercise** also releases fat-burning peptides that are at work for several hours, which also makes us happy.

Humor and laughter change my point of view instantly. Have you ever been very mad at someone and then they do something that makes you smile? All of a sudden, the anger vanishes. Laughing and smiling are magic (Figure 10-3).

Changing your facial muscles by turning the corners of your mouth up, as if smiling, increases blood flow to the brain, and "happy" peptides are released. This happens even if you are not really feeling happy (Klein, 1989). If you are feeling bad physically or mentally, spend time with a four-year-old, turn on a funny movie, watch kittens playing, anything to make you laugh.

Refrigerator wisdom:

The arrival of a good clown exercises more beneficial influence upon the health of a town than twenty donkeys laden with drugs.

Thomas Sydenham, 17th century physician

Seven days without laughter makes one weak.

Spending time in **nature** always seems to improve what I'm thinking and feeling. Sometimes that means taking five minutes to lay on the ground in the front yard or sit with my back against a tree out behind the nursing school. And then there are the long visits, the vacations, time to vacate the mind (Figure 10-4).

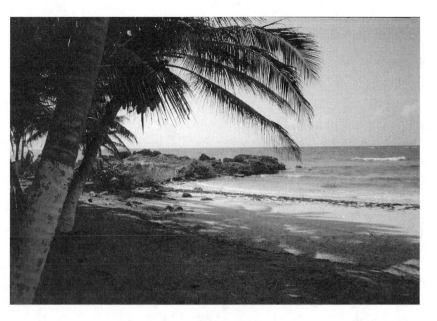

Figure 10-4

In those deep immersions in the world of natural rhythms, for long periods, I remember the way. In a study of 12,000 men over nine years, those who took a vacation almost every year were 20% less likely to die from any cause and 30% less likely to die from heart disease (Gump and Matthews, 2000). The young of most species spend much of their day playing. One purpose of **play** among children and adults is the acting out of fear, aggression, and grief to learn to feel them and deal with them. Play also makes us laugh, loosens us up, which loosens the information flowing in us as peptides. Play lets us take ourselves lightly. As we become grownups, we begin to play less and less. I wonder if there is a relationship between playing and aging? When I'm with Eli, he often wants to play "let's pretend." Imagining takes us to new places in our thoughts. A cardboard box becomes a spaceship traveling at warp speed to planets in another galaxy.

MEETING OUR NEEDS

Meeting our needs usually involves some external activities and some internal activities. When our needs are not met, we often feel angry and frustrated. Meeting our needs changes our feelings to satisfaction and curiosity. All of us have needs. When Eli was about three he would wander around the room saying, "I need someping." Feelings of discontent alert us that one, or all, of our needs are not being met. Many of us have learned that it is selfish to have needs, or that we don't deserve to have our needs met. This is simply wrong. We all deserve love and happiness. If these needs are not being met, we do *whatever* it takes, even being unkind or becoming ill, to meet them. For example, Ellen and David have a basically happy marriage. David doesn't seem to hear many of the things Ellen tells him. She begins leaving him notes. Finally she begins to get frustrated and angry, asking him if he is hard of hearing. David asks, "What is wrong with you?" Ellen screams, "I need for you to listen to what I tell you. What I say is important." Suddenly she feels a great release accompanied by tears. Her feelings immediately change when she expresses her need for respect. David is very sorry, not realizing he was not listening.

Recall that Erickson's nursing theory, Modeling and Role Modeling, describes how one of the primary roles of the nurse is to help clients meet their needs. Unmet needs contribute to disease in the bodymind. A client's needs are not met until the *client believes* they are met (Erickson, Tomlin, and Swain, 1983).

All humans have five basic needs according to Dr. William Glaser. These needs are love and belonging, fun, freedom, power or respect (feeling like people listen to us), and survival (Glaser, 1994). Glaser's theory is called control theory because he believes that we must feel like we have control in life so that we can meet our needs. Criticizing someone is the quickest way to make them feel out of control. When we feel out of control our first reaction is usually to become defensive, then angry. If we notice these emotions, it is a signal that one or more of our needs are not met. We can then change our behavior to meet our needs.

We all form a picture in our minds of what our Quality World looks like when all of our needs are met. Your Quality World is made of quality moments. When you notice yourself feeling wonderful, take note. This is a quality moment. Notice what you are thinking, feeling, and doing that created this moment. All of your behaviors are trying to make your world look like the pictures of your Quality World. If your world does not match your internal Quality World, you feel dissatisfied, which leads to depression or anger. To regain a sense of control, you must either replace the pictures in your Quality World with new ones that are attainable, or change aspects of your total behavior to make your external world match your internal view of a Quality World (Figure 10–5).

Often the behaviors we must change are our patterns of communication. Few of us learned how to communicate effectively, especially in situations where we feel fear. There is only love and fear at the bottom of all other emotions. First we feel fear, then hurt, then sadness, then anger, then depression. When we are angry, or depressed, asking "What am I afraid of?" can be very revealing and healing. Very often we are afraid of not being loved.

On a Personal Note

Jonathan and I have been together for 25 years. I am convinced one lesson we are here to learn together is how to communicate our feelings and needs, especially when we are angry and afraid. It took me eight years to become conscious enough in stressful encounters to even know what I was feeling. I would often go unconscious, fall asleep, or "just not hear things." We began learning about communication and consciousness in relationships. After I knew what I was supposed to do, it took another five years to figure out when I should do it. I knew that things went from good to awful in five minutes. Something was happening, but I had no idea what it was.

With intention and effort, I discovered I was afraid to express my feelings and needs. I began forcing myself. The world did not end. Sometimes I'm able to notice the signals telling me that I'm about to go unconscious, and sometimes I don't. I'm getting better though. The more I try, the more I succeed. I always feel a great release of emotion and very often, amazing changes occur.

These questions are helpful in discovering and meeting our needs.

- Are you frequently feeling angry, sad, or fearful?
- What needs are not being met?
- What behaviors are you doing to meet your needs?
- Are they getting the results you want?
- What other behavior can you choose to meet that need?
- What other picture can you choose?
- When I think of these changes, what am I afraid of?

Priceless Thought-Changing Gems for Any Occasion

1. Turn the corners of your mouth up several times a day, especially when you don't feel like smiling. Look at yourself in the mirror, and smile at yourself. It's so ridiculous, even thinking about doing it always makes me laugh. I carry a small mirror with me for emergencies.
2. Get into the habit, especially in stressful situations, of intentionally taking three deep sighs.

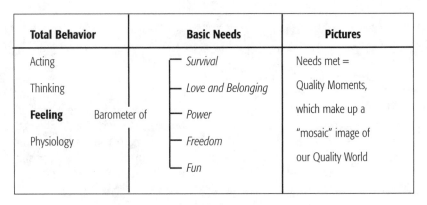

Total Behavior		Basic Needs	Pictures
Acting		⌐ *Survival*	Needs met =
Thinking		⊢ *Love and Belonging*	Quality Moments,
Feeling	Barometer of	⊢ *Power*	which make up a
Physiology		⊢ *Freedom*	"mosaic" image of
		⌐ *Fun*	our Quality World

Figure 10-5   The Three Parts of Control Theory (© 1993 by Jonathan Walker. Used with permission.)

Intentional Internal Maneuvers for Changing Thoughts and Feelings

In the following techniques, we intentionally bring our awareness to the present and use these exercises for change.

TAKING A MOMENT TO BREATHE

In addition to using the breath to help us notice what we are thinking, we can intentionally use it to change our TF. We mention breathing often because it is the most powerful and readily accessible ally we have for creating the world we experience.

Most autonomic nervous system functions of the body, like heart rate and digestion, are not easily under our direct conscious control. The breath, also part of the autonomic nervous system, usually moves automatically, but we can easily become aware of it, and change its speed and depth. The breath is a bridge allowing us to connect our conscious aspect and subconscious aspect (controls body function) to begin the healing process. By directing the exhale to a tight or painful area, we can use the breath to direct our attention to areas of the body that need relaxation and healing.

The movement of breath, through the connections of the olfactory nerve in the nose, affects the pituitary gland, hypothalamus, and limbic system in the brain (Rama, Ballentine, and Hymes, 1990). Remember from Chapter 9 that the pituitary gland affects most of the other glands in the body. The hypothalamus governs the autonomic nervous system, affecting all automatic functions, and changes nervous input from the five senses to chemical output to the body. The limbic system governs memory and emotions. It may be through these connections that breathing affects the stress response, and the health of the body.

During the stress response our breathing changes to shallow chest breathing. If we unintentionally form a habit of this shallow breathing, we continually recreate the stress response. Intellectual activity, fear, anxiety, and depression also lead to shallow breathing. If we are continuously engaged in these activities, we have air deprivation. This habit leads to slower metabolism, decreased immune function, decreased physical energy levels, and a build-up of toxins in the body.

We breathe differently when we are experiencing each emotion. If the feeling is: anger, the inhale is shallow, the exhale is panting; fear, the breath is rapid and shallow; sorrow, the breath is spasmodic and broken; joy, regular inhales and exhales, chest cavity relaxes (Chopra, 1993). **Consciously changing the rate and depth of breathing changes what we are feeling.** When we are relaxed, our breathing is deep and slow from the diaphragm, the muscle under the ribs. The abdomen expands outward with the inhale, and comes in with the exhale. Intentionally breathing in this way helps to lower high blood pressure and relieve stress. Oxygen levels to the body increase. Anxiety, headaches, depression, and muscle tension decrease (Rama, Ballentine, and Hymes, 1990; Davis, Eschelman, and McKay, 1995).

Breathing also creates changes in the amounts and kinds of peptides that are released from the brain. Many of these peptides are endorphins which elevate mood and relieve pain. All peptides can be found in the respiratory system, perhaps explaining why we can intentionally use the breath to affect pain, healing in the body, and experience altered states of consciousness (Pert, 1997). As continual, relaxed breaths encourage the flow of peptides, they also release emotions held in the bodymind. When we find ourselves at an emotional impasse, a few deep breaths can unblock stuck or hidden emotions that we need, and want, to become aware of. I especially use deep sighs in times when I am feeling intense emotion. It is amazing how a few deep breaths bring a sense of calmness, or sometimes, tears of release.

PROGRESSIVE RELAXATION

In *Basic Science in Nursing Arts*, Day (1947) recommends teaching clients progressive muscle relaxation as a measure to help them relax and sleep. "If all other measures fail to induce sleep, the nurse may have to resort to a sedative."

Edmund Jacobson, an American physiologist, first described progressive relaxation in the 1920s. In this technique, we intentionally use our thoughts to become aware of and release muscle tension. You will be amazed at how differently you feel after squishing your face up, and then completely releasing it. When you are finished, your whole body feels tension free. This simple tightening and releasing helps you remember what the muscle feels like to be relaxed. After a little practice, you can learn to quickly mentally scan the body wherever you are, notice areas that are tight, and immediately release the tension. Soon the muscles will get accustomed to being relaxed, and they will get your attention when they become tight.

We discussed using physical cues to help us become aware of our thoughts. We can use tightness or pain in a muscle as a physical cue to bring our awareness to the muscle. Here is an opportunity to notice your thoughts. Are your thoughts contributing to muscle tension? When muscles are tight and constricted, so is the flow of peptides, and so is the easy movement of TF. As the muscles relax, our thoughts begin to move more freely, bringing new, creative ideas to our consciousness. Try tightening and relaxing a tense muscle or two, and notice the difference.

Steps of Progressive Muscle Relaxation

1. Sit or lie in a comfortable position.
2. Focus on your right foot. Move it around a little. As you inhale, tighten the foot. Hold the tightening for three to four seconds, and then relax it with the exhale. You can also focus on your foot and notice if there is any pain or tightness in it. Take five slow, deep breaths in a comfortable rhythm, like deep sighs, and direct your exhale to the foot. As you release the air, release the pain or tension in the foot.
3. Next focus on the right calf. Repeat the steps above.
4. Repeat the steps for the following areas. Right thigh, left foot, left calf, left thigh, right hip, left hip. Abdomen, chest. Lower back, mid back, upper back. Right hand, right arm, left hand, left arm. Right shoulder, left shoulder, neck, face.
5. Now as you are connected with your body, and it is relaxed, begin to take connected, relaxed breaths. Choose whatever pace and depth are comfortable for you. Notice the inhale and exhale. Begin counting your breaths. See if you can reach 10.

IMAGERY

Imagery is intentionally using our TF to create a picture in the mind of what we want to happen, either in the outside world or within the body. Imagery helps you enter your bodymind network. When you create vivid pictures in your mind, the brain and body often can't tell whether the image is created by your thought or whether it is a real situation being perceived with the senses in the outside world. Have you ever began thinking about a food that you love to eat, and started salivating? When you think about standing on the edge of a high cliff, do you get butterflies in your stomach? Our TF let the body know what is expected of it. When we create an image with our thoughts, the body tries to create the appropriate changes that correspond to the image (Siegel, 1986; Pert, 1997).

Sometimes we must hold images of the desired changes in the mind frequently, over a long period of time, to bring about the desired changes. Sometimes, however, imagery creates change in the body instantly. In one study, people were sitting still in a chair and asked to imagine that they were running a marathon. Their heart rate increased, muscles contracted, and they began sweating, as if they were actually running the race. Their body attempted to make internal changes to match the mental image (E. and A. Green, 1977; Brigham and Toal, 1990).

We can use imagery to change our TF to stop the stress response, relax, and create health in the body. With imagery we can decrease heart rate, blood pressure, sleep problems, and the length of labor. Anxiety, fear, chronic muscle tension, pain, and the discomfort of childbirth can be reduced. Blood flow, gastric processes, and temperature can be controlled. Use of imagery can speed healing and recovery from surgery, injury, or skin conditions such as warts and psoriasis (Sobel and Ornstein, 1996). For other bodymind benefits, see Figure 10-6.

Giedt (1997) discusses imagery as an independent nursing intervention. She suggests that mental images may be the true language of the body. Many aspects of immune function, such as natural killer cells, Salivary IgA, and lymphocyte function, can be enhanced with relaxation and imagery in people with no disease process, and in people with cancer. Nurses can guide a client, describing a relaxing situation, as the client forms the image in his mind. Nurses can also teach the client to use imagery on his own to create physiologic and psychological changes. Giedt also makes excellent suggestions describing how the nurse can conduct research using imagery.

Client Population	Benefits
New, first time mothers	Decreased anxiety and depression during first four weeks after birth (Rees, 1995)
Terminal cancer	Increased life expectancies (LeShan, 1994; Cousins, 1989; Achterberg, 1985; Simonton, 1978)
Nursing home residents	Improved immune function (Kiecolt-Glaser, Glaser, and Willinger, 1985)
Clients waiting to have colon surgery	Less anxiety before surgery, afer surgery–less pain medication, bowel function returned faster, slept better (Tusek, et al., 1997)

Figure 10-6 Bodymind Benefits of Imagery.

Using Imagery in Nursing

I work in outpatient surgery. One day Mr. B was my patient and I was preparing him for surgery and asking him if he had any questions. He was very afraid and didn't want to go. I told him I had taken a class where I learned that imagery can help people relax and asked if he'd like to try some. He said, "Sure, anything." I asked him to go to his favorite place, a place where he felt safe and comfortable. He told me about the flowers, the trees, the weather, the road, the location, and the breeze near the lake he was imaging. I handed him a pencil and said, "Take this to surgery and when you feel afraid, hold it and think of this moment." Mr. B came through surgery just fine. Later he found me and said, "You know I never would have believed it but that pencil helped me remember my safe place. I wasn't afraid." He still comes to see me.

Lou, R.N. for 35 years

How to Do It

There are many ways to practice imagery. Some people set aside a special time each day to practice. They: (1) Find a time when they will not be disturbed for at least 10 minutes. (2) Sit or lie in a comfortable position. (3) Practice progressive relaxation as previously described to relax the tension in the body. (4) Notice the breath, observing the inhale and exhale. (5) Then begin whatever type of imagery they want to use. **Imagery is most effective when we include all five senses, plus movement and feeling.** We often need to repeat the images frequently. Right before falling asleep is a very good time to use imagery because the active mind is turning off, and the subconscious mind takes the image to work on it. How many of us watch the news or television before bed? Choose with care what you program into your mind right before bed.

Some people listen to a tape of guided imagery where you picture in your mind what the person is describing on the tape. Some people practice their imagery as they are driving in the car, exercising, cooking, or anytime there are a few spare moments. The eyes do not have to be closed. In the beginning some people use a photo to help them firmly establish what they want to image. You can make a collage of magazine photos and put it on the refrigerator. Once you get used to doing it, imagery can be practiced anytime and anywhere.

The image does not have to be realistic. For example, some people with cancer imagine the cells of the immune system to be sharks swimming around and eating the cancer cells, or a knight destroying them with a sword. If there is pain, a cool, calm river can flow through the body, washing the pain away. For the healing of a cut, a shoe is laced up tight. For depression, a strong, warm sun breaks through the dark clouds. An image I find works great in my massage practice when someone has a tight area is to tell them to imagine it as an ice cube. As they take each breath, they imagine the exhale is melting the ice into a warm puddle.

Two types of imagery are: (1) Process imagery—picturing the steps unfolding that will lead to what you want. (2) End result imagery—picturing your goal, what you want, already happened. The two can be combined. For example, if you want a particular job, process imaging is seeing yourself doing all the steps necessary to prepare you to do this job well, whether physically, mentally, or emotionally. End result is imaging yourself doing that job. See Figure 10-7 for suggested ways to practice imagery.

In the safe place mentioned in Figure 10-7, you can invite your inner-self, advisor, a teacher, or Higher Power to visit you. There are many forms an advisor can take. If you are not comfortable with the form that comes, send it away and ask for another. You might ask for understanding and/or advice, or what you might do to create healing. You can ask for the best way to change a behavior or heal a relationship. The answer often comes very quickly. It may come in words, pictures, or sounds.

When I want to relax, I'm in a hammock between two palm trees on the beach south of Tuulum in the Caribbean. I'm in the shade, sipping a cool beverage, the breeze is blowing, and the waves lull me into Ga-Ga land.

Situation	Suggestion	Benefit
Upcoming stressful situation	Rehearse it in detail in your mind, what you want to say, in the situation where you will be	Creates confidence and control in the actual situation, helps realize potential pitfalls
Pain	Imagine muscles becoming soft, flexible, and moving easily; see self enjoying riding in a car without pain; see self easily doing an activity if can't do it now	Less fear of movement, confidence, grater flexibility and less pain
Disease or less than normal function of area of the body	Get an anatomical picture of the area in a perfect state and put it in a visible spot, imagine that part of your body looking like that and performing its function perfectly; focus your attention on the area, send it energy or light and ask it what message it has for you	Engages the body's internal healing systems to bring about the changes you envision, gives feeling of control and input to the healing process
Stress, fear, anxiety, confusion	Imagine yourself in a safe place, one you've been to or one you create in your mind, include all 5 senses	Comfort, security, control, relaxation, peace, a place to return to away from the chaos of life

Figure 10-7 Ways to Use Imagery.

MEDITATION

The purpose of most meditation is to interrupt the random flow of thoughts that we typically have, and intentionally focus the mind. It is the mind's job to think, analyze, and organize, so we must give it something to focus on. Some forms of meditation help us focus our attention on what we are doing in the present moment. Other forms focus on the repetition of a word, phrase, or behavior. Meditation helps us remember that we direct the mind. The mind is not designed to control us.

There are many kinds of meditation including the Relaxation Response, Mindfulness Meditation, and meditation practices of different spiritual traditions. We have found that meditating for even 5 minutes provides a break from the hectic TF of life. Meditation can be as simple as sitting in a chair, setting a timer for five minutes, and letting yourself think only of things and places you love. This interrupts thoughts that may be producing a stress response, gives the body a break, and gives you an opportunity to choose different thoughts. When the stress response is halted, the peptides reestablish their natural, harmonic flow that encourages health. In this time of inner stillness, we can closely observe our thoughts, and very quickly become conscious of our feelings.

Relaxation Response

The Relaxation Response can be easily learned, practiced, and taught, and brings about many beneficial effects in the bodymind. Herbert Benson, M.D., is a pioneer in the study of the connection between the mind, body, and spirit. His interest in this area began in the late 1960s when some of his students who practiced Transcendental Meditation invited him to observe their physiology as they meditated. He hooked them up to equipment and made a groundbreaking discovery. Their blood pressures and heart rates dropped, and then returned to normal when the meditation was over. By consciously altering their mental state, they altered their physiology.

By 1975, Benson had developed the Relaxation Response and began researching its effects. He found that regular practice of this technique could reverse the stress response as well as having myriad beneficial effects on the bodymind. A prominent feature of the technique is that it decreases the body's need for oxygen, allowing all systems of the body to slow down and rest (Benson, 1996).

The Relaxation Response is now taught and researched at the Mind/Body Medical Institute at Harvard Medical School in Boston by Dr. Benson and his colleagues. A similar program has been started at the Memorial Herman Healthcare System in Houston, Texas. Institutions can receive training and become affiliates of the Harvard Mind/Body Institute.

The above results were achieved by practicing the Relaxation Response for 10 minutes, twice a day. It is very simple, there are no harmful side effects, and the

Benefits of the Relaxation Response

Decrease to normal, or eliminate
infertility
pain
muscle tension
insomnia
side effects of treatment for cancer and
    AIDS
cardiac arrhythmias
blood pressure
cholesterol
breathing rate
heart rate
anger
hostility
anxiety
depression
drug, alcohol, and cigarette abuse

Increases to normal
restfulness
concentration
immune function
ability to cope with stressors
alpha brain waves (associated with
    creativity and meditation)
feelings of well-being and hopefulness

benefits are widespread. Benson does not recommend setting a timer. For myself, I found that at first my mind would not allow me to take the time unless it could be assured that I would not "waste too much time" and go over my 10 minutes. So, I set a timer. It took a month of constantly bringing my attention back to my repetition before I began noticing that the thought train had slowed down and sometimes come to a halt. I began experiencing the space between thoughts.

Relaxation Response

1. The **repetition** of a word, sound, phrase, or simple activity chosen by the individual. If the person cannot be still and close their eyes, a repeated muscular activity such as knitting or focusing on the feet hitting the ground when walking, will work.
2. When, or if, you find yourself thinking about something else, **bring your attention back** to the repetition.

Mindfulness Meditation
1. Focus on your breath to bring you to the present moment.
2. When a thought comes into the mind, observe it.
3. Simply notice any feeling associated with the thought.
4. Then, bring the attention back to the breath.

The Relaxation Response is very simple, yet very powerful. Many people find a quiet place, close their eyes, and sit in a comfortable position. They focus on the breath, noticing the inhale and exhale, not forcing it. These steps are helpful, but not necessary.

Mindfulness Meditation

Jon Kabat-Zinn has taught Mindfulness Meditation for 13 years at the University of Massachusetts Medical Center's Stress Reduction Clinic. People report a decrease in anger, hostility, depression, and medical symptoms, regardless of diagnosis. It can reduce pain and improve mood, helping people live in the present moment rather in the fear that they will never be free of pain. In a study of people with psoriasis of the skin, those who listened to a tape of someone guiding them in doing Mindfulness Meditation had a clearing of skin lesions 30–40 days sooner than those who did not listen to the tapes (Kabat-Zinn, et al., 1998).

Mindfulness Meditation can be done while sitting, or performing any activity of daily life. This technique is relaxing, interrupts the stress response, and so changes our TF. It helps to train us to be conscious in the presence of our TF, whatever they may be (Kabat-Zinn, 1993).

FREEZE FRAME

Freeze Frame (FF) is a very effective technique that is designed to be used *during* a stressful situation to help us become aware of our thoughts and choose a new response (Childre, 1994). It combines breathing, imagery, and consciously choosing our feelings. When practicing FF we "freeze" the current scenario and shift our focus of attention away from it for a few seconds. This can be done during a conversation while someone is talking to you. First of all you must recognize that you are having a stressful feeling. Then, focus on the heart area and remember and reexperience a specific time when you felt a positive, fun feeling. This shift interrupts the mental and physical aspects of the stress response in the moment that it is happening. Return your focus to the current situation and ask your heart for the most efficient response to the situation. Focusing on heart-centered feelings allows you to have a different perspective of the situation, and so choose a more effective action.

When FF is practiced regularly, immune system function increases (Rein, Atkinson, and McCraty, 1995), anxiety decreases (Rozman, et al., 1994), heart rhythms improve, the autonomic nervous system comes into balance, and blood pressure decreases (McCraty, et al., 1995; Tiller, McCraty and Atkinson, 1996). These studies are described in greater detail in Chapter 12.

At Motorola, administrative staff, engineers, and factory workers participated in a study for six months using FF. At the end of the study, the 28% who were hypertensive had normal blood pressures, there was a 26% reduction in burnout, and a 36% reduction in physical stress symptoms. Participants said that they felt less anxious (18%) and hostile (20%), and more empowered (93%) and content (32%) (Barrios-Choplin, McCraty, and Cryer, 1997).

CHANGING FROM A PESSIMISTIC TO OPTIMISTIC EXPLANATORY STYLE

Explanatory style is what we tell ourselves about, or how we explain, what happens in our world. Changing the way you explain what happens in the world changes your feelings, and so what you experience (Seligman, 1990). Recall from Chapter 9 that a pessimistic explanatory style can lead to poor health and less success at work and relationships. People who are helpless typically have a pessimistic way of explaining what happens to them, meaning (1) they see bad things that happen as permanent, (2) pervasive-affecting all things in life, and (3) that they are their fault. For example, if they drop a glass on the floor, they think, "I can't believe I'm so stupid. I can't do anything right." A group of researchers at the Mayo Clinic found that when people had explained the world in a pessimistic way for 30 years of their life, they had a significantly increased risk of early death (Muruta, et al., 2000).

With an optimistic way of viewing life, when a bad thing happens, we tell ourselves, "It will be over soon. It's only this one situation, and accidents happen." Bad events are explained as (1) temporary, (2) specific to the event, and (3) not usually our fault. We learn each of these styles of explaining what happens in the world when we are children from listening to how people close to us explain the world. To see what your explanatory style is, listen to what you tell yourself when bad, and good, things happen. For examples, see Figure 10-8.

To adopt an optimistic explanatory style, change what you tell yourself to reflect that most bad events are temporary, only affect a very small part of your life, and are usually not your fault. Replace thoughts of constant worry with helpful thoughts that are realistic and help you enjoy life. When you look in your heart at your view of life, is there a Yes or No?

A SHIFT OF PERSPECTIVE

Stepping Outside the Box

Sometimes, to get a new perspective we must take a step outside of our comfortable box of what we think we like, and who we think we are. This can sometimes be done by moving our physical body. Moving across the room to a different chair, in a different light, allows us to contemplate a problem in a new way. Moving outside to a beautiful spot brings amazing insights. Without changing our physical position, we can travel on the inside, stepping, and sometimes

When Bad Things Happen

Pessimistic	Optimistic
Permanent	*Temporary*
I'm always exhausted.	I didn't get enough sleep last night.
We never have any fun.	We haven't made time for fun things lately.
Pervasive	*Specific*
I'm so stupid.	I'm not very good at math.
I'm a terrible nurse.	I'm better at home health nursing than hospital
TV is useless.	nursing.
	This TV show is useless.
Personal	
It's all my fault.	*External*
I'm not a good nurse.	Everyone involved played a part.
	I was given too many patients to care for.

When Good Things Happen

Pessimistic	Optimistic
Temporary	*Permanent*
I was lucky this time.	I always do well at tennis.
This weather won't last long.	We have great weather here.
Specific	*Pervasive*
I look OK when I get dressed up.	I look great.
She speaks well to a small group.	She is a good speaker.
External	*Personal*
The lighting in this picture was good.	I take good pictures.
It was an easy recipe.	Thank you. I enjoyed making it.

Figure 10-8 Optimistic and Pessimistic Explanatory Styles.

jumping outside of our thought boxes. We move to a new point from which to view. For example, from the point of view of being in an airplane, a big city looks like tiny lights. From another view, people are having coffee and cleaning floors.

When we feel stressed and overwhelmed, we often don't know where to begin to find a new view. We can guide the mind with a few questions to lead us out of the box (See Figure 10-9).

When a situation looks really bad, it is helpful to ask yourself, "What is the worst thing that could happen?" If it did, what would you do? We often discover that the worst thing would not really be that bad.

A New View

Do I want to leave the situation?

Yes   No

Do it.   Can I change the situation?

                Yes   No

                How?   1. How can I look at it differently

                Do it   2. What actions or behaviors can I add to my

                                 life to meet my needs?

Copyright Marsha Walker, 1996

Figure 10-9 Finding A New View (© 1996 by Marsha Walker. Used with permission.)

> *Refrigerator wisdom:*
> We must welcome the night. It is only then that we see the stars.

Have you ever found yourself thinking, "I really don't like my job, but I can't quit." Our sister Diana was an EKG technician at a large hospital in Houston, Texas. She and her husband owned a home, had large bills, and much stress. They worked different shifts, and their lives were quickly headed downhill. They stepped out of their box. They quit their jobs, moved to a small town in central Texas by a lake. She has always loved dogs, and so decided to learn dog grooming. Now she has her own business and is very happy and spiritually fulfilled. She says dogs are so much more fun than people.

> *Refrigerator wisdom*
> A deadend is just a place to turn around.

One day when Eli was five we were walking through a parking lot. He exclaimed "Look at that angel!" "Where?!" I practically yelled. He pointed to the back of a Toyota van. To Eli's eyes, the Toyota insignia was an angel. When I viewed the car through his eyes, I could see the angels, too. It made me wonder how many other angels I could see with eyes that don't have a box.

Seeing with New Eyes

Have you ever heard or read a word or phrase that opened up a whole new view? These moments often slip by unnoticed. If we begin to watch for them, they seem to happen more and more.

One day we were talking to our friend, Scott, about how rough our day had been. He said, "It's just Life." Now when it seems that another stressful event simply

Take a moment and try this exercise, if you have a situation you want to change.
1. Imagine a situation in your life that you really want to be different, but you believe it is impossible.

Now, suppose a miracle occurred, and the changes you had wished for actually happened.

What would this situation look like?
How do you feel?
2. What would my job, body, relationship, etc. look like if I could have fun being in it?

Imagine the scenario and how you feel.
What things would have to change to make it this way?
What actions can I take that would cause these changes?
What's keeping me from doing these things?

could not happen in one day, we look at each other, shrug, and say, "Life." The multicolored tapestry of it all. One day I was driving in the traffic and found myself repeatedly saying, life, life, life, li, feli feli fly fly, fly. At the moment I began to fly, I stepped out of my thought box. What if Life is a game that we play to learn. To enter a body, we must agree to forget everything we know about who we are, and how the universe really works. In the first five years of life, we are taught that all things are separate, discrete entities. We must believe this to learn our lessons and truly enjoy the 3D amusement park that is life, with all the tastes, touches, sights, smells, and sounds. Without 3D bodies you can't enjoy a chocolate malt in quite the same way. Yet, these delights have a way of filling all our thoughts if we aren't careful, becoming our whole world, as the rides in an amusement park create the illusion that they are real. As we grow, we feel an inner urge, a knowing that there is something more. This knowing brings us full circle, remembering that all is connected, and love is all that is real. Wouldn't this be quite an amazing game?

Some of these shifts are so abrupt and transforming that we can't ignore them. A hole is poked in our old view, and light comes streaming in. According to Avram Goldstein, a pioneer in PNI, there is a sudden release of endorphins that flood the brain during the ahh-hah or thrill.

One night we were sitting in Dirty Nelly's, a wonderful Irish pub on the river walk in San Antonio, Texas. They serve pints of great dark beer, unlimited peanuts, and you can throw your peanut shells on the floor. All of a sudden a voice from within said, "Just this one lifetime, can you trust? Can you trust that if you help people and have fun, you will be fine?" I felt like I had been shocked. I had never thought of the idea of not having to worry about a retirement account, a house payment, or future career decisions. What if I did trust? It opened up a whole new world of possibilities I am still contemplating.

Have you ever sat around with friends, and each person describes in how ever much detail they want, what they would do if they won the lotto? Eyes glitter and begin looking at new horizons.

Some movies create the ahh-hah shift. Movies are very powerful because they suspend the everyday thinking mind, allowing their message to affect the subconscious mind. They also stimulate the entire PNI network. A few of these movies are *What Dreams May Come,* the *Star Wars* series, *Thirteenth Floor, Sliding Door, The Truman Show,* and *Matrix.*

Thrill gives a new view of the world. If you find yourself wondering where the thrill has gone in your life, try getting eight or nine hours of sleep for a few days in a row. When we don't get quite enough sleep, all we can do is maintain. We don't have the energy to notice the exquisite beauty of the rainbow on the soap bubble or the light playing on the leaves. Thrill comes from feeling the dance in all things. Our dog, Jasper, sometimes races through the house at top speed, in and out and through the rooms. You can tell by his face, it is purely for the thrill of it. When Eli was three, he came running into the house screaming, "Hurry! Hurry! Come look." I ran outside. He pointed to a pill bug rolled up in a ball. Child eyes see wonders and feel the thrill in everything.

Getting in Touch with Thrill

1. What have you experienced lately that was so exciting that you just couldn't wait to tell someone?
2. What is it that you love about vacation?
3. What is so much fun, that just thinking about it is thrilling?

Why does a snail who has all he needs on the ground and carries his home around on his back, take the time and energy to crawl up a flight of stairs to our deck? Why would he then crawl up the legs of the table to sit on the railing? Perhaps in the world of snails, as in the world of humans, there are those who in their own small ways, step out of the box and do something, just for the thrill of it.

Every time we move outside our box, the mosaic of who we are and who we can become is enriched.

SUMMARY

The ultimate source of happiness is in our mental attitude. Even if you have good health, material facilities used in the proper way, and good relations with other human beings, the main cause of a happy life is within. Anything and everything is a possible cause of frustration and unhappiness. This leaves us with only one option: to change our own attitude.
                                                            —*the Dalai Lama (1998)*

The techniques suggested in this chapter are some we have used in our own lives. With lots of intention and work, we are beginning to notice what we think and feel, even during the tough times. We are frequently able to choose responses that are different from our past, patterned reactions, ones that are heartfelt and caring. Even if we fail, the more we try, the more we succeed. Every time we are able to make that leap, choose something new, it is thrilling. There is hope.

If you practice these techniques, you will realize you are not your TF. You will begin to connect with who you are on the inside. As we connect with our own heart, we prepare the way to connect with others.

In these last two chapters, we have learned how to use our TF to create desired connections within our own body to aid physical healing. These techniques also help us create a mental landscape that allows us to begin to experience the reality we want. Choosing our TF during a massage creates a relaxed, balanced state in our own bodymind that enables us to give the best massage we can. In addition to creating connection within ourselves, massage acts as a bridge for connecting with another. In the following chapters we explore connection with others. In Chapter 1 we discussed touch, both physical and nonphysical, as ways of connecting. We now continue our discussion of nonphysical touching by exploring energy, the human energy field, and healing. Knowledge of the human energy system helps us understand how we can connect with others energetically using our hands and our TF, enhancing the massage we give.

PUTTING THESE IDEAS INTO PRACTICE

1. Describe one personal situation in which you often go "unconscious," and what new responses you want to choose.

2. Recall a time when you stepped out of the box and describe the new view you saw.

3. Create a plan for your client population to help them with stress producing TF, choosing from the techniques in this chapter.

CHAPTER 11

The Energy Field, Spirituality, and Connection

A human being is a part of the whole, called by us "Universe;" a part limited in time and space. He experiences himself, his thoughts, and feelings as something separated from the rest—a kind of optical delusion of consciousness. This delusion is a kind of prison for us, restricting us to our personal desires and to affection for a few persons nearest us. Our task must be to free ourselves from this prison by widening our circle of compassion to embrace all living creatures and the whole of nature in its beauty.

—Albert Einstein

OBJECTIVES

1. Describe three characteristics of the human energy field.

2. Discuss four ways in which our thoughts and feelings affect our energy field.

3. Discuss the reasons why using light, color, sound, and music increases the healing potential of massage.

4. Explain how addressing the energy field during a massage increases the quality of the connection between giver and receiver.

5. Discuss three characteristics of our world that suggest our connectedness to each other and a Higher Power.

6. Discuss four health benefits of including spirituality in one's life.

7. Describe four techniques for increasing our awareness of our connection with Spirit.

The chapter on PNI looked at how our thoughts and feelings (TF) create connections within our bodies. These connections contribute to stress or relaxation. As we give a massage, the state of our bodymind conveys these messages to the receiver, affecting their experience of the massage. In this chapter we begin to explore another way we can use our TF to connect with others. TF are forms of energy. This chapter discusses energy, the individual human energy field, and the energy field that connects us all. We begin to see how our TF affect our own energy field and so the fields of others.

Why do we include this topic in a book about massage? Most importantly, when we work closely with people, whether giving a massage or any other nursing intervention, the energy fields of giver and receiver are constantly interacting, affecting each other. Using our TF to intentionally direct that interaction greatly benefits the healing of both. Secondly, we introduce several energy-based therapies that enhance the massage experience and can also be used as independent interventions. We briefly discuss how we can use our hands to assist the energy field of another, and our own, to come into balance. Helping the energy to resume its natural flow helps the muscles release tension. Learning to detect imbalances in the client's energy field can direct us to where they need massage the most. Light and sound, both being forms of energy, will also be discussed briefly as additional tools to increase the healing potential of massage.

After learning about individual field interaction, we turn to the energy field that connects us all. This exploration of connection leads to a discussion of spirituality and its relationship to massage and healing. Learning about the energy field as a medium for connection also provides foundational information for practicing steps two and three of HeartTouch (Chapter 12).

In the beginning of nursing, Florence Nightingale included spirituality and Higher Power in nursing and healing. Nursing has embraced energy field interaction since the 1970s when Martha Rogers, one of the first nursing theorists, proposed her Science of Unitary Man (now Human Beings) to describe and predict nurse/client interaction for healing. Todaro-Franceschi (2001) discussed energy as a bridging concept for nursing science comparing the views of Nightingale, Levine, and Rogers. Also in the early 1970s, Dolores Krieger, Ph.D., R.N. and Dora Kunz founded Therapeutic Touch (TT), a technique teaching nurses to detect and balance the energy field of the body. Over the last 30 years, many nurses have conducted research exploring the theory and practice of therapeutic touch in a variety of nursing settings (Wilson, 1995; Madrid and Winstead-Fry, 2001).

EVERYTHING IS AN ENERGY EVENT

The following pages summarize a few principles in physics to help us understand what energy and energy fields are, and how fields interact. If these ideas interest you, see Appendix B for a more detailed discussion.

We, and all things in the universe, are made of atoms which are made of subatomic particles. Subatomic particles are constantly moving. Each subatomic particle has either a positive, negative, or neutral charge. Each moving charge produces a vibrating field around it. This field produces a force that affects any other particle, or field, near it. All of the chemical reactions in our bodies that are necessary for healthy functioning happen through the interactions of subatomic particles and their energy fields. When a charge moves through a mass, a moving field is produced around it. We are a mass, our nervous system is a constantly moving charge, and so we have a moving field around us.

The equation most of us have seen, $E=mc^2$, means that energy and matter continually transform into each other at very high speeds. Subatomic particles constantly travel at very high speeds, so all matter, including us, has a physical aspect and an energetic aspect. We are, at the same time, individuals interacting, and fields of energy interacting.

In physics, the Law of Resonance states that any vibrating body is affected by all forms of vibration. Since we are made of vibrating subatomic particles/energy packets, we are affected by forms of vibration such as light, sound, and the healing energy from the hands. Thoughts and feelings are also vibrations with which we affect our own bodies, others, and the world.

Physics also tells us that because of our energetic nature and that of all things in the universe, there really are no separate entities. Instead of focusing on separate individuals, the focus is on interactions. The theory of interconnectedness tells us that once two individuals, whether subatomic particles or humans, have established a connection, they are connected energetically for a long time. We are all part of an interconnected network of interaction.

The uncertainty principle says that we choose the reality we experience by what we choose to focus on. When we select one point of view, we immediately eliminate many other possible realities that we could create for ourselves. We literally change the world by how we look at it, and what we tell ourselves about it.

Have you noticed that the passage of time, whether it seems long or short, depends on what you are thinking. Five minutes waiting for an ambulance to arrive seems like forever. Five minutes doing your most favorite thing goes by in a flash. Reality changes according to what we focus on. Time is created by one thought following another. The more thoughts we have, the faster time seems to go. The fewer thoughts, the slower time passes. Between thoughts, when there is no thought, there is no time. There is only experience, or being. When we are just experiencing, time is irrelevant. When we again look at a clock, many hours may have passed, or just a few minutes. Reality changes with a shift of our focus of attention.

Have you ever called someone dear to you on the phone, and they say, "I was just going to call you"? Have you noticed two dogs staring at each other, and jump up at the exact same second and begin to play? Have you ever seen a cat watching something up in the "air" that is invisible to our eyes? There is much more to our world than most of us have been taught. We are much more than a three-dimensional body. We are all connected in deep and profound ways that we are just beginning to realize. Of course plants and animals think we are a little slow catching on because they have always known about energetic connection, and use it to communicate every day.

From the study of physics and subatomic particles, we learn that it is our nature to continually connect, and it is our nature to continually transform, moving to fully experience our true self.

We may therefore regard matter as being constituted by the regions of space in which the field is extremely intense . . . There is no place in this new kind of physics both for the field and matter, for the field is the only reality.

—Albert Einstein

Matter, which is you and me and all three-dimensional things, are regions where the field is extremely intense. We are beings of energy.

THE INDIVIDUAL ENERGY FIELD

Our adventure as an energy being is similar to a long distance commute home on the freeway. The weather is great, the traffic is flowing along smoothly. Your thoughts wander to many different things. Before you know it, you are half-way home. Space and time seem to have been altered by where you focus your attention.

You entered a state of flow. You are part of a larger movement, the traffic all moving together down the road. Suddenly someone passes you, and you notice thick, black smoke billowing out of the tailpipe. Your full attention becomes riveted on the person in the car. They won't look at you. Finally, you honk and signal them to the side of the road. You both get out and run for cover. You take them to the nearest phone, and stay until help arrives. After exchanging phone numbers, you hug good-bye. You again enter the flow of traffic. After awhile, you are back in your thoughts. You have always been on your way home. You just decided to stop for a detour to interact, communicate, and help.

Each person is a particular energy pattern, a unique condensation in the flow of the constantly moving universal energy field. There is no time or space, only movement and consciousness. When we decide to focus more and more on an individual interaction, we manifest a physical body to experience a particular kind of very important interaction with others who have done the same thing. The more we focus on the individualness, the more that is all that fills our awareness. We begin to believe we are the body, and others are separate. After some heartache, joy, service, and love we move once again back into the universal field, and become one unique pattern, moving and flowing. We chose an adventure for a while, as we chose to stop and help the person with car trouble. Just as the traffic was still moving by, we are always one with the field, and we are still on our way home.

We are now going to focus on the individual energy field while always remembering that as we are individuals in one moment of focus, we are part of an interconnected energy network in the next. In our nursing practice, in massage, and in our lives, we are constantly affecting and being affected by the energy fields of others, if we can even speak of "others." To encourage healing as much as possible we need to know a little about how the individual energy field works and how we can intentionally affect it for healing. Plants, animals, and people all have individual fields, and in this way we can communicate with and help each other.

Plants

In the 1940s Semyon and Valentina Kirlian discovered Kirlian photography. They built a very unique type of photographic equipment which detects a glowing, or luminescence, that is emitted by, and surrounds all living things. They could take two leaves that looked exactly alike and tell which one was diseased because the field around it was dimmer. When a corner of a leaf was removed, the glowing outline, or field, remained in the same shape as if the leaf was still there.

In Tompkins and Bird's (1973) well-documented book, *The Secret Life of Plants,* you learn that plants are connected to humans and all living cells through their energy field. Your life will never be the same once you read it. One of many fascinating accounts describes the experiences of Cleve Backster, America's foremost lie detector examiner in 1966. He was an expert at reading lie detector machines, interpreting the graph made by the machine to determine people's emotions. One day he decided to attach the electrodes to a plant in his office to see if it responded to water being poured on its roots. The needle began to jump, creating a graph very similar to the ones produced when people felt emotions. He then decided to burn the leaf that had the electrodes attached. As soon as he got the picture of a flame in his head, *before he even moved to get a match*, the plant started causing the graph to go crazy. He had discovered that plants can tell what people are thinking and feeling, and that they have emotions! Plants are very sensitive to the touch, thoughts, and feelings of people, animals, and other plants. Plants can't reach out with their arms so they touch us with their energy.

Even though we have felt a disturbance in the energy field of a plant that was injured, we had no idea that plants consciously choose their feelings and care about the well-being of people. If they can affect electromagnetic equipment to create a desired effect, I wonder what kind of effect they could have on our world, if they took a mind to. We may be sustained by plants in many ways much more important than the sustenance of the physical body. Adding plants to our homes and healthcare settings may encourage healing more than we realize.

Animals

In the 1940s, Harold Burr, physician and anatomist at Yale University, found that all living beings, even cells, have electromagnetic fields around them just as particles do in physics. Cancer could be detected by changes in the field before any clinical signs were observed (Burr, 1972). Kirlian photography shows an energy field around roaches, lizards, and all living things. These photographs show that before the body becomes ill, it begins to increase the energy flowing through it, especially to the affected areas. If the increase is not enough to restore health, changes in the energy field begin to occur, such as dimness and breaks in the field. Doesn't this seem like an inexpensive, non-invasive way to detect the very beginning of imbalance so we can prevent illness from developing?

Several articles in the magazine, *Dog World* in 1992 and 1993, discussed the use of acupuncture by veterinarians. After giving a dog an acupuncture treatment, the vet took Kirlian photographs of the dog's paw print, and saw an increased energy flow which led to increased health. One veterinarian found that after the dog received acupuncture and his energy level rose, the dog would transmit some of his energy back to his owner by touching him. They found that in people and dogs, the giving and receiving of energy was often done by touching.

In many cities, animal therapists (accompanied by their person) visit hospitals and nursing homes. Friedman and Thomas (1995) reported that pets improved the health of people with heart disease and increased their chances of survival after surgery. Our experience of the healing power of animals is mostly with dogs. One day I decided to sit on the floor with our dog, Sophie, for as long as she wanted me to. When she saw I was not getting up, she curled into a ball in between my legs with her head on one leg and her back along the other one. She took a deep breath and let her body sink into mine. I began to feel a strong, warm energy permeate by body. With my hands and legs touching her, it was like she was giving me an energy treatment. Finally, after about 15 minutes, the energy stopped, she looked at me, and got up and walked away. I felt extremely blessed.

All of us who have had the honor of being loved and trusted by an animal, know that they are truly a gift. Sharing a home with them is a rare treat if we open our eyes and see who they are, and open our hearts and let them in. It's hard for almost anyone to stay in a bad mood around a wagging tail or a purring little motor. They teach us about living in the moment, play, patience, forgiveness, and unconditional love.

The Human Energy Field

Jonathan's mother had her leg amputated at the knee. She would complain that the foot that was gone still hurt. He gave the phantom foot a massage, rubbing the area in space where the foot would have been. She said it relieved the pain. I'm sure some of your clients have told you about their phantom pain. Perhaps he was helping to balance the energy field that was still there.

Instead of a person being a body surrounded by an energy field, we are energy fields of varying frequencies. For example, if you take steam and cool it (slow its vibrational frequency), you get a more "solid" form, water. If you continue to lower the vibrational frequency, you get ice. So it is with us. The aspect of us that vibrates at the highest frequency is our spirit, or essence. As the vibrations slow down, we have the energy field, and slower still is the physical body. Disease in the body is a lower vibration still, being more constricted and condensed. It is all vibration.

We can increase our vibrational frequency through TF of love and happiness, touching, meditation, and prayer. Eating healthy food, breathing clean air, drinking pure water, and relaxing in nature raises our vibration. Sometimes changing our vibration creates healing in the body and sometimes it does not. Each soul has a purpose, lessons to learn. We do not know what they are for another. Most of us are only just learning to go inside and listen to what our own lessons are. If healing of the physical body is not in the plan, balancing of the field can help to raise the spirit in the heart and mind.

HOW DO WE KNOW THE HUMAN ENERGY FIELD EXISTS?

The human energy field can be detected by Kirlian photography. You may have seen a picture of an aura, or the colors of the energy field around a person's body. Remember, this is a snapshot of just that one moment. Our TF change the vibrations, and so the colors, in our energy field from moment to moment. I once had the opportunity to place my fingertips on a Kirlian device. Figure 11-1 is a photo showing the energy coming from my fingertips with no particular intent or thoughts in mind.

One way of knowing its existence is through the description of people such as Dora Kunz (1991) and Rosalyn Bruyere (1994) who can see the field and how it changes as we feel and think. There are techniques to learn to see the field if you are interested (Brennan, 1987). You can learn to feel the field yourself, and experience it firsthand by learning Therapeutic Touch, Healing Touch, or other energy-

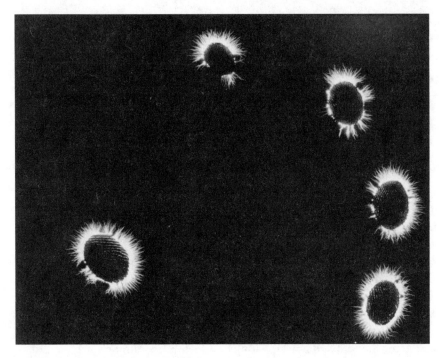

Figure 11-1 Kirlian photograph of the energy field around finger tips.

based therapies. Another way to decide whether the field exists is to read about it. Richard Gerber, M.D. (1988) offers an excellent account of energy fields, chakras, and many kinds of energy healing, with impressive research.

Dr. Valerie Hunt has taught at Columbia University and UCLA and has done ground-breaking biomedical research on the human energy field (Hunt, 1995; Bruyere, 1994). In the 1970s, she received a grant to study Rolfing, a type of deep tissue bodywork. She placed EMG electrodes on the body of subjects and connected them to recording machines. Regular, high frequency electrical energy patterns were emitted by the energy field that had never been recorded and were not muscle, nerve, heart, or brain waves. Rosalyn Bruyere, founder of the Healing Light Center in California, was asked to observe the energy field as the subjects were Rolfed. She was unaware of what was being recorded in the observation booth by the computers. As Bruyere reported changes in the field, the machines were recording exactly what she reported. Each color had its unique wave pattern. When she saw orange in the field, the frequencies recorded were of red and yellow, which combine to make orange. Different emotions felt by the giver or receiver created wave patterns in their field that corresponded to the wave pattern of certain colors. Love caused the field to turn pink, some red frequency mixed with white.

All changes that took place in the body seemed to take place first in the field, including changes in blood pressure and heart rate. The giver and receiver's fields interacted throughout the session. Hunt believes that these same field interactions occur in all successful bodywork sessions, including massage. By the end of the session, many of the patterns in the giver's and receiver's fields were the same. This study suggests the importance of our TF when touching a client in massage, or any other nursing intervention, since what we think and feel creates patterns in our field.

WHAT IS THE FIELD LIKE?

Different "experts" describe the field in different ways, depending on how they see it. Since it is all energy, always moving and changing, and is influenced by our TF, each individual perceives the field somewhat differently. People who see the field agree that:

1. There is a field.
2. It has areas of different frequencies within it.
3. It is always moving.
4. It has many colors.
5. It has chakras (spinning wheels of energy).
6. It is affected by TF.
7. We can affect it with our hands.

A book we found very helpful was *The Personal Aura* by Dora Kunz (1991) who saw energy fields since she was a child. It describes her perception of what the energy field is, what it looks like, and how we affect it with our TF. We had the honor of studying with Ms. Kunz in 1978 and 1979. Light sparkled from her eyes and love from her heart. She also co-authored *The Chakras and the Human Energy Fields* with S. Karagulla, M.D. which discusses the relationship between changes in the energy field and illness.

According to Kunz, there are different aspects, or layers, to our energy field, each with its own vibrational frequency. Radio waves all travel through the same space to your radio. They can function independently because each wave is traveling at a different frequency. It is the same in our energy field. Each aspect of the field vibrates at a different frequency. The aspect closest to the physical body, about 2", is the **etheric** aspect, and is silver blue in color. It is the blueprint of what is happening in the physical body, and balancing this aspect helps to balance the physical body. It transmits a stream of energy from the universal field, or healing energy of the universe, to the body. The next aspect is the **emotional,** or astral, that extends to about 1 1/2 feet from the body. The patterns of the energy of our emotions move in this aspect of the field. The third aspect of the field is the **mental,** 1 1/2–3 feet from the body, in which the patterns of the energy of our thoughts flash around. The mind affects and is affected by this layer. The fourth is the **spiritual,** causal, or intuitive aspect of the field that carries the Self's intention to be. It is Universal Consciousness focused in the individual self. Some say it is the soul. Wisdom, insight, inspiration, intuition, and direct knowing come from the vibration in this field. It is not constrained by time and space, and does not disintegrate at the death of the body like the other layers. The Greeks called it Augoeides, meaning "the luminous radiation of the spiritual Self, of which incarnate life is but the shadow" (Karagulla and Kunz, 1989; Kunz, 1991).

Our energy field allows us to exchange energy with others and with the Universal Source of Healing Energy. The body needs this energy (sometimes called prana or chi) to function at its greatest potential. This constant movement and exchange of energy creates health and well-being of the bodymind. One way this exchange of energy takes place is through the chakras.

The Chakras

Chakra means spinning wheel. In the energy field, the chakras look like spinning whirlpools. These clockwise spinning whirlpools are energy transformers. They are able to take the energy from the Universal Field which vibrates at a high frequency, and slow it down progressively in each layer of the field so that each layer, and finally the physical body, can use it (See Figure 11-2). This energy feeds and nurtures the field and the body. Like breathing, energy also moves from the body, out through the chakras, back to the Universal Field. There are seven main chakras, however there is a smaller chakra at each joint of the body.

When we are healthy and happy, the main chakras are about 3 inches in diameter and spin in a clockwise direction. If you were looking at a clock placed on someone's body, the hands move in a clockwise direction. This is how the energy moves in the chakras. It is the same on the front and back of the body. If a chakra moves counterclockwise, back and forth in a line, or in a very small circle, that area needs some energy balancing. Each chakra corresponds to an area where there is a concentration of peptide receptors along the spine. As you recall from Chapter 9, endorphins and other peptides are made and received by these sites. This means our emotions have great influence on these areas and the chakras, and these areas (and the chakras) have an influence on our emotions. Each chakra also corresponds to the closest endocrine gland and nerve plexus, supplying energy to them and organs that are nearby. For centuries, Eastern cultures have believed that each chakra contributes in a different way to physical and emotional health.

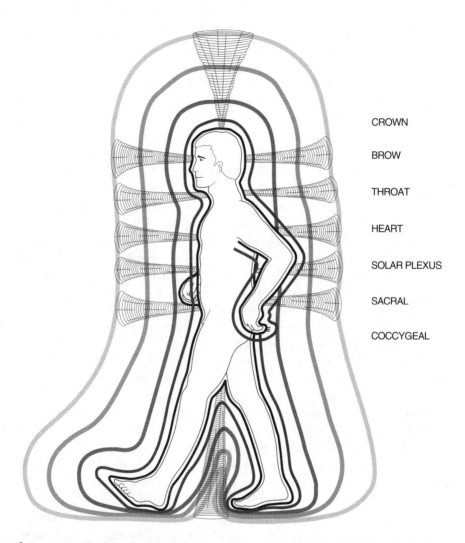

CROWN

BROW

THROAT

HEART

SOLAR PLEXUS

SACRAL

COCCYGEAL

Figure 11-2 The chakras in relation to the layers of the energy biofield. (Reprinted with permission from Janet L. Mentgen, Program Administrator, Healing Touch.)

THE ENERGY FIELD AND HEALING

The patterns in our energy field are associated with the transformation of the bodymind and spirit. Certain patterns in the human energy field suggest a time when interventions may be most healing. Chaos theory in physics explains some of these patterns within the human energy field, and is now being applied to nursing, weather, and many interactions (Forrest, 1999; Newman, 1999; Walsh, 2000). We usually think of chaos as negative. It may not be negative at all, but a pattern that we have just identified with uncomfortableness. We often feel restless when it is time for a change. Disease and conflict are signals that we need to change to move to our next higher level of health and relationship. A system is two or more interacting entities, such as people in a business or relationship, forces in the weather, subatomic particles, or two energy fields. An open system is when there is input to, and output from, the system. Chaos is the apparent disorder of open systems, as though they are trying to fling themselves into a higher order of being. When energy is added to a system, a disturbance is created, and a transition to a higher order often happens. The disturbance interrupts the natural process of deterioration, or entropy. Chaos arises in any situation when a certain level of complexity is reached (Prigogine and Stengers, 1984). Gleick (1987) says that the more chaos or disturbance there is, the more complex is the solution to the chaos; however, with that solution, there is a larger jump to a higher order.

When this level of complexity, or ridge of chaos, is reached, it is a vulnerable time when energy input from other systems can greatly affect the system. There is an increased likelihood of resonating with, or entraining to, other vibrations. Even small disturbances, or input, can rapidly alter the entire system. There can be sudden illumination of consciousness, changes in the body for health or illness, and decisions made that can alter the course of our lives.

This pattern, or ridge of chaos, can be detected in the human energy field as a spiral pattern. If the human field has few chaos patterns, it has a limited capacity for different reactions to stimuli (Hunt, 1995).

How can we use this information about chaos? When we feel confused or frustrated, instead of viewing it as negative, we can view it as though we are standing on the edge of understanding, the ridge of chaos. The solution, a new experience, a new life is a moment away. At this time, it is particularly important to be around vibrations that affect you in a positive, desired way. With just a little input of energy, a disturbance is created that helps us dance and jump to a new, higher level of order and insight. That input can be many things, including massage, an experience in meditation, or a walk in nature. A conversation with a friend, or with God, can bring a sudden insight. Sleep, a good meal, or the right book might be that input. We suddenly have a completely different perspective on what actions to take to solve a problem, how we view the world, and who we are.

We are beginning to see that all aspects of who we are from physical to emotional to mental to spiritual are affected by vibration, and depend on each other vibrating in harmony for most efficient functioning. Our eyes and ears bring us information about our world through the vibrations of light and sound. The electrons around the atoms of every cell vibrate. The chemical processes between atoms occur via exchanges of energy. Peptides carrying information throughout our body can only attach to receptors on cell walls if they vibrate in harmony. Our energy field and chakras are vibrating energy patterns. Recall that anything that vibrates is affected by other vibrating sources.

Doesn't it make sense then that the vibrations of thoughts, feelings, energy from the hands, light, and sound affect these vibratory dances? If disease is a "slow" vibration, would rhythmic, faster-moving vibrational frequencies in the bodymind create healing?

Tools for Balancing the Energy Field

There are many excellent books on the energy field and how to maintain and restore its health. The energy-based therapies we use in our practice lean toward simplicity. Because energy is constantly moving, the fields change moment to moment with our feelings, thoughts, or what we had for lunch. Because we don't know exactly what each person needs, we use and teach techniques that provide the receiver's field with a source of energy that it can use to balance itself. The following techniques can be used alone, or in combination with other nursing interventions. You can also use them in your personal life. We include them in this book because we find they enhance the receiver's experience of massage.

THOUGHTS AND FEELINGS AFFECT THE ENERGY FIELD

The TF we have affect all aspects of the energy field, including the chakras. Our beliefs of how TF affect the energy field most closely resemble those of Dora Kunz, whose views will be discussed in this section. The emotions we feel affect the etheric field directly affecting all aspects of health. Feeling continuous hostility or anxiety causes the energy transmission to the body from the field to be erratic. Fear and depression decrease the energy flow to the body, especially affecting the kidneys. Chronic tension depletes our energy reserves making heart attack and kidney problems more likely. When we are calm and happy, energy flows evenly and rhythmically from one field to another, and to the body (Karagulla and Kunz, 1989; Kunz, 1991).

The emotional, or astral, field is very impressionable, responding quickly to our emotions. Feelings are currents of energy that become patterns in the field. Different feelings are represented in this field by different colors and images. If we continually feel the same feelings, whether "bad" or "good," the patterns remain in the field. They give rise to the same feelings again, and so a cycle develops. Feelings, whether positive or negative, are reinforced or strengthened, by energy coming from the universal field. Changing feelings that do not help us allows the patterns in the field to change, and vice versa.

The mind finds expression in the mental field. The everyday mind integrates and interprets sensory data and perceives relationships. The abstract mind finds meaning, unities, and new ideas. There are two aspects of the everyday and abstract mind (1) integrating and assimilating data, originality, finding meaning; (2) false reasoning, self delusion, separation, worry. We choose which aspect of mind fills our thoughts. Colors in the mental field indicate our interests. The mental field holds ideas as patterns of energy. When we have a strong image in the mental field, the field easily transfers the idea to the mental field of others, which is how ideas are spread. If we hold rigid thoughts, we keep ourselves from being able to attract, adopt, entertain, and understand new ideas.

The mental and emotional fields greatly affect each other. If the mind does not have to deal with emotional stress, it assimilates information very well. Insight originates in the causal or spiritual layer, is developed rationally by the mind, and is registered and stored in the brain and body. The mind depends on the body for physical expression. The interaction between the emotional and mental fields may play a role in the effect of imagery on the body, and therefore, healing. When we hold an image in the mental field it creates a pattern of energy that is strengthened if emotion is added. These patterns affect the etheric aspect of the field that has a direct effect on the body. Since the receptors on the cell walls send and receive vibration as they choose which peptides to connect with, patterns in the energy field may affect these peptide/receptor dances.

TF are very powerful for creating movement in the chakras. Chakras, being connectors from the field to the body and being associated with endocrine glands and nerve plexis, may be the path that TF travel from the field to the body and to conscious awareness. The most effective way we have found to help people balance their chakras is by asking them to focus on the area and hold the image in his mind of a clockwise whirlpool of energy. Usually within seconds, the chakras will begin spinning in the desired way. Each chakra is associated with different TF (See Figure 11-3). When the chakra moves in a healthy way it is easier to feel the associated feeling. Conversely, when we intentionally feel these feelings, the chakra is strengthened.

Remember from PNI that when we become aware of our emotions and let them come in and move through, the healthy flow of peptides in the body is maintained. We have just learned that if we allow emotions to move through us, the fields continue to vibrate and move in harmony. Information is transmitted throughout the body via the emotion peptides. Information is transferred through the energy fields via vibrating frequencies. Emotion is a vibrational frequency. What if emotions create patterns of movement in the field which then creates these same patterns of movement in the peptides because they are moved

Chakra	Associated Thought, Feeling, Activity
First (Base of spine)	Trust that there will be enough
Second (Sacral)	Passion, desire, creativity
Third (Solar plexus)	Personal will, courage, ability to forgive and release, a disturbance here makes it hard to control feelings
Fourth (Heart)	Love, compassion for all beings, balancing it balances all chakras, balance chakra three and four in all healing work
Fifth (Throat)	Sensitivity to vibration, reaching out, communicating
Sixth (Brow)	Integration of ideas and experience, expands through imagery and visualization
Seventh (Crown)	Spiritual aspect, all ranges of consciousness, expands through meditation

Figure 11-3 Thoughts and Feelings Associated with Each Chakra.

by emotion? Emotional energy may be the carrier of information throughout the field, as well as the body, affecting health and happiness.

The health of the chakras and the field is greatly affected by patterns of TF that we repeat over and over. If we hold in "negative" emotions for long periods, continuing to feel them, the movement of energy in the fields is disrupted. Our ability to receive healing energy from the Universal Field is restricted. This decrease of energy flow adversely affects the health of our physical body, our ability to choose new TF in response to situations, and our awareness of our connection to Spirit. Feelings of love, happiness, and forgiveness allow the energy in the field to move in a rhythmic pattern that creates health in the bodymind.

The field sends these "negative" or "positive" patterns out into the world, and attracts similar patterns from the world back to us. Once again, here is a way we can create our reality. Have you heard the saying, "What goes around, comes around"? If you have found yourself experiencing uncomfortable situations over and over again that you do not want, examine the TF you are regularly having. They are creating patterns of energy in your field that are like magnets, bringing to you the experiences that have always come as a result of those TF. Entertain TF of what you want in your life. You will send out new patterns of energy, and attract a new life to you. If you are happy with what is coming your way, notice what you are thinking and feeling and by all means, keep that thought. We attract people and situations to us to show us our good and bad. From this mirror, we can choose which patterns, words, thoughts, feelings, behaviors, we want to keep and which to change.

USING THE HANDS TO BALANCE THE ENERGY FIELD

Receiving a good massage helps the field become balanced. There are many other techniques for using the hands to help the energy field to balance itself, including Therapeutic Touch, Healing Touch, Reiki, and Polarity therapy, to name a few. They all use somewhat different techniques with the hands and have somewhat different philosophies about how much the giver directs and manipulates the healing energy. Some techniques do not touch the body at all, but just work within the energy field. All energy therapies work with the same human energy field and they all intend to help the receiver's energy field rebalance itself so that healing can happen. If one technique especially attracts you, look into it further. Always follow your heart.

Therapeutic Touch

Therapeutic Touch is only partially about healing others. Equally—perhaps even more importantly—it is about an inner journey. It is important to acknowledge that the empowerment in Therapeutic Touch comes through the therapist's quest for a liaison with the Inner Self.

—Dolores Krieger

In the early 1970s, Dora Kunz and Dolores Krieger created Therapeutic Touch (TT) and began teaching Krieger's nursing students at New York University how to do it. Since Krieger's first research study in 1973, much research has studied the effects of Therapeutic Touch (Wilson, 1995). When people receive TT, 90% have a profound relaxation response with decreased respiration, warmer extremities, lower voice, and decreased anxiety and pain.

Practitioners also benefit from practicing TT, including increased intuition, significant improvement in lifestyle, improved health, and prevention of burnout. They also feel a greater spiritual quality in their lives and more altruistic feelings and compassion for others. Quinn and Strelkauskas (1993) found that TT enhances immune function in both practitioners and recently bereaved recipients.

In 1991, Daniel Wirth reported some most impressive findings (See research box). He studied the effects of TT on wound healing in a double blind, control group study.

Thousands of nurses and people from all walks of life have now learned TT and practice it in hospitals and homes. The beautiful thing about TT is that it is easy to learn and practice, and is extremely effective. All it takes is being present

The Effect of Non-Contact Therapeutic Touch on the Healing Rate of Full Thickness Dermal Wounds			
Day	0	8	16
Wound Size			
Test	58 mm²	3.9	4
Control	58 mm²	19.34	5.8

On day 16, 13 of the 23 test subjects were completely healed. 0 of the 23 control subjects were completely healed.

Significant difference—.001

—Daniel Wirth, M.S., J.D.

in the moment, having the intent to help the person feel better, and the willingness to assist their body to heal itself.

Almost all of us are born with the ability to use our hands to feel energy field. We are just never told that we can, or taught how to do it. We can learn to feel when the energy field is moving in a healthy, balanced way, and when it is not moving. We can learn to help restore healthy movement to the field (See Figure 11-4). In our 20 years of teaching TT, 95% of everyone in class can learn to do it

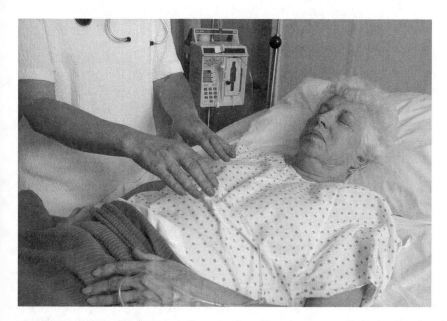

Figure 11-4 Therapeutic Touch and other energy-based therapies are very effective in promoting relaxation and relieving pain and discomfort. Directing and modulating of energy in non-contact therapeutic touch.

in about three hours. The more you practice, the more sensitive your hands become, and the easier it is.

We believe all of us are pathways for the healing energy of the universe, nature, or God. When we have a caring intent to help another and ask that the energy flow to help them, it comes through us to them. You may ask, "Can't they ask God and get it directly?" Of course they can. It just seems that when two or more are gathered for loving and healing, it seems to be more powerful.

Krieger's *The Therapeutic Touch* (1979) explains in detail how to do TT, or you can take a workshop. Healing Touch Level I teaches Therapeutic Touch as one of its techniques. The Nurse Healers Professional Association can also help you find a teacher in your area. (For contact information, see Appendix A.)

Steps of Therapeutic Touch

1. Center and ground yourself. *Centering*—bring your full attention to the receiver, wanting to help them, letting all other thoughts pass out of your mind. Centering can be taking a few deep breaths, meditating, or saying a prayer. *Grounding*—connect with the stable, nurturing energy of the Earth.
2. Assess the energy field—use the hands to notice areas in the field that are not moving. They feel different from the rest of the field—warm, cool, tingling.
3. Unruffling—long sweeping movements with the hands to establish movement in the field.
4. Directing and modulating—return to areas discovered in step 2 and hold your hands over them or unruffle them. Allow energy to move to the client, assisting his field to rebalance itself. We ask that his body take the universal healing energy and use it in whatever way is for the highest good of all concerned. Some people touch the body (contact TT) and some do not (noncontact TT).
5. Closure—knowing when to stop, reassess entire body to see if the field feels balanced.

Therapeutic Touch, at its core, is the offering of unconditional love and compassion. We're here for service. We're here to love other people.

—Janet Quinn, PhD, RN

Healing Touch

Healing Touch is a system of many different energy-based therapies founded around 1978 by Janet Mentgen, R.N. She has the same gentle, healing quality as Dora Kunz and Dolores Krieger. Many who learn and practice Healing Touch are nurses, many are not. *Healing Touch* is an excellent book describing the different Healing Touch techniques, benefits, and research (Hover-Kramer, Mentgen, and

Scandrett-Hibdon, 1996). Janet Mentgen formed the Colorado Center for Healing Touch, and schedules for workshops can be found by contacting them (see Appendix A).

LIGHT AND COLOR AS HEALING TOOLS

Chapter 4 discusses the use of light, color, sound, and music in creating a relaxing environment for massage. The next two sections discuss benefits these modalities offer in addition to relaxation. Light is energy waves traveling through space. It is made up of all of the colors, each color being a wave traveling at its own unique frequency. We see this when sunlight hits a prism in the window, and rainbows dance around the room. Being vibrating frequencies, light and color affect the health of our energy field. As we learned earlier, all chemical reactions in the body occur by photons, or particles of light, being exchanged within cells. We are light in our deepest essence. Doesn't it seem natural that light and color are necessary for health?

Light

In massage, low lighting is most relaxing. However, since light is a form of energy, we want to discuss some of its healing qualities. Since the early days, nurses have used heliotherapy or ray therapy to improve patients' health (Harmer, 1924; Tracy, 1938; Nightingale, 1957; Libster, 2001). One technique was giving light baths by moving patients outside in the sun.

Most species have always lived outside, including humans, being nourished by the light of the sun. It has only been in the last 50 years that people spend most of their time indoors. How do you feel when you lay outside in the sun for a few minutes, especially in the spring with a cool breeze blowing? Sunlight is full spectrum light, composed of all wavelengths, including all the colors, ultraviolet (UV), and infrared frequencies. Dr. John Ott, past director of the Environmental Health and Light Research Institute, has done fascinating research demonstrating the effects of full spectrum light on the health of plants, animals, and people. He believes many of our health problems are due to lack of exposure to the full spectrum. Fluorescent lights are deficient in red and blue, which the sun is strongest in. Regular light bulbs are also deficient in blue light (Ott, 1988).

The exposure to UV light that creates healthy results can be very short. Problems come when our exposure causes the skin to turn pink. To begin to see some of the benefits of UV light, expose the skin to two minutes of sunlight per day, with no lotion, avoiding 10 a.m.–2 p.m. Allow the eyes to look at sunlight (not the sun) with no sunglasses or UV tinted glasses. Research suggests that lack of sunlight may be causing many of our chronic illnesses, including problems with the heart and immune systems (Kime, 1980; Ott, 1988; Lieberman, 1991).

Think about it. Many of us get up, go to the garage, get in the car, drive to work with UV tinted glasses and car windows, get out in the parking garage, go in, stay in for 8 hours, come home, all with UV protection, and stay in until we go to sleep. Even when we go out, we wear UV lotion, UV glasses, and hats to shade the eyes. It is conceivable, especially as we get older, that we never have sunlight enter the eyes and almost never touch the skin.

Be sure you spend a little time outside each day. If you care for children, the elderly, or people who cannot get outside on their own, help them to an ample portion of full spectrum light each day. Sunlight is best, or full spectrum fluorescent bulbs. Not all fluorescents are full spectrum, so ask for them especially.

Color

All of the colors combined together make up white light. Each color vibrates at its own frequency, with red being slowest and violet the fastest.

One of our greatest sources of delight is watching the sun come through the prism hanging in our window. Prisms project vibrant color all over the room and allows you to actually hold a rainbow in your hand. Just as it is important to eat a variety of vegetables, it is important to expose ourselves to a variety of colors. Because each color has a different vibrational frequency, each one has a different effect on the energy field and the body. There are excellent books that discuss the physical and emotional effects of each color, including research studies (Ghadiali, 1933; Babbitt, 1967; Burroughs, 1976; Lieberman, 1991).

As mentioned in Chapter 4, the warm end of the spectrum (red, orange, yellow) is stimulating. If you want to use just one color to encourage the healing of the physical body, use green, and of the emotional self, magenta (red and violet). The cool end (turquoise, blue, indigo, violet) is calming. No coincidence our world was originally mostly green and blue. See Figure 11-5 for effects of each color.

To bring color into your life, eat colored food, and have colored pieces of cloth where you can see them. Wear colored clothes. To see the effect, dress for several days in black, brown, or gray. Then try blue shades for a day, then red or yellow, then green. Collect colored stones and have live flowers around you. Bring artwork, colored curtains, and colored light bulbs into your surroundings. Imagine a client, or yourself, surrounded by a ball of colored light. The color will then permeate and affect the energy field and body.

If there is a color that you dislike intensely, it usually holds a key to healing of the bodymind. Incorporating it into your life can bring balance to your field. It can stimulate emotional memories and associations about a particular illness or situation that can be unpleasant at first, but instrumental to healing. This principle has been used with anxiety, depression, phobias, migraines, obesity, and drug and alcohol abuse (Lieberman, 1991).

Color	Benefit
Red	Stimulates the sympathetic nervous system, increasing circulation, blood pressure, respiration, excitement, and anxiety.
Orange	Helps the body to expel toxins and relieves constipation, gets anything that is clogged up, moving again.
Yellow	Increases absorption of food, stimulates the nerves, eyes, ears, and mental processes.
Green	Overall physical healing, good for everything to do with the body, including muscle problems, cuts, bruises, and disease.
Turquoise	Burns, insect bites, and skin problems.
Blue	Very relaxing, stimulates the parasympathetic nervous system, lowering blood pressure, tension, and respiration
Indigo (deep midnight blue)	Aids immune function, sleep, and pain relief.
Violet	Enhances meditation, spiritual connection, immune function.
Magenta (combination of red and violet)	Balances the heart and emotions.

Figure 11-5 Benefits of Each Color.

SOUND AND MUSIC

Sound also moves through space in waves of energy. Sound is to music as light is to color. Each different note or tone of music is a different frequency of sound. Because sound moves in waves of energy, it also affects the energy field and bodymind.

Sound

The Bible says, "In the beginning was the Word, and the Word was with God and the Word was God." Many cultures, including the Tibetans and American Indians, believe there was a word that brought the world into being. For the Sufis it was "Hu", the Chinese, "Kung" and the Eastern Indians, "Om."   A fascinating video, *Of Sound Mind and Body,* explores Dr. Hans Jenny's experiments demonstrating the effect of sound on matter. In this video, sand is spread on a metal plate. When the sound "Om" is chanted, vibrating the plate, the sound waves of "Om" cause the sand particles to move into a mandala pattern. With other sounds, the sand particles begin streaming around in a spiral pattern. Some sounds cause the sand to form a shape that looks like the spinal column.

Recall that the subatomic particles that make up all things in the universe are vibrating patterns of energy. It is possible to see how sound created the forms we call the world.

The planets, receptors on our cell walls, and the subatomic particles in all things of the universe, all vibrate. The energy fields of each individual vibrate in harmonious rhythms. All of these vibrations produce sound. They affect each other with sound, and are affected by sound. The DNA, the molecule in each cell that tells the cell how to work effectively, is affected by phonons (Hobza and Zahradnik, 1988). Phonons are quanta, or packets, of energy created by sound. According to Deepak Chopra, M.D., in Ayurvedic medicine of India, disease occurs when the vibration of the DNA, mind, and body are not synchronized. Making the sound "Om" can bring them into balance.

Toning is one of the most effective ways to use sound to help the body heal because we use our own voice to create the sound. The body will make the sounds it needs to heal itself, if we let it. To practice toning, open your mouth and let whatever sound come out that naturally wants to come. Tones resonate with areas of the energy field, creating needed release of constricted patterns, and strengthening enlivening patterns. Toning affects all vibrating structures within the body as well (Keyes, 1973).

Words are very powerful, not only for communicating ideas, but the sounds of the consonants and vowels vibrate the body in different ways. In his school of wisdom, Pythagoras would not let his students speak for the first five years. When they did, they could better understand the power of the word in creating and healing. I'm sure you have experienced that the tone of words is often more powerful than what is said. We are usually unconscious of the tone of our words, yet it is this subtle aspect of conversation that creates feelings. The vibrations of the feelings cause both people to vibrate in harmony, allowing them to share sadness, anger, love, excitement, or peace. Try a day without speaking to bring your awareness to the music of your words, and that of those around you.

We must be aware of our sound environment. It can increase or decrease stress, relaxation, and health. Surround yourself with sounds that make you take a deep breath and relax. We begin to ignore sounds in our world if they are there long enough, but they are still affecting the bodymind. Keep in mind that we need periods of silence just as we need periods of darkness. Have you ever been away from town and noticed your ears pounding as they get used to silence? Treat yourself to a walk in a wilderness area sometime, away from the sounds of civilization. We go backpacking, and when we are in the silence, we feel our awareness begin to move out from the body, expanding into the silence. In the wilderness, with no man made sound, the hum of nature as a very subtle, ever present song can be heard.

Music

Have you ever been feeling pretty relaxed, sitting in your favorite chair and suddenly you hear loud, booming music with a very strong base rhythm? The heart starts pounding, you become very energized, and sometimes irritated. Music also soothes the soul and heals the body. We have all experienced feeling stressed, angry, and closed off from the world. We happen to hear some beautiful music on the radio in the car, and our mood completely changes.

Recall the Law of Resonance that says when two vibrating objects come close together, they begin vibrating at the same frequency. Vibrations produce repeated patterns, or rhythms. Stronger rhythms entrain, or change, weaker rhythms to match the stronger frequency. We have seen that the subatomic particles in our atoms vibrate, the receptors on cell walls vibrate, our heartbeat creates a rhythm. All of these are affected by the vibrations of music.

Music that is 60 beats per minute, like Baroque music and Mozart's Largos, synchronizes the heart rate to the rhythm of the music, and can reduce the heart rate from 72 to 64–68. Alpha brain waves, which are seen during relaxation and meditation, are induced by music that is 60 beats per minute (Spintge and Droh, 1992). From what we learned about stress, anytime the body is relaxed, the stress response is interrupted, benefiting numerous functions in the body.

From 1977–1985 Ralph Spintge, M.D. (1992) did many research studies with 50,000 people looking at the effects of music on the body. With dental surgical patients he found that within 10 minutes of starting the music, the stress response in the endocrine and cardiovascular system decreased. The experimental group had decreased pulse, blood pressure, and ACTH. In other studies he found that cortisol was decreased (enhancing immune function) and beta endorphins (enhances mood and decreases pain) were increased. He found that the most important factors were: (1) the person selected the music, (2) there were no extremes in rhythm or melody; and (3) instrumentals were best.

Premature infants listening to music gained weight faster and were discharged five to seven days sooner, saving an average of $4,800 per infant (Caine, 1991). Music also decreased the numbers of heart attacks in ICU's, clients needed less pain medicine post-operatively, and there was less anxiety in children waiting for surgery. There are countless studies documenting the effectiveness of music for physical, mental, and emotional health. Music is most helpful when it is begun before a procedure and continued throughout (Furman, 1996).

Music seems to be most effective in changing mood when we first listen to a piece that is similar to the mood we are in, synchronizing ourselves with the music. For example, if you are stressed, choose fast rhythms at first. After several minutes, change the selection to one that sounds the way you want to feel. Specific selections of music inspire specific moods at work and home (Lingerman,

1983; Merritt, 1990). If you want an easy way to tune yourself, your chakras, and their corresponding areas, sing the song: Doe a deer, a female deer. Doe, Rae, Me, Fa, So, La, Tee, Doe, or CDEFGABC. This is the scale of the seventh math chakras, with Doe (first chakra), Rae (second chakra), etc.

What can you do to get "in harmony" with another? Listen to the same music, chant together, sing together, or play music together. Breathe in the same rhythm, laugh together, discuss something you both feel the same way about, or just sit in silence together.

In *The World is Sound,* Joachim-Ernst Berendt (1991) points out fascinating correlations between musical scales, harmonies, and melodies, and the makeup of the physical world we live in, from our DNA, to each element in the body, to the makeup of planets. In the 1600s, Johannes Kepler found that the movements of the orbits of the planets produce vibrations and sounds that are in harmony with each other. Life on Earth is affected by the sounds, the vibrations, coming from space. The tones of the visible planets cover eight octaves which is the identical human hearing range. The spin of the electrons around the nuclei of atoms produces sounds. Carbon is one of the most important components of life. The six electrons spinning around the nucleus of a carbon atom produce a tone scale of CDEFGA which is the tone scale produced by the spinning chakras (plus B), beginning with C at the base of the spine. It is also the predominant chord of the Gregorian chants.

Listening to a recording of the sounds from space recorded by Voyager, we expected to hear mostly silence. Instead there were clear rhythmic patterns and musical tones. Perhaps from our electrons, to our DNA, to our nervous systems, to our spirits, we are hearing and responding to the music of the spheres. It may be the energy that inspires us all to dance the dance of life.

"All things . . . are aggregations of atoms that dance and by their movements produce sounds. When the rhythm of the dance changes, the sound it produces also changes. . . . Each atom perpetually sings its song, and the sound, at every moment, creates dense and subtle forms."

A Lama in Tibet who referred to himself as a 'master of sound'
—Alexandra David-Neel, 1936

BEING IN NATURE

As little kids, many of our mothers told us, "Go play outside, it's good for you." Most of us feel better after we take a walk around the block. There is more to the enhanced sense of well-being we experience after being outside than the effects of exercise alone. The Earth has the ability to nurture us if we let her. She has the ability to decrease our feelings of stress, and bring our frazzled inner-rhythms into coherence, or harmony, within minutes. How? When we are in nature, we are surrounded by living things. Even most deserts and areas of the Arctic are teeming with life. Microbes are everywhere. The more abundant the trees, birds, and plants, the easier it is to feel the healthy, living energy field exuding from everything. When we walk among them, their harmonious rhythms entrain ours, causing us to resonate with a more rhythmic, calm vibration. The Earth's ionosphere, the electromagnetic field around the Earth, has a vibrational frequency of about 7.8 Hz. (cycles per second). When we are meditating, or feeling calm or creative, our brain waves are in the alpha frequency of approximately 7–13 Hz. (Goldman, 1992). The Earth can entrain our bodies into relaxation, and connect us to each other, if we tune in to her.

Try lying down on the ground on your back for about 10 minutes. You will feel your tension drain away into the Earth where she can transmute it into life-giving energy once again. Why do people go to the ocean or sit beside a creek for relaxation and rejuvenation? Water is living, moving. Our bodies are mostly water, approximately 85%, so it is very easy for us to resonate with it. People often ridicule "tree huggers." Try sitting with your back against a tree, or hugging one. Trees are deeply grounded in the Earth and exchange energy with the heavens. Your energy begins to resonate, being deeply grounded and reaching skyward. Have you ever stood amongst the redwoods of California? Some of them are 2,000 years old. There are circles of them you can stand in the middle of. They have been there, friends, for two centuries. When you stand in their midst, you have no doubt that these beings are powerfully, consciously, affecting you, and others, for great distances. In their presence, we felt awe and great reverence.

Applications of Energy-Based Therapies

Many healthcare facilities have sun rooms. Plants, pets, and flowers are increasingly found in nursing homes. Children's hospitals are often painted in rainbow colors. Laurel Emryss writes and plays harp music for people who are dying. Energy based therapies that use the hands to balance the field are used in many healthcare facilities.

Since the 1970s more than 100,000 people have been trained in Therapeutic Touch and Healing Touch. About 43,000 are healthcare professionals, half of whom practice it in their lives, professional and private. TT is taught in more than 100 colleges and universities, and in more than 75 countries. It is a nursing intervention that is a treatment for the nursing diagnosis, "energy field disturbance," recognized by the North American Nursing Diagnosis Association (Carpenito, 1995).

Nurses at Toledo Hospital Cardiac Critical Care Unit in Toledo, Ohio, were working with a client who had coronary artery bypass surgery, and was having complications. He was having trouble breathing due to pain, and was taking maximum doses of pain medication. Doctors were having no success. One of the nurses gave him a Healing Touch treatment. The next morning he was walking in the halls with no pain, did not have to use oxygen, and was taking deep breaths. He was discharged the following day (Villaire, 1999).

In 1999, Seton Hospital, one of the hospitals of the Daughters of Charity in Austin, Texas, approved TT, Healing Touch Level I, and Holistic Touch (their own form of energy therapy) as interventions for healthcare professionals in their hospital. As of 2001, clients at Columbia-Presbyterian Medical Center in New York can receive energy-based therapies if they request it through the Columbia Integrative Medicine Program headed by cardiologist, Mehmet Oz.

Lou told us this story of how she used a combination of energy-based therapies in the neonatal intensive-care unit.

"I have been a nurse for 35 years in the OR and pre- and post-surgery. I decided to learn about holistic nursing through the Holistic Nursing Series in the CE department at the University of Texas School of Nursing in Austin, Texas. After taking several workshops in the series, I found out that my son was going to be the father of twins. On April 11, 1996, I came to one of the workshops and told everyone the twins had been born very premature, at 25 weeks. Jacob weighed 1 lb. 9 oz. and Kristin weighed 1 lb. 11 oz. The doctors told us that the twins had very little chance of living, and if they did they would have multiple physical and mental problems.

Being their granny, I decided differently. The class I took that day was called 'Using Energy to Enhance Nursing Practice.' We learned to use energy therapies, such as Therapeutic Touch, music, sound, color, and light in healing. I asked the teacher and my classmates to help me think of how I could use what we had learned that day to help the twins. We all formed a circle, visualized the twins, and focused our thoughts on them, sending them love and seeing them healthy. They all gave me the red stick'um dots from their name tags as physical reminders that they were all thinking about me and the twins. I put them on the twins' incubators.

The neonatal unit had a "No Touch" policy. Both babies had bilateral chest tubes, feeding tubes, and were on ventilators. They had no finger or toe nails, no eyebrows, eye lashes, or nipples. They were covered with hair. At day five, Jacob's colon ruptured and an emergency colostomy was done. The doctor gave him almost no chance for survival.

I created a protocol for my babies and taught it to the family and nurses. The red dots from the class at UT remained on the cribs. When people were washing their hands, they washed away all negative thoughts about the babies' prognosis. Only positive, healing thoughts were allowed near the babies. Therapeutic Touch was done on the babies. Everyone in the family would center, ground, and image the twins being two years old and running through the bluebonnets, chasing their dog at their home in the country. We would assess the field, unruffle, and clear any congestion from the field. We held our hands in the energy field over the babies' lungs and abdomens which were the greatest problem areas. We imaged energy as a stream of light and love coming from God, flowing through us and going into the twins. We kept our hand over areas where we felt a drawing or pulling of energy. It felt like a flowing movement, like warm water bubbling and going through my hand to each baby. We smoothed the field with a gentle stroking motion of the hand. The babies were more relaxed after the session, their respirations were slower, and they turned their heads toward the person doing the energy work. We visualized soothing colors, greens and blues, surrounding and permeating the twins, and sang Amazing Grace to them. After the sessions, their elevated blood pressures and amounts of insulin needed dropped.

Finally I convinced the nurses to let the family touch each baby's foot with one index finger. At first, the foot was rigid, then it became soft and relaxed. Respirations slowed, the babies' color changed, and they began to turn their heads toward voices. The family always talked to the babies. There was always soft music playing in the nursery. I made them pillows that stayed in their cribs with music boxes in them that played Brahms lullaby. Their hats were bright colors. Rainbows, as well as brightly colored drawings by the nurses, were on their cribs. I continued to come to the monthly workshops, never knowing if the babies would live another day.

Not only did Jacob survive the surgery, but both twins began to make progress. I convinced the staff to let the family hold the babies. We began to give short massages on their feet, shoulders, neck, and back. The twins began to gain weight more rapidly, and muscular and neurological progress was noted. Finally, they came home.

At two and a half the twins were saying the ABC's, singing Mary Had a Little Lamb, and were perfectly normal in every way. The doctors say it's a miracle. Grandma believes it was a lot of love and the extras she learned in class.

Kristin and Jacob are now running through the bluebonnets and chasing their dog at home in the country."

As a species, we are growing. We are realizing, and knowing in our hearts, that we are not the body alone. We are spiritual, energy beings. When we are out of balance, we need more than drugs and surgery. We need light, sound, touch, and love. We are manifesting this knowing by a real change in our healthcare establishment.

THE ENERGY FIELD AND MASSAGE

It is certainly possible to give a great massage knowing nothing of the energy field. However, we have learned in this chapter that we have an energy aspect as much as a physical aspect. Massage helps to balance the energy field. Recall, when we continually have "constricted" TF, muscles become tight. When we hold onto these kinds of TF, corresponding energy patterns persist in our energy field. As massage loosens the tension in the body, TF change, and corresponding patterns in the field are energized, making it easier to let go of the associated thought or feeling. We can more easily entertain new thoughts. The relaxation brought on by the massage creates new energy patterns and healthy movement in the field.

Just as a massage helps to create harmony in the energy field, balancing the energy field greatly enhances the experience of a massage. We integrate energy-based therapies into the massages we give in several ways. When we are preparing to give a massage, before we begin any interaction with the receiver at all, we first center and ground. As previously mentioned in Chapter 4, centering and grounding brings our awareness, calmly and clearly, to the moment. We can be fully present for our client. We can also best choose our thoughts, words, and actions. From the point of view that client and nurse are two fields interacting, it becomes clear why it is so crucial to monitor our TF as we massage. Just as our hands affect their muscles, our TF affect their energy field. The vibrations of our TF vibrate our own field. Their field begins to resonate, or vibrate, in synch with ours. Their TF and physical body are affected. In the same way, their TF affect our field. If we keep our energy exchange with the world open, we are not affected by the unbalanced energy of others. Letting feelings in and out, reaching out to people who nourish us, and being in the wholeness of nature encourage the movement of feelings—and so energy—through our fields.

After centering and grounding, we do an energy assessment (the second step of TT) on the front and back of the body if possible. After practicing assessing the energy field of different people, it takes 30 seconds or less. An energy assessment points out the overall tension in the body, and which areas we want to be sure to include in the massage. Sometimes the areas the client says are painful may not be the origin of the problem. An assessment can pick up the area of cause, as well as symptom. We find that including unruffling (Step 3 of TT) at the beginning of the massage allows the muscles to begin to soften and release tension. After the massage we do another assessment. If any of the imbalances are still there, we do energy work on the area, or more massage. At the end of the massage, unruffling increases the sense of relaxation. Sometimes resting the hands on an area that is still a little tight and allowing healing energy to flow into the area, helps it complete the releasing process.

Using light and sound also contributes to the relaxation of the bodymind during a massage. When we feel a tight muscle as we are giving a massage, we visualize that area permeated with green light because it is the healer of muscle and tissue ailments. We add blue or indigo for relaxation and pain relief. If the person wants music, we ask them to choose something that is relaxing to them. For more details on the use of color and music in the massage setting, see Chapter 4.

From one point of view, when we massage, we are touching the skin of another. Our hands are kneading the muscles, nerves, and tissues encouraging them to release, let go, and relax. From another point of view, we are fields of subatomic particles spinning at great speeds, constantly interacting by giving off and receiving packets of light patterns. Two light beings move into each other, share information, and move apart again, both different, and hopefully better, than before they met. Both points of view are as true as if you ask yourself, "Do I see a whir of movement, or a hummingbird's wing?" Do you see a waterfall or a droplet of water? When you watch a movie do you see a million little lights flashing on a screen, or do you see people laughing, crying, and living life? Our bodies are but a captured moment in time, a frame of the movie, slowed down for closer observation and enjoyment.

THE UNITY OF ALL THINGS

When elephants cry, we are all wounded.
As eagles return to the skies, we all fly once more.

Perhaps one of the most valuable lessons we learned from this section on the energy field is that there is no separation. Have you ever developed a really close relationship with someone and over time you notice that similar events are happening to you both, at almost the same time? Connections we make with others, especially if they contain much time spent together or strong emotion, are energetic connections that can last a very long time, over great distances. When we think of being connected to someone, we usually think of us as two separate beings, sharing a feeling in common, a child in common, or a house in common. What we have learned in this chapter helps us see that not only are we connected to others, but we are one with others. As energy beings interacting, we merge. Just as a subatomic particle and a field are two aspects of one entity, we are each an individual and at the same time one with all other individuals, including plants, animals, and the Earth.

As we continue to expand our view of who we are as energy beings, we see that all entities, everywhere, interacting, create a field that is a network uniting us all, from the microbes to the stars.

It is useful to divide the world into separate objects to conduct our daily affairs, but this separation is not an actual characteristic of reality. It is an abstraction devised by the discriminating and categorizing intellect. Everything is a part of everything else at a very fundamental level.

When the mind is disturbed,
the multiplicity of things is produced,
but when the mind is quieted,
the multiplicity of things disappears.

—Werner Heisenberg, physicist

We are not, and never will be, alone. We are not healthy as isolated entities. We seek connection. Connection leads to meaning in life, and transformation. Everything in the universe is designed to work together if we are to reach our greatest potential. When we massage another, we are not two separate entities. We are connected much more deeply and profoundly than just hands on a body.

We are vibrating, dynamic beings capable of much more than we have ever imagined. According to some, there are not even really individuals. There is only a whole, that is interacting.

And what is this whole?

The discovery that space is not a vacuum is seen as one of the most important findings of modern physics. Particles come into being in, and vanish again into the "void." Particles (matter) cannot just appear from nowhere, therefore there must be a field of energy from which the particle arises. This suggests that space is "alive," a moving field of interacting energy. The void pulsates in rhythms of creation and destruction. The existence and fading of particles are ways in which the void moves (Capra, 1983). There seems to be a universal field of energy, from which matter arises and into which matter once again returns.

Because humans are one with this inseparable whole, and humans are intelligent, this implies that the whole is also intelligent (Chew, 1968). A leader in nursing, Margaret Newman, describes a person as a unique pattern of consciousness within a field of absolute consciousness. Absolute consciousness is love (Newman, 1999). David Bohm, a prominent present day physicist, proposed the theory of implicate order which studies the relationship between consciousness and matter. He saw mind and matter as mutually enfolding projections of a higher reality which is neither matter nor consciousness (Capra, 1983).

We are now going to humbly explore our connection with this universal field, this higher reality.

SPIRITUALITY, HEALING, AND MASSAGE

In this chapter, as we continue to explore massage as a bridge for connecting, we see that as beings of energy, as we massage another, we are connecting in a deeper way than just touching with the hands. Our energy fields interact. As we learn about energy fields, we see that not only are there unique, individual fields, but there is a universal field connecting all things, everywhere. If we are going to look fully at how massage creates connection, we must explore this universal field. This path leads us to spirituality. There are several reasons to include spirituality in this book:

1. Spirituality is part of the HeartTouch intervention (Chapter 12) which helps us give a massage with heart.

2. Spirituality involves connection, which massage seeks to create.

3. Spirituality improves health, a goal of nursing and massage.

4. Nurses are asking for more ways to include spirituality in their practices, and giving massage with heart is one way.

Can spirituality bring meaning to a nurse's daily work, or to the life of a dying client? What is the role of spirituality in massage? This section explores these questions.

What is Spirituality?

First, what do we mean by spirituality? An individual's view of spirituality is a most deep and personal experience. According to Webster's dictionary, spirituality is the quality or state of being spiritual. Spiritual means related to, or affecting the spirit, joined in spirit, and relating to sacred matters. Spirit is defined as an animating principle held to give life to physical organisms, a supernatural being, or essence, the immaterial intelligent or sentient part of a person, and the activating or essential principle influencing a person. For some, it is difficult to even discuss this mystery in words. Because of its vital role in health and well-being, we are making a humble attempt. As nurses, we realize that we must address not only the body and mind of our clients, but also the spirit.

For some, spirituality is connecting with the inner self in solitude. Often people find spiritual fulfillment by gathering together in places of worship. For some, it includes a feeling of love and connection to others. Spending time in nature is a spiritual experience for others. Spirituality is often defined as a sense of self-transcendence, occurring through a connection with others and/or something greater than ourselves. Communing with Higher Power is spiritual to some. For many of us, spiritual fulfillment is some combination of the above.

In this book, spirituality does not refer to any one religion. Spirituality focuses on the common ground between people. People can focus on their spiritual nature whether they have particular religious beliefs or not. The word "God" elicits many feelings and thoughts within us, depending on what part religion or spirituality has played throughout our life. People use many different names and have many different meanings for a Higher Reality. Higher Power, or any of these names, when used in this book do not refer to darkness, evil, or the devil. As we mentioned in the introduction to the book, when we speak of Higher Power, we refer to that which helps us know truth, love, light, connection, healing, and intention for goodness. Some of these names include Nature, God, Spirit, the Divine, Organizing Principle of the Universe, the Absolute, Goddess, Allah, the Tao, Universal Mind, or the One. Where you see the word God or Higher Power, please substitute whatever name you use to refer to the universal source of life, light, healing, and love.

So, what is spirituality? Connection with Higher Power, finding meaning in life, transcending the daily personal self and feeling connected to others, and having a feeling of hope.

CONNECTION WITH HIGHER POWER

Jews, Christians, and Muslims have developed remarkably similar ideas of God, which also resemble other contemplations of the Absolute. When people try to find an ultimate meaning and value in human life, their minds seem to go in a certain direction. They have not been coerced to do this; it is something that seems natural to humanity.

—Karen Armstrong, *A History of God*

As we look at cultures the world over, the concept of a Higher Power, and coming to know that Power through prayer has been in stories and ancient texts as far back as we know. Many of these stories describe how a connection with the Divine brings healing of mind, body, and spirit. Many spiritual traditions speak of a Higher Reality or Higher Power, as being omnipresent, or everywhere, just as the universal field of physics connects all subatomic particles, everywhere. We may have a continual connection with God, arising from God and returning to God, as the subatomic particles emerge from, and fade into, the universal field.

Different cultures express connectedness and oneness with the Divine in unique ways (Ornish, 1998).

1. Hindu—Thou art That, the Universe is Brahman
2. Christian—(Jesus)—The Kingdom of God is within
3. Buddhist—(Buddha)—All are Buddhas
4. Islam—(Muhammad)—Wherever you turn is God's face, he who knows himself, knows God

Could it be purely coincidence that, even before television and satellite dishes connected the globe, the vision of God came to the mind and heart of people so separated by great distances?

Herbert Benson, M.D., founder of the Mind/Body Health Institute in Boston, says that we are very likely "hard-wired for God." When we contemplate God, the neurochemistry in our brains creates a very peaceful and calming experience that is beneficial to our health. If faith, prayer, and contemplating God makes the body healthier, then those who do these activities will live to reproduce. These behaviors will be passed on as necessary to survival (Benson, 1996).

In a study at the University of California at San Diego, Ramachandran suggests that there may be neural circuits in the temporal lobe of the brain that are involved in mystical experiences and God. This portion of the brain seems to be naturally attuned to ideas about a supreme being (Hotz, 1997).

Eugene d'Aquili, professor of psychiatry at the University of Pennsylvania and Andrew Newberg in the nuclear medicine program, concluded a two year study of the brains of people practicing Buddhist meditation also suggesting that an intuition of a transcendent reality may be hard-wired into the human mind. Feelings of calmness, unity, and transcendence correspond to increased activity in the brain's frontal lobes. The amygdala of the brain generates a sense of religious awe when certain religious gestures, such as bowing or making the sign of the cross, are performed. Religious practices stimulate the brain, creating perceptions of higher states of consciousness. Both parts of the autonomic nervous system (sympathetic and parasympathetic) are activated at once by meditations that focus on repetition (as in the Relaxation Response), whether repeating a word while sitting still, or when moving, as in the religious whirling of the Sufi tradition. During these activities, people say they experience "oceanic bliss," the absence of boundaries between beings, the absence of a sense of time flow, and the experience of a Divine Being (d'Aquili and Newberg, 1998).

Is it possible that the One wants us, and all beings, to know Her/Him/It? Perhaps for this purpose our brains contain special areas to guide us to the experience of communion with the Divine. The body is healthier and the mind more peaceful when we fill our minds and hearts with God.

Although many scientists still want to keep spirituality and science separate, many physicists are coming to the conclusion that this universe may well have been created by a Creator. There is so much evidence supporting the Big Bang theory of how the universe came into being that most scientists now take it for granted. The chances that all the variables could have converged at just the exact moment to create the Big Bang have been calculated at 1 chance in 1 with 60 zeros after it. I have no idea what that number is called, but it is huge. In other words, it is very highly unlikely that it happened by chance. Therefore, a Creator is likely.

It's better to see God in everything than to try to figure it out.

—Neem Karoli Baba, revered Indian sage

CONNECTEDNESS TO OTHERS AND MEANING IN LIFE

We have all felt alone. Feeling we are separate creates sadness, fear, and illness. We may feel a physical or emotional separation from loved ones or friends. We may not feel part of the group at work. We often feel confused when we don't feel connected with our inner self, our true nature. Belief that we are separate from God creates a profound sense of loneliness.

Part of feeling spiritually whole is feeling that life has some kind of meaning. Meaning in life comes from feeling connection with our inner self, and connection with others. When we feel connected, we feel accepted, heard, and loved. As you recall, social support, or having someone you can count on, talk to, cry and laugh with, is one of the most crucial factors to creating long-lasting health. We all want someone to tell our story to. When we help others, we also feel connected, and that life has purpose. Most of us find great comfort in knowing we are a beneficial, integral part of a whole. Feeling part of a whole gives us the idea that there may be a greater plan, and this also gives meaning to life. We transcend our ordinary view of ourselves and our life when we connect to something greater.

When we look at a subatomic particle as matter, each particle is separate. From the point of view that it is an energy packet, all is energy interacting. The universal field is the interaction of energy packets. If we believe that we are only a body, it is very easy to feel separation. We are not just a body. We are energy, spirit, always, continually connected to, and interacting with, each other. Always one with the Divine. Sometimes we forget our connectedness. From our point of view we often feel so far from God. From God's point of view, we have never left.

We feel most closely related to others when we see things we have in common. Brothers and sisters may have the same eyes or toes, indicating they are family. Cultures share common foods, language, and customs, indicating they are "family." Everything in this universe is made of the same four subatomic particles. We are all related, we are all family.

Just as we see the same patterns in faces between parents and children, we see the same patterns repeated over and over again in myriad situations throughout the world we live in.

The Branching Pattern

Think of how many times you see movement occurring in a branching pattern, where there is movement from a wide area flowing into smaller branches (see Figure 11-6).

This branching pattern is seen in the root system of any plant, coral under the sea, and the Mississippi River delta viewed from space. Our lungs branch into bronchi and alveoli, our blood vessels branch into capillaries, and the leaves in plants have branching veins. Isn't it interesting that plants use this branching system to get nutrients from the soil and the air, and our "branches" are in our lungs and our "roots" in our intestines?

The Mandala Pattern

The mandala pattern symbolizes wholeness. In the East it is used as an aid to meditation and worship, and it is the pattern of many stained glass windows in cathedrals. We see the mandala pattern in snowflakes, the cross section of a lily stem, a thistle flower, and the diatom—a tiny one-celled water creature. Recall that when sand is spread on a metal plate and OM is chanted, vibrating the plate,

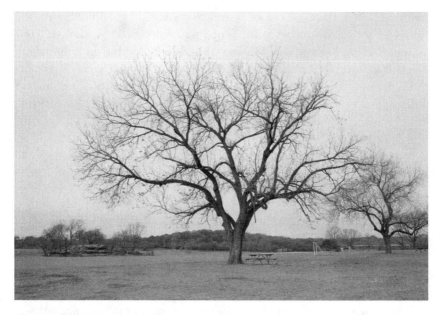

Figure 11-6 Branching pattern.

the sand particles move into a mandala pattern. Recall that spiritual traditions in India believe that OM was the sound that organized the matter of the world, bringing it into being.

Spirals

The indigenous people of New Zealand, the Maori, believe that the spiral symbolizes a sense of relatedness and oneness with all parts of the universe, from rocks to stars. Many American Indian cultures use a spiral pattern called the Mother Earth Symbol to signify emergence and rebirth. This same symbol appears on 3,000-year-old coins from Crete in the Mediterranean that signify fertility, the Labyrinth, life and death (Doczi, 1994). Coincidence?

Spirals have been carved into prehistoric stones believed to be used to connect with the Divine. If you notice architecture, pottery, jewelry, wrapping paper, and candles you will see the spiral. Many seashells and snails are spirals, and the patterns on a peacock's tail feathers grow in patterns of two spirals moving in opposite directions.

Our DNA, the blueprint of each cell, is two interacting spirals. Our finger and toe prints are spirals, as is the cochlea of the inner ear, and the axonemes of our red and white blood cells. Recall that the chaos pattern in physics indicates that the system is getting poised to move to a higher level of functioning. This chaos pattern is a spiral pattern.

The hair at our "soft spot" on our heads is in a spiral as is our Milky Way galaxy (Figures 11-7 and 11-8).

Is it possible that all the similarities we see are just a coincidence? In atoms, electrons turn on their axis as they move around the nucleus, like the Earth turns on its axis as it orbits the sun. The electromagnetic field around the Earth and the alpha brainwave of a relaxed person are both approximately 7.8 cycles per second. Could it be a coincidence that many living things including goldfish, roaches, mice, dogs, and humans need choice in their environment to have healthy immune systems?

Could it happen by chance that the patterns described above are seen so often in so many varied aspects of our world? Repeated pattern is not random. Repeated pattern is a design. A design means there is a Designer, or Designing Principle. Perhaps as the energy of this Designer moves through humans and the Uni-verse as sound, light, and love, these patterns are left upon us, and our world, so that we recognize that everything in this universe is part of one big family, and remember the way home.

Spirituality and Healing

One reason to address spirituality in massage is because it helps us remember our connection. Another reason is that it increases the healing potential of the massage. Our spirit feels the need for healing when we feel the pain of separation. Just as the neck and shoulders send a pain signal to wake us up when we have forgotten to move from the computer, our spirit sends depression, sadness, loneliness, and despair to wake us up when we have forgotten to be still and connect.

What heals the spirit? Spiritual healing is reconnecting. Sometimes that reconnection creates physical healing. Sometimes our life once again has meaning, our thoughts turn to helping others and having fun, and we feel hope and love. For some people spiritual healing happens at church, in the hospital, or when singing, painting, massaging, or dancing. For others, spiritual healing happens in quiet prayer, in nature, or reading meaningful writings. For an account of spiritual healing, see Appendix C.

In 1987, Sir John Marks Templeton established the John Templeton Foundation with a quest of finding out all he could about God. He says he has never been so enthusiastic, or happy. In 1997 he said in the *Palm Beach Illustrated,* "I helped more than a million people to become wealthier in my business, but I did not notice that it made them happier. . . . Only if you're on a solid basis, spiritu-

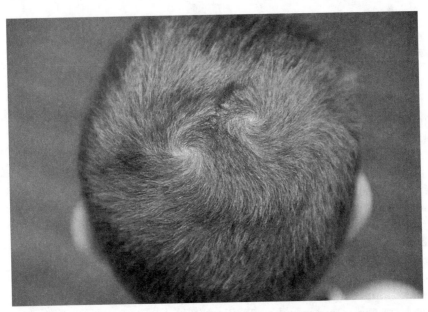

Figure 11-7 In ways we have yet to discover, we are related to magnificent celestial giants light years away.

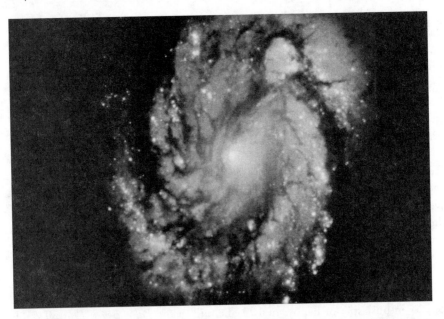

Figure 11-8 Spiral galaxy. (Hubble Heritage Team, AURA/STScI/NASA. Reproduced with permission.)

ally, are you likely to be permanently happy." He offers $15 million yearly to researchers of all faiths to discover the connections between spirituality and healing such as: What is consciousness? How do God and the cosmos relate? and How does prayer work? He funds universities for adding courses on spirituality and healing to their curricula (Witt, 1997).

In the spring of 1998, I attended a Spirituality and Healing in Medicine conference sponsored by Harvard Medical School. There were 700 attendees who were nurses, ministers, psychologists, physicians, and many others all wanting to hear the latest ideas and research about how spirituality affects healing. For contact information, see Appendix A. There is now a Mind/Body Institute in Houston affiliated with the one in Boston. Dr. Benson's group is available to help any hospital interested in establishing such an institute.

As you can see, a light is being focused on spirituality and healing. Reported in the *Journal of the American Medical Association,* religious involvement has been found to be a protective factor against many illnesses. It is suggested that religion and spirituality are essential, not optional, components of patient care. In 1994 only three medical schools taught courses on spirituality, and as of 1997 there were 30 (Levin, Larson, and Puchalski, 1997). Articles on spirituality in nursing practice appear in a wide variety of journals such as *Applied Nursing Research, Journal of Holistic Nursing,* and *Journal of Cardiovascular Nursing,* to name only a few. Many cultures have never doubted the role of a Higher Power in healing. Scientific inquiry is now entering the age-old quest to understand God.

Studies now indicate that whether we go to church, have faith in God, believe we will be healed, or pray at home, religious/spiritual activities help the body and mind heal (Matthews and Larson, 1995). According to a Gallup poll in 1990, 96% of Americans said they believe in God, and 75% pray at least once a day. Of 212 studies examining the effects of religious commitment on healthcare outcomes, 160 (75%) demonstrated a positive benefit of religious commitment. Religious commitment includes one or more of these factors:

1. Attendance in a place of worship
2. Prayer
3. Intimacy with God
4. Religious programs on television
5. Religious and other volunteer activities
6. Financial contributions to ministries
7. Feeling religion has importance and meaning in your life
8. Scripture and other devotional reading

These factors decreased alcoholism, psychological distress, heart disease, emphysema, cirrhosis, and state and trait anxiety in people with cancer. People tended to live longer.

Several studies demonstrate the cost benefit of spiritual practices. Heart surgery clients randomly assigned to a chaplain intervention showed an average two day shorter length of stay than those with usual care resulting in about $4,200 cost savings per client (Bliss, McSherry, and Fassett, 1995). Hospital stays are nearly two and a half times longer for older clients who are not religious compared to older clients with any kind of religious affiliation (Koenig and Larson, 1997).

Religious beliefs and activities can have a beneficial impact on emotional coping when people have cardiac bypass surgery, depression, hemodialysis, hip replacement, gynecological cancer, and breast cancer (Larson, 1998; Pressman, et al., 1990).

In a study of 232 people who had open heart surgery, people who had strong religious beliefs were three times more likely to survive than people without religious beliefs. These results were seen *after accounting for the social support* gained by being with people in church (Oxman, Freeman, and Manheimer, 1995).

In a sample of 1,718 people, those who attend religious services at least once a week have stronger immune functioning than less frequent attendees. The specific immune factor measured (interleukin-6) affects AIDS, osteoporosis, Alzheimer's disease, diabetes, and other serious illnesses (Koenig, et al., 1997).

We may not yet know exactly what the scientific reasons are for these findings, but we know the findings do exist.

Spirituality in Nursing

The entire June 1998 issue of the *Journal of Holistic Nursing* was devoted to the spiritual and holistic views of Florence Nightingale. Nightingale's strong spiritual beliefs guided and permeated her entire life, including the development of nursing. In a wonderful collection of her writings, we get a glimpse of her thoughts about spirituality:

> "What is Spirituality? Feelings called forth by the consciousness of a presence of higher nature than human. In accordance with God's law, human consciousness is intending to become one with the consciousness of God. For what is Mysticism? Is it not the attempt to draw near to God, no not by rites or ceremonies, but by inward disposition? Is it not merely a hard word for "The Kingdom of Heaven is within"? Heaven is neither a place nor a time. There might be a Heaven not only *here* but *now*. . . . Where shall I find God? In myself."
>
> Cited in Calabria and Macrae, 1994

Modern nursing had its roots in the work and teachings of Ms. Nightingale. It is no wonder that caring for the spiritual needs of people is an inner yearning many of those drawn to nursing. Helen Erickson suggests nursing interventions to help clients meet the spiritual needs of feeling hopeful, making meaning of life, and receiving unconditional acceptance (Erickson, Tomlin, and Swain, 1988). Jean Watson explicitly addresses the soul, and emphasizes the spiritual dimension of human beings and its importance in healing. She discusses transcendence as the actualization of one's spiritual essence. Margaret Newman says that a person is a unique pattern of consciousness within a field of absolute consciousness. Absolute consciousness equals unconditional love, and health is movement toward that consciousness (Sarter, 1997). These are only a few views on the role of spirituality in nursing.

Spirituality has been discussed and researched in nursing literature for some time. Patients' perceptions of their spiritual needs were: meaning and purpose, love, trust, hope, forgiveness, and creativity (Carson, 1989). In a study of people who were HIV positive, those who were spiritually well, according to a Spiritual Well Being Scale, were able to find meaning or purpose in their life and were hardier. When people are hardy, they are better able to resist the negative effects of stress (Carson and Green, 1992). Hope is often maintained by having religious belief, support from family and friends, belief in miracles, and involvement in work or vocations (Hall, 1994). Goldberg (1998) found spirituality in the nursing literature to include, physical aspects (touch and healing), emotional aspects (hope, love, meaning, and religion/transcendence), and focus on relationships. In Nursing Administration Quarterly, Krebs (2001) describes the benefits of spirituality and prayer for clients and suggests ways nurses can integrate spirituality into a busy nursing practice.

Establishing a spiritual connection with a client and helping them meet their spiritual needs is meaningful to the nurse as well as the client. True connections, even if only for a few moments, make life worthwhile. They are what we all seek. How do we begin to connect with our inner spirit, the spirit of others, and with God? Sometimes we must just have faith that the right words will come when they are needed.

Refrigerator wisdom

When you come to the edge of all the light that you know,
and you are about to step off into the darkness of the unknown,
Faith is knowing that one of two things will happen:
there will be something solid to stand on
or you will be taught how to fly.
    —Drs. Jordan and Margaret Paul in *Conflict to Caring*

1. Establishing a sense of trust
   caring attitude
   touch (Chapter 1, 6, 7)
   technical competence with tasks performed
   special attention to unique needs (Chapter 9, 10)
   nonverbal communication—maintain eye contact, body positioning that faces them
   listening
   soft tone of voice
   doing what you say you'll do
2. Finding meaning and purpose in life, in suffering, illness, and in death (Part III) by:
   A. Fostering connectedness with:
      inner self, values (turning inward), the external environment, nature, a
      Higher Power, people, pets, and a greater purpose in life
   B. Prayer and/or discussions with others about spiritual feelings
   C. By receiving and giving love (ch. 12)
   D. Touch, massage, energy-based healing (Ch. 6, 7, 11)
   E. Helping the receiver, or self, find hope by:
      Knowing others care, seeing self in the future, pointing to a future source of love,
      health, order, possibilities and powers beyond the current situation.
      Making choices in life that establish a feeling of control (ch. 9, 10).
3. Being present
   A. Listening to the whole story, understanding, respecting personal beliefs, giving
      undivided attention in a calm, unhurried manner
   B. Surrounding other, self, with love and acceptance, practicing HeartTouch
      (Chapter 12)
   C. Touch, massage (Chapter 7, 8)
   D. Compassion—listening for their needs, allowing suffering to be expressed
4. Offering to pray with and/or for the client (chapter 11)
5. Discussing/teaching massage, meditation, prayer, Relaxation Response, imagery,
   HeartTouch, Mindfulness Meditation with patient and family (Part III)
6. Setting up visits with clergy

© 1998 Marsha Walker (Used with permission.)

Figure 11-9 Enhancing Spiritual Well-being in Self and Others (© 1998 by Marsha Walker. Used with permission.)

We offer suggestions about how to enhance spiritual well-being and connection in Figure 11-9, as compiled from literature on spirituality and our own personal and professional experience.

Some nurses do not feel comfortable discussing spiritual needs with clients for personal reasons or because it has not been part of their nursing training. Follow your heart. In some situations, you may find that you and the client feel most comfortable using touch to create a spiritual connection. Here is an excellent moment for massage. The practice of "laying on of hands" can also be used even if you don't want to do a specific energy-based therapy. Ask the client's permission, and place your palms on the body, either on an area of pain or disease, or just resting on the feet or an arm. Center and ground yourself and ask that the Divine, the Healing Energy of the Universe, move through you to the client to help them in whatever way is best for all concerned. Take relaxed breaths, let your body relax. If you feel intuitively to move your hands to a different area, do so. You and/or the receiver may feel your hands getting warm. The session can last for one minute or as long as you have. You can be silent or pray aloud. Nurses can also teach this technique to families of clients and other nurses.

In a workshop we teach on Spirituality in Nursing, we often start by having the giver just rest her hands on the receiver's body to experience the power of touch for creating spiritual connection. A nurse might try this exercise with a colleague or client in appropriate situations in the work setting. One person lies on a massage table, bed, or sits in a chair surrounded by the rest of the group. The person on the table is asked what areas of his body would like attention. After taking a moment to enter a meditative, or prayerful, state of mind, everyone in the group places their hands on the person's body. Each person in the group allows their heart to guide the placement of their hands. Everyone has the intention to help the receiver heal in whatever way is best for her or him. The giver is asked to entertain caring TF for the person on the table. Each person in the group takes a turn as receiver.

The experience as giver and then as receiver, is remarkable. As givers, people have varying responses, including feeling intuitively guided and realizing the reason they came into nursing was to help people directly, in ways like this. They say that at first they felt strange, not "doing" anything except touching and caring, but then began to notice that something was happening without their direction. They could feel heat or energy passing through their hands to the other person, and some felt a connection with a Higher Power.

Receivers said the hands of the giver often got very warm, and this made them feel comforted and relaxed. Some had emotional experiences because it was the first time in a long time they had been touched solely for the purpose of helping them feel cared for. Some felt relief of pain or tension, and others felt a clarity and calmness of thought. Some said that at first they found it hard to just lie there and receive the attention, but later began to feel held by warm arms allowing them to explore feelings of self-worth.

At the end of the class, one of the nurses told us she had recently been diagnosed with several brain tumors. She had been doing many therapies including touch, prayer, and energy-based therapies. She was scheduled to have a CAT scan, and then surgery the next day. After the group work, she was beaming with tears in her eyes as she said, "I knew I was supposed to be here. The love and support I feel is just what I need. I'm going to be OK." I heard from her the next week. The surgery had been canceled. The pre-surgery CAT scan had shown that several tumors were gone and others were smaller. She had been laughing and dancing all week.

Paths of Connecting with Spirit

Recall our discussion of the Relaxation Response and Mindfulness Meditation in Chapter 10 as ways to help us become aware of, and direct our thoughts. We discussed how being in nature can balance our energy field. These techniques also help us connect with our own spirit within, and the Divine. Using these techniques, we can train ourselves to enjoy longer and longer periods of being awake and aware in the present moment, and open the door for communion with Spirit. Prayer is also a way that many people connect with the One. You will notice that we see our old friend, the breath, once again. Spirit comes from *spiritus,* defined in Webster's dictionary as breath. Breath is defined as spirit and animation, suggesting a relationship between conscious breathing and connecting with Spirit. Appendix C offers a meditation that helps to create spiritual connection.

RELAXATION RESPONSE

Recall that in Dr. Benson's research, the benefits of the Relaxation Response are achieved by two steps: (1) focusing on a repetition whether a word, phrase, or movement and (2) returning to it when the mind wanders. In the 1970s when Herbert Benson began to explore this new phenomenon, he decided to look to the world religions who had forms of meditation to see if there were any commonalities in their meditation practices. He found that in the Hindu tradition there was the repetition of the word Om. In a sacred Hindu text called the Upanishads from the seventeenth-century B.C., it is written that if one wishes union with God, focus on the breath, and repeat a word or phrase with each exhale. In the Jewish tradition from 4–5 B.C., it is written to repeat the "name of the Seal" with each outward breath. In the Christian tradition from 2–4 A.D. people would kneel and repeat the word Jesus with each exhale. In Shintoism, numbers are counted with the exhale. In Islam, there is a repetition of Insha' Allah. Buddhists repeat Om, ma-ne, pad-me, Om (Ohm, mah-nay, pahd-may, Ohm). In the Sufi tradition, spiritual practices include spinning, sometimes very slowly for hours to connect with the Divine (Benson, 1996).

So, to connect with God, many traditions incorporate repetition (whether a word, action) and/or a focus on the breath. Both of these focus our awareness so that we don't get lost in the movie of our thoughts. Many people report that while they are practicing the Relaxation Response they feel a divine, or spiritual presence. Becoming conscious in the moment, letting thoughts go, and focusing on repetition, seem to create conditions under which it is easier to feel the presence of the Divine.

MINDFULNESS MEDITATION

Recall from Chapter 10, that in Mindfulness Meditation, when a thought arises, you notice it, observe it without analyzing it, and return your focus to the breath, or your chosen object of focus. Mindfulness Meditation, also called Insight Meditation, is about 2,500 years old. It is a Buddhist practice for cultivating greater awareness and wisdom by being awake in each moment, which allows you to live that moment as fully as possible. With continued practice of this meditation, people report a change in the quality of their awareness, an inner balance of mind, insights, and profound experiences of stillness and joy. People begin to experience a trusting connection to others, a sense of being part of the greater flow of life, and a sense of oneness with the world (Kabat-Zinn, 1993).

BEING IN NATURE

When people in many cultures ask how to connect with Spirit, they are told to go sit in nature until they hear the word of God. It is often easier to hear the voice of the One in the stillness of nature away from the sounds of the city, electricity, and other people. Observing the repeated patterns in nature is one way to learn about the Designer. After sitting in one place in a natural setting for 20 minutes or so, the plants, animals, and the Earth begin to trust you. They become curious, extending their energy to explore and connect. Soon they embrace you as part of the natural order and harmony that is their world. The mind becomes quiet. Treasures reveal themselves.

By experiencing Her image or reflection in the beauty, spontaneity, stillness, and movement of nature, we get to spend time with, and come to know the One.

A Meditation

In the rustle of the leaves, we hear the whisper of God.
In the perfume of the flowers, we smell the fragrance of God.
As the stream rushes over and around rocks, we hear the laughter of God.
In the touch of the grasses, we feel the hand of God.
When we look up to the treetops and down to the bottom of the river, we look into the face of God.
As we sit on the Earth surrounded by life, we are cradled in the arms of God.

—Marsha Walker

We feel the wind, but we can only see it by noticing how it blows the leaves, the water, or the sand. Such is God.

PRAYER

Prayer is recognized in many cultures as a way to connect with the Divine. What is prayer? Prayer is each person's unique, deepest connection between their inner being and Higher Power. It may be jubilantly twirling and dancing with God. It may be entering into the stillness and being with the Absolute. According to the Princeton Religious Research Center, 90% of the people in the United States feel that God loves them. In *Time* Magazine, 82% of Americans believe in the healing power of prayer, 77% believe that God can intervene to cure those with a serious illness, and 73% believe that praying for another can help cure their illness (Larson, 1998). These statistics reveal that a large percentage of Americans believe that their thoughts can help create a change in their own, or another's bodymind, even at a distance, when they connect with God. Recall from our discussion of the power of belief, 60–90% of the illnesses we experience show marked improvement depending on the strength of the person's belief in the method of healing, whether it is a drug, sacred stone, or prayer. Our belief is very powerful in bringing about change. Considering the power of belief, if prayer is important to a client, perhaps it should be included in any program to improve their health.

I imagine some of you have prayed for a client, family member, or yourself, and feel very strongly that it helped. When I pray with,, and for, clients, they seem to feel more comforted than before. One of the most healing things I can do for a client, and myself, is to take a moment and come together with God.

The National Center for Complementary and Alternative Medicine has classified prayer as a spiritual treatment modality in the category of mind and body control (Dunn and Horgas, 2000). Prayer is frequently used as a nursing intervention (Lewis, 1996; Dossey, Keegan, and Guzzetta, 2000).

For approximately 20 years, the Spindrift organization has been conducting research that shows that prayer works. Their studies examine the effects of prayer on a variety of living systems including molds, seedlings of plants, and people. To determine if any type of prayer was more effective than any other, they looked at directed and non-directed prayer. Directed prayer has a specific goal in mind, such as to increase blood flow, to get a certain job, or heal an illness. Non-directed prayer has no specific outcome in mind, praying for what is best for the individual, or "Thy will be done." In their studies the non-directed approach was somewhat more effective than the directed approach (Dossey, 1997). The important point is not which is better, but that they both work. Use whatever method fits your personality, beliefs, and situation. For contact information, see Appendix A.

Many studies examine the healing power of prayer. In one study, a cardiologist, Randolph Byrd, wanted to see if prayer had an effect on people with heart

Prayer and Back Pain

I injured my back about 15 years ago in a horseback-riding accident where I fell off of a horse and slammed onto the concrete. Nothing was broken, but there has always been a pull and a strain there that never went away.

I'm a dog groomer and recently I've been doing a lot more bathing. and so I have a lot more pressure and stress on my back. One day I bent a certain way, my whole back caught, and I could barely straighten up. That next morning it hurt so bad I could not even move. I couldn't get up off of any chair I was sitting on. I couldn't stand up. When I tried to walk it was just so excruciating. I would just cry. This lasted for at least two solid weeks. I went to a chiropractor every day. It helped a little bit. The next morning it still hurt so badly I could not move. I sat and prayed to God every night and listened to my healing tapes. Every morning I got up and it still hurt. I continued to pray and praise God. I realized that my work was going to have to change. I kept asking God what it was that He wanted me to learn.

One day I called a friend and I said, "I want to get together and pray. I can't do this anymore. I know that I'm going to be healed." I believed it completely in my heart. We sat in the park and we prayed. She put the Bible on my back and we both prayed. And I was saying, "I accept this healing. I am a child of God. And I totally believe that I will be healed." I had my hand on my friend's knee and she said I started gripping it so hard, and my whole body was shaking. And at this time I was crying—not from pain—but from this incredible joy that I can't even explain. My friend had her hand on the Bible we put on my back and said her hand felt like it was being sucked to the Bible like a vacuum cleaner hose. At that point she said she felt a very strong energy coming through her hands from the Bible. My back and body felt like they were pulling something from the Bible. After this, when I started shaking I kept saying I claim this healing and then I just expelled a breath and when I did I stopped shaking and sat there for a little—we prayed a little more. I stood up and the pain was completely gone. I mean completely gone. And so I prayed even more and thanked and praised God and the next morning I got up—nothing. No pain. Not any at all. From that time on I have picked dogs up and even slipped with them. Not only did God heal the recent pain that I had, but He healed the old injury as well. I do truly believe that it is a miracle.

—Diana M.

problems. He conducted a randomized, double-blind study where 393 patients admitted to a coronary care unit were assigned to either a group receiving prayer or a control group receiving no prayer. The people doing the praying were given first names and descriptions of the condition of those they were praying for. The ones praying were of many faiths, and were told to pray in whatever way they felt comfortable. The results were very impressive. The people in the group that was prayed for needed five times less antibiotics, were three times less likely to develop pulmonary edema (the lungs fill with fluid), none needed to be connected to a ventilator, and fewer died. Twelve people who were not prayed for needed breathing support (Byrd, 1988). With results like these, it seems that all interested clients might benefit from prayer. In a replication of Byrd's study, Harris et al. (1999) found that the prayer group had better CCU courses as derived from blinded, retrospective medical chart review, compared to a control group.

Dunn and Horgas (2000) found that prayer was used by 96% of community-dwelling Elders as a self-care modality to cope with stress, and it did not differ across income, religious affiliation, or age. Those who used prayer were significantly more optimistic and self-reliant.

Recognized healers who use the laying on of hands, acknowledge the role of prayer and God in healing. Agnes Sanford wrote, "When we pray in accordance with the law of love, we pray in accordance with the will of God." Ambrose and Olga Worrall wrote: "In true prayer our thinking is an awareness that we are part of the Divine Universe." (LeShan, 1974).

Massage and Spirituality

The art of massage has much in common with the arts as we commonly think of them, such as dance, sculpting, music, and painting. Certainly performing massage is much like a dance. When we learn to dance, there are specific steps we must remember. When we first begin to dance, those first moves may be the only ones we use in our performances. With practice, we relax and begin to improvise. So it is in massage. We discover, by letting go and following, that we are responding to the rhythms of our body intelligence. We become sensitive to the receiver's body and how it responds to the massage. The massage becomes a continual interaction, leaving ourselves and the receiver changed and energized for the better.

As in sculpting, our hands glide through the receiver's tissues shearing off the superfluous and excessive tension carried within them. What is removed vanishes into the air revealing the relaxed and graceful person who was already there, encased in their once rigid resistance.

Giving a massage is much like performing music by playing an instrument. When we first touch the instrument, we may be unfamiliar with the way it feels and somewhat awkward when we try to produce the sound we want. We may feel much the same when we begin to practice our first few massage strokes. If our first few attempts are somewhat uncomfortable, we adjust our stance and the pressure and speed of our touch. But soon we gain facility, and the sounds we hear from the receiver will be pleasant ones indeed. Familiarity with learning the basic routines, as in playing the scales on an instrument, will lay the groundwork for future improvisation. In massage, as in musicianship, patient mastery of the fundamentals may be difficult for students who hear the music in their heads and know what it should sound like, wanting to hasten to improvisation before the basics are mastered. Your patience in the beginning will be rewarded when you enjoy and treasure your first experiences of hearing music pour from your hands.

Like the painter, you are working with light. Your hands and fingers are moving through a rich and intricate network of photons of light in the form of muscles, tissues, nerves, and cells. For the sensation of your hands to register upon the canvas of your receiver's brain and nervous system, millions and millions of microscopic chemical reactions have to take place each and every moment. For these minute chemical reactions to fire and transfer along those miles of bioelectrical pathways, countless millions of electrons within the cells will have to heed a new call. They leave their subatomic orbits and join a different orbit to which they are compelled and drawn. Each time they jump to a new path, a tiny gleam of light (photon) is released. One long, slow stroke of the hands up alongside the spine sets off a subatomic display of light and pattern at the very heart of the body's being. Like the painter, you are a bringer of light and color, stirring up a thousand tiny prisms, so that beauty and grace may have a more restive and accommodating canvas from which to shine.

What is it about some paintings that cause us to stare in awe for long moments as we are transported beyond the canvas and paint into another world? Why do we feel compelled to touch and explore some sculptures as they beckon to us? As we are carried within and away by music, how can it cause us to begin swirling, or shed many a tear? Why do we feel transformed after receiving a massage?

It is Spirit. The artist becomes a vehicle for Spirit to move into the physical/mental/emotional plane and connect with us, reminding us who we truly are. In massage, Spirit comes through the touch of the hands, the look in the eyes, the tone of the voice, and the vibration of the energy fields of giver and receiver as they merge. Whether it is through massage, art, song, or dance, Spirit comes to replace TF of the day with those of meaning, inspiration, and love.

SUMMARY

In Chapter 9, we learned how our emotions move peptides that convey information connecting all systems of the body. In this chapter, we learned that we are connected to others near and far through our individual energy fields. Our fields are mediums through which emotions travel and connect us. Now we have an even deeper understanding of the power that our TF have on our own bodies and that of those we massage. As our exploration of connection expands, we realize

422   CHAPTER 11

that we must consider the role of spirituality in nursing and massage. In this chapter we come to see that massage is a reflection of life. It's all about movement, rhythm, and connection.

What can we do to give a massage that creates a spiritual connection? How do our TF actually affect the health of our clients? What role does love play in the spiritmindbody? How do we touch with our hearts? In the remainder of this book we learn to give a massage with heart. Part III has provided information and techniques that create a foundation from which to practice the HeartTouch technique while giving a massage, and in many situations in daily life. As we learn Heart-Touch in the next chapter, we discuss the benefits of heart-centered awareness and techniques for entering the heart space. We also explore what we consider to be the most important part of massage, of healing, and of life—the sharing of love.

PUTTING THESE IDEAS INTO PRACTICE

1. Learn to assess the energy field. Every day for one week choose a situation in your life where an individual (person, plant, animal) or yourself, has an injury. Move your palm over the area slowly several times with your eyes closed and see if you feel any difference between the injured area and healthy area. You may feel heat or a magnetic pull.

2. Think about your area of practice and imagine situations in which you might use the tools for balancing the energy field.

3. Take a moment and write down your own personal definition of spirituality.

4. Over the next week, choose three clients and incorporate spirituality into your interactions with them.

HeartTouch: Love as Connector

With single mindedness, the master quells his thoughts.
He ends their wandering.
Seated in the cave of the heart
He finds freedom.
The way is not in the sky.
The way is in the heart.

—Buddha, the *Dhammapada*

OBJECTIVES

1. Explain the difference between physical and nonphysical touching.
2. Describe the three steps of the HeartTouch technique, and three situations in which you might use it.
3. Discuss the role of focusing on the breath in Heart-Centered Awareness, and the benefits of intentional heart focus to the health of the bodymind.
4. Discuss the value of giving and receiving love in the healthcare setting.
5. Describe a time when you felt a distant connection with another, and discuss the beneficial use of distant healing in healthcare.
6. Discuss the relationship between intentional heart focus, love, Higher Power, and healing.

Through the years of giving massage, we began to realize that our massage was evolving. We began to feel more peaceful afterward, and our clients began to tell us it was a healing experience for them. As we began to teach massage workshops we wanted to help others have a similar experience, so we carefully observed just what we were doing during a massage so that we could try to convey it to others. We discovered several steps that we were including in each massage that transformed a group of good techniques into something special. We decided to call this technique HeartTouch (HRT) because that is exactly what it is, a touching of hearts.

In this chapter, we offer this technique to you. Part III is about connecting, within ourselves and with others, and how massage is a bridge to aid in that connecting. HRT is a combination of all that we have discussed in Part III. Each of the first three chapters of Part III stands alone as a valuable tool for healing. When taken together, they create a very powerful pathway for discovery and transformation.

In HRT, we not only connect with our inner self in a way that improves our own health, but we use our conscious intention to connect with and affect the health and well-being of others. If you practice HRT while giving a massage, it becomes much more than a routine of techniques. HRT adds a special quality to any nursing intervention. A family member can also use this technique to connect with a loved one while sitting beside their bed.

In this chapter we first look at the foundation of HRT. We then take each step and discuss its importance in the healthy functioning of the Spiritmindbody, including research.

EARLY DISCOVERIES

When we looked closely at what we were doing as we gave a massage, we discovered a heart-hand-heart circle. We noticed that how we were feeling influenced how we touched the receiver. And how we touched the receiver influenced how they felt. We began to pay attention to this heart-hand circle.

What We Feel Influences How We Touch

We all have many opportunities to touch people in a day. The touch can be holding a hand, helping a child into the car, giving a shoulder massage, picking up an arm to take a blood pressure reading, or turning someone who is sick in bed. People often form their deepest and most lasting impressions about who we are by how we touch them. Imagine what it would be like if you were in a hospital bed and couldn't see, talk, or move your body? If someone rubbed your back, could you tell if they cared about you by the way they touched you?

We found that when we were feeling certain feelings we touched the receiver in different ways. Distraction, worry, anger, and disapproval often cause the fingers to be rigid and not fully in contact with the receiver's body. Movements of the hands and fingers are often quick and hard. One movement does not flow easily into the next. Although none of us ever intend to communicate these feelings to others through our touch, it happens.

If you notice you are feeling any of these feelings, take three or four breaths to bring you to the present so you can intentionally choose the thoughts and feelings (TF) you want to convey to the client through your hands. When we intentionally feel appreciation, peacefulness, joy, acceptance, and love, our hands are warmer, and the touch is gentle. All of the fingers are in full contact with the skin. All movements are slow. One motion gracefully follows another.

When most of us see a newborn, we automatically feel tenderness and love. Our hearts melt. How do you touch a newborn baby? All of your conscious awareness focuses on that baby, and how you touch it. You are fully present in the moment, touching very slowly and softly, sometimes with only one finger. You touch it as if it is so fragile and most precious. All of us want to be touched this way. There is a place within us that is forever fragile and vulnerable, and needs to feel safe and loved. This kind of loving touch, if only for a moment, reaches that place, and we feel connected.

How We are Touched Influences What We Feel

The way our hand touches another creates feelings in their heart. In addition to physical touch, we touch others in non-physical ways—thoughts and feelings also touch our hearts.

PHYSICAL TOUCH

Receiving physical touch affects us in the heart and causes us to experience emotion. When we are touched with love, that love fills the heart (Figure 12-1).

Physical Touching Creates Feeling

For a moment, imagine each of these different kinds of physical touching, and notice the feelings they cause you to have:

The breeze against your face in the springtime
Bare feet on a soft rug in the morning
Wearing a tie or pair of shoes that is too tight
Hitting your head on the corner of the cabinet
Lying in a tub of warm water
Holding hands with the one you love the most
The smooth coolness of ice cream on your tongue in the summertime
The hug around your neck of a precious child

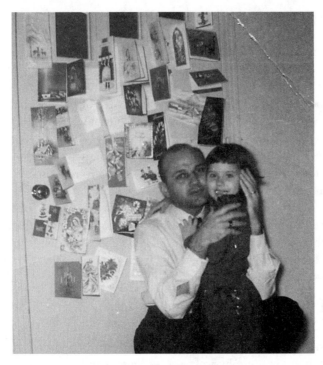

Figure 12-1

Slow, gentle massage strokes create feelings of safety and comfort. Fast, hard strokes can cause feelings of uneasiness, agitation, or mistrust. Touch brings feeling into our world based on what we have learned to connect or associate with that touch. Touch also stimulates the thoughts, brain, nervous system, glands, and muscles to change in ways that cause us to feel.

TOUCHING WITH THE HEART

Non-physical touching also causes us to feel emotion. Touch is given and received with the heart through a word, a look, a pause in a conversation, or a feeling sent our way. No physical touching is necessary. This touching of the heart causes our bodies to have physical responses that are as strong as those caused by physical touch. We say we are "touched" when something wakes up a feeling inside us. Tears flow in response to a kind action directed our way. The heart races when we are touched by people in love, even when they exist only in a book or movie. We are touched, or moved, when we hear music, smell a room that reminds us of Grandma's house, a friend sends a card during hard times, or a spouse has dinner ready for you after a hard day. When another feels moved in their heart by our touch, they often reach out to connect with a hand, or their heart, giving back to us. And so the heart-hand circle goes.

Feelings of the heart are communicated in many ways, sometimes over great distances, and even across the expanse of time. Florian told us this story.

"This is my story about my first sickness. It must have been 1937, so I was 12. What do I remember most? Who came to the hospital to see me. I had scarlet fever. Two big men came and put a quarantine sign in front of the house. "Do not enter. Quarantined. Contagious." They wrapped me up in a white sheet and put me in an ambulance. I left all my brothers and sisters for the first time. There were 11 of us. Where am I going? They hauled me off to the welfare hospital. There was no such thing as medical insurance. We couldn't afford it with 13 mouths to feed. I guess the guy upstairs probably looked over us. I stayed there probably almost two and a half months. I had been there three weeks and nobody came to see me.

One day blood just started rolling out of my nose. I didn't have a button. The hospital wasn't equipped to have a button for the nurse. So I hollered and hollered. By that time, the bed sheet was almost saturated with blood. Finally the nurse came in and put two Q-tips in my nose. I looked like a walrus. But, two days later my oldest sister Angie came up. I can still see her face as she looked through the little window in the door. Nothing like it. It's how you feel inside. It's a bond. Some kind of magnetism. She brought me a fire engine truck just as red and beautiful as can be, with white wheels on it. Another two or three weeks went by and that was the only toy I had. First time you realize you have a family and you miss your brothers and sisters. Nobody could come in or go out. And you lose that bond. You think you're happy and you won't miss your family until something like that happens.

When I walked out, it was like a different world. The trees were blooming. Everything was beautiful. Absolutely fantastic. And when I told that to Angie on her 80th birthday, she said, "You remember that?" I said, "Boy, like it happened yesterday." You can remember the big things, possibly, if you try."

The Touch of Spirit

We began to notice another kind of touch in our massage sessions—the touch of spirit. What is it that sparkles out from the eyes? What do we so miss when a loved one dies? When two people feel safe with each other, hearts open and spirits venture out. This can happen during a massage. Those looks, those touches, those words filled with spirit touch our hearts most deeply, creating connection. There is another kind of spiritual connection that began to happen in some massages. As we focused on feeling love for the receiver, we noticed a connection with

Higher Power. This kind of touching is also accompanied by emotion. When touched by the Divine, the heart, body, and mind are filled with love. The touch of Higher Power comes as a whisper in the ear, a hand on the face, a stirring in the heart, and brings us to this moment to be loved, and to love.

After noticing our massages for awhile, we began to see a pattern in those massages that felt special. During the massage, we kept our focus on how our hands were touching the client, trying to replace stray thoughts with life-giving thoughts. We found something to love, or appreciate, about the receiver as a whole, deserving person. This loving energy was visualized as surrounding and permeating the client's body and energy field. A connection with Higher Power was made, asking for healing that would most benefit the client. This pattern became HeartTouch.

When trying to find the best ways to teach this to others, we searched the literature to see if anyone talked about using love and/or connection—with or without Higher Power—to assist with healing. We found a few techniques, along with some research, that incorporated one or more of these ideas, but in different ways (Childre, 1994; Laskow, 1992; LeShan, 1974). From our personal experience and this support from the work of others, we feel HRT may be beneficial to you.

HEARTTOUCH

HeartTouch is an internal maneuver that can be used anytime you want to create a connection with another, whether you touch physically or not. It can be completed in one minute at the beginning of an interaction, and can be used continually throughout. HRT can be practiced sitting in a hospital room with a loved one, in the rush hour traffic, or during a difficult conversation. It can be used as you are washing your hands when you enter a client's room, as you are changing a dressing, or when you give a massage.

HRT contains three steps: (1) Heart-Centered Awareness, (2) Loving-Touch, (3) and Connection with Higher Power (Walker, 1998). As the chapter unfolds, each step will be discussed in detail, including research and benefits to health and well-being. If you don't believe in a Higher Power as defined in Chapter 11, practicing the first two steps of HRT will still bring benefit to you and your client. Although research has not yet been done on the complete HRT technique, we present research studies that relate to each step, supporting the effects we notice in practice.

As we continue to practice HRT, we find that it leads us down a path of discovery and transformation involving:

The Breath as a Guide

The Heart as a Doorway

Love as the Key

HEART-CENTERED AWARENESS

From what we have discussed about PNI (Chapter 9) and Techniques for Changing TF (Chapter 10), you will see how practicing Heart-Centered Awareness (HCA) benefits your physical and emotional well-being. It also creates a balanced, coherent state in your bodymind as preparation for sending love and appreciation to the receiver in the Loving-Touch step.

HCA has three steps:

1. Centering—Take a few slow, deep breaths and bring the focus of your attention to the moment, letting go of all thoughts except being present to engage in the current situation.

2. Picture a small circle of light moving from your head, down your neck to your heart area. Once at your heart area, with each breath, allow the circle to grow.

3. Remember a situation where you felt loved, or were with someone you loved. Allow yourself to be in that situation, hear the sounds, smell the smells, see the sights, and feel the feelings.

The Breath as a Guide

We can go for weeks without food before the body dies. We can go for days without water. Take a moment and take a deep breath, and hold it. How long did you last? I didn't even make it for a minute. We can't ignore the breath, it happens continuously. The breath probably plays such a paramount role in the Spirit-mindbody so that at some point we will discover its role as a guide. What does a guide do? It leads us by focusing our attention on where we are, and what is important. The breath focuses our attention in the moment, helping us center. Since we are always breathing, it is easy to focus on when we want to use it to change what we are thinking and feeling.

Chopra (1993) suggests that the breath connects the organism to consciousness as the junction of the mind, body, and spirit. We can consciously control the breath with the mind, and the breath affects the body in myriad ways. Continual movement of the breath contributes to continual movement of prana, or chi, the life energy flowing from Spirit to every aspect of life. Balanced prana affects the physical body by creating a responsive nervous system, proper formation of tissues, strong immunity, and physical vitality. Balanced prana also contributes to sound sleep, mental alertness, enthusiasm, and spiritual realization. Depleted prana is directly linked with aging and death.

Recall that breathing in different rhythms changes our TF. Breathing slowly and deeply creates TF of calmness and clarity. One of the most amazing revelations I have experienced about the breath is that consciously changing my breathing pattern alters what I am feeling. What a wonderful tool! I have noticed that if I am nervous, stressed, or angry my breath is very shallow, and there are long pauses between breaths. When I remember to use those feelings as a wake-up call, I consciously change my breathing to deep, slow, and regular. I become conscious of what I'm thinking and feeling, and can choose from there.

We have found that the breath is also a built in guide to help us remember our connection to Spirit. As mentioned previously, one definition of spirit is breath. The breath is an ideal guide between the everyday world we all live in, and the inner world. By focusing on the breath, it can lead us past the obstacles and diversions of thought that the mind brings into the path. Following the breath with our awareness will lead the mind to stillness. As the mind dwells more and more in stillness, we awaken to the inner reality that is present all the time; the reality that fuels our being with nourishment, light, play, meaning, curiosity, and love. As we dwell more and more in this inner reality, we remember how we are meant to live in this world, and who we really are. "Be still and know that I am God." Psalms 46:10.

This exercise will give you practice in becoming conscious of your breath and directing it. It can be practiced for a few seconds, or as long as you wish. After you become familiar with it, it can be done driving a car, lying in bed, or in any situation.

Getting Acquainted with Your Guide

One of the easiest ways to begin to get in touch with your breath is to take 10 slow breaths, like gentle sighs, inhale and exhale. Notice the air as it passes in and out of your nostrils. See if you can make it through 10 breaths without the mind carrying you away. Continual, slow breaths bring us to the moment. Try practicing this several times a day for one week. Then try to finish 20 consecutive breaths.

The Heart as the Doorway

When we put our attention on the breath, it helps us become calm, present, focused, and centered. We can then follow our guide to the heart. Continuing with HCA, imagine a small light on your forehead, and follow it to your heart area. As you inhale and exhale, the circle of light grows. You are now resting in the heart, the seat of power. What you think and feel in this place greatly affects your physical body, and the ease with which you are able to handle stressful situations. The heart, not the mind, is the place of wisdom and understanding.

"As a man thinketh in his heart, so is he." Proverbs 23:7.

THE POWER OF THE HEART

The heart is the main power center of the body. The rhythm of the heartbeat produces an electromagnetic field that is approximately 5,000 times stronger than the field produced by the brain. The field of the heart can also be detected 8–10 feet away from the body using a magnetometer. The same electrical patterns generated by the heart can be detected in our brainwaves (Song, Schwartz, and Russek, 1998). The electrical signal of the heart can be detected by placing an electrode anywhere on the body, such as the toe or ear lobe, indicating that it permeates every cell in the body. The electromagnetic field of the heart is affected by the feelings we are having (Childre and Martin, 1999).

The heart communicates with the body and brain through chemical and neural messages. John and Beatrice Lacey (1970) were among the first to research the relationship between the heart and the brain. During the 1960s and 70s, they found that the heart talks to the brain. The heart sends signals through the nervous system to the brain that affect what we perceive through our five senses and how our muscles react; in other words, how we perceive and react to our world. These signals affect brain output to the autonomic nervous system (automatic functions) that affect blood vessels, organs, and glands in the body. Signals from the heart are also sent to the cortex of the brain, the center of higher thought and reasoning. In 1974, Gahery and Vigier found that by stimulating the vagus nerve, a pathway from the heart to the brain, the brain's electrical response was half its normal rate.

From the science of neurocardiology, Armour and Ardell (1994) found that the heart also has its own nervous system that operates and processes information independent of the brain or nervous system of the body. This nervous system inside the heart integrates incoming information from the brain with sensory information originating from within the heart itself. Based on this integration of information, signals are sent to the heart muscle that affect its function. An interesting question arises. What might be the source of this sensory information originating from within the heart?

The heart also communicates with the brain and body by secreting hormones. One hormone called atrial natriuretic factor, or atrial peptide, affects blood vessels, the kidneys, adrenal glands, and regulatory areas in the brain. Some studies suggest that it affects immune function and inhibits the release of stress hormones (Childre and Martin, 1999).

From the above information, we see that the heart has a profound effect on the brain and body. Can the heart be influenced, perhaps through our feelings, to affect all of these areas in ways that are beneficial, or detrimental, to health?

INTENTIONAL HEART FOCUS

As early as 1628, Sir Wm. Harvey spoke of the effects of TF on the heart. He said, "Every affection of the mind that is attended to with pain or pleasure, hope or fear, is the cause of an agitation whose influence extends to the heart."

Most of us in the Western culture have been led to believe that the mind is the center of understanding, and it is the mind that we should turn to when deciding what to do in any given situation. The mind is an excellent tool; however, if the situation involves emotion, relationships, or spiritual quest, the heart is the place to turn. Even our daily language connects the physical heart and feelings. When we feel love, we say our heart is overflowing. We say we are heartbroken when we are desperately disappointed over a situation. "Bless your heart" is used both when someone is having a hard time, and when they have done something wonderful. When we feel very moved, we often put our hands over our hearts.

Just as we talked about physical touching and non-physical touching, we also have a physical heart and a non-physical heart that is an energy center, or electromagnetic field. Focusing on the area of the physical heart helps us enter the energetic, or spiritual heart. From this inner place, we can connect with the heart of another. In this place, we also hear what to think to best create physical and mental harmony within ourselves.

The Institute of HeartMath was founded in 1991 by D. L. Childre to find out what the heart really is, and the role it plays in our health. He has put together a team of researchers to measure the qualities associated with the heart that he believes are love, care, compassion, and appreciation. Very interesting research from the Institute of HeartMath suggests that when we focus our attention on the heart and the surrounding area, and consciously feel emotions, we can affect the heart, and so the rest of the body. They suggest that heart focus may create a coherent state in the body and mind that creates a shift in perception allowing greater self awareness. Their research indicates that the electrical field of the heart is where love enters the human system. The DNA molecule seems to function as an antenna, receiving frequency information from the heart. Transformation takes place according to how much you follow your heart in your moment to moment attitudes and decisions. Perhaps feelings of love, by creating balanced rhythms in the heart, can affect even the DNA of each cell.

The following research explores the power of intentional heart focus using Freeze Frame (FF), a technique developed at the Institute of HeartMath. Recall from Chapter 10 that in FF you focus your attention on the heart area and remember a positive or fun experience. The changes noted in the following research occurred only when the feelings were truly felt. The same results were not found if the person just thought about the feeling.

McCraty, et al., (1995) were the first to demonstrate that positive emotions can significantly influence heart rate variability (HRV). HRV is an non-invasive test to distinguish between stimulating (sympathetic) and relaxing (parasympathetic) regulation of the heart, and is an indicator of the health of the cardiovascular system. The heart functions most efficiently when there is a balance between sympathetic and parasympathetic input. When the HRV is high, the heart is flexible and able to change its rate easily to adapt to a new situation. For example, when you are resting, the heart rate is very slow. If all of a sudden someone pounds at the door, you are startled and jump up to see who it is. Your heart immediately begins beating very fast. It must be able to change its rhythm very flexibly to accommodate your life. The heart rate must be able to change in response to feelings, thoughts, and physical activities. When the heart rate variability is low, it is predictive of cardiovascular disease, high blood pressure, and sudden death from heart attack and congestive heart failure. Low HRV is also associated with diabetic neuropathy, decreased hormonal responses, and rejected heart transplants. Emotional states such as major depression, panic disorder, anxiety, and worry are related to low HRV. Through the baroreceptor system (a nerve pathway) connecting the heart and the brain, our heart rhythms affect the brain, influencing blood pressure and our ability to make decisions, problem solve, and be creative.

In one study, 24 men and women volunteered to participate, were trained in FF, and randomly assigned to two age and gender matched groups. Then, for five minutes, one group recalled an event that still produced feelings of anger, and the other group recalled feelings of appreciation. Anger created: (1) a decrease in HRV (decrease in flexibility of the heart to change), (2) an erratic pattern between sympathetic and parasympathetic (inefficient heart functioning), and (3) increased stimulation to the heart. The heart sends these messages of imbalance to the brain, influencing our thoughts, the way we perceive our world, and the functioning of the entire body. Appreciation created: (1) increased HRV, (2) increased balance between stimulation and relaxation to the heart, (3) increased blood pressure control, (4) balanced rhythmic pattern between sympathetic and parasympathetic input (efficient heart functioning). The heart sends these messages of balance to the brain, influencing our thoughts, the way we perceive our world, and the functioning of the entire body. All of these then move toward greater clarity and coherence.

Rein, Atkinson, and McCraty (1995) tested the effects of compassion and anger on salivary IgA (S-IgA). Increased S-IgA indicates increased immune function. For 15 minutes, two groups experienced care and compassion (CC) [one group was self induced (FF) and one externally induced (watched a video)], and two groups experienced anger and frustration (AF) [self induced (recalled experience) and externally induced (video)]. In both the CC and AF groups, only the self-induced method significantly increased S-IgA.

The 30 participants were then age and sex matched and randomly assigned to control, CC, and AF groups to determine the long-term effects of these emotions on S-IgA. The CC group used FF, and the AF group used self recall. The feelings of anger and compassion were both felt *for only 5 minutes!* With care and compassion, immune function increased above baseline for six hours. Total mood disturbance, such as tension/anxiety, anger/hostility, fatigue, and confusion decreased, with participants reporting feelings of love, appreciation, and tranquillity.

With anger and frustration, immune function was decreased below baseline for six hours. Total mood disturbance significantly increased, with participants reporting frustration, aggravation, and resentment. They had increased headaches, indigestion, muscle pain, and fatigue that lasted for three to six hours. No significant changes were noted in the control group.

Rozman, Whitaker, Beckman, and Jones (1995) found that when HIV positive individuals practiced FF for six months, they experienced significant decreases in: (1) state and trait anxiety and irritability, (2) behavioral and emotional symptoms, and significant increase in: (1) hardiness (feelings of control, commitment, and challenge), (2) general well-being, and (3) physical vitality.

Tiller, McCraty, and Atkinson (1996) studied the effect of FF in the laboratory and the workplace on autonomic function (parasympathetic and sympathetic balance). Twenty participants were trained in FF and connected to ECG (electrocardiogram) electrodes. In the lab, baseline measurements were made and were taken during a 5-minute session of consciously focusing on a loving state. There was a significant increase in baroreceptor activity (increased blood pressure control) and parasympathetic activity (relaxation).

The group in the workplace wore a Holter monitor to record HRV, practiced FF during stressful situations, and made a recording when they began practicing

FF. Feeling love and appreciation created increased HRV, baroreceptor activity, as well as parasympathetic activity, and decreased sympathetic activity (decreased stimulation) in the workplace under real-life stressful situations.

The researchers also found that emotions such as appreciation, love, and compassion create a distinct mode of cardiac function called entrainment where the heart rhythm is very ordered, and entrains, or synchronizes the brain and other areas of the body with itself. There are areas of the body called biological oscillators that have cells that produce rhythmic oscillations or beats. These areas include the heart, areas in the brainstem that affect breathing, the baroreceptor network that affects blood pressure, the digestive system, and areas of the brain affecting the muscles and nerves. When the heart is beating in this very ordered way, it is able to entrain other body oscillators and create a synchronization, or frequency lock. **Focused attention on one oscillator can change its rhythm, and so change the others.**

When the heart is functioning in the entrainment mode, the brain's electrical activity (EEG) is brought into entrainment with the heart rhythms at a frequency of about 0.1 Hz (cycles per second), exhibiting balanced sympathetic and parasympathetic activity. Breathing and blood pressure also become entrained. It seems that with increased baroreceptor activity, which involves the vagus nerve, there is increased entrainment between the heart and the brain. This may explain the change in the function of the cortex of the brain and the heightened intuitive awareness. People report longer periods of clarity and exuberance along with decreased depression, anxiety, and fear. Massage also stimulates the vagus nerve (Field, 1998), perhaps explaining why massage can balance blood pressure and respiration, decrease physiological arousal, and create a perceptual shift to a calm, clear, mental/emotional state.

These studies suggest that we can intentionally, with our TF, affect the messages the heart sends to the brain. We can also use our TF to create a coherent, synchronized vibrational frequency between all of the biological oscillators in the body.

Bottom Line of Heart-Centered Awareness

Practicing HCA creates a resonance throughout a person's own body. In HCA, use the breath as a guide to bring your attention to the present moment, then to the heart area. Feelings of appreciation and love while focusing on the heart create a balanced heart rhythm that entrains the brain, breathing, and other body oscillators. This creates coherent convergence—synchronized vibration, or frequency, throughout the body. Feeling love, even for a short period, creates a connection within ourselves that leads to greater relaxation and health.

The best and most beautiful things in the world cannot be seen, or even touched. They must be felt with the heart.

—Helen Keller

LOVING-TOUCH

Loving-Touch (LT), the second step of HRT, builds on the information pertaining to PNI (Chapter 9) and energy/spirituality (Chapter 11). In this step, we connect with another. In HCA, love creates a resonance, or similar frequency, between areas of our own body. In LT, the love creates resonance between ourselves and another person. We know that the heart generates the strongest electromagnetic field produced by the body, and that this field becomes more coherent when we intentionally feel love. We learned that the vibration of one person's field produces similar vibrations in another person's field. When people touch, the pattern of the ECG from the heart of one person can be seen in the EEG pattern of the brain of the *other* person. These measurements, although weaker, can be detected when the two people are up to four feet apart! (McCraty, Atkinson, and Tomlinson, 1998). So, in LT we create a connection with the client through the energy of the love we feel in our heart, whether we touch or not.

Loving-Touch has two steps:

1. Allow thoughts of all things about the client that you may not like to fall away. Accept the person as a worthwhile human being. Notice something about them that you can appreciate and/or love. No matter who they are or how they act, love the child that is somewhere inside.

2. Send feelings of love from your heart area to the client. If you are touching them physically, imagine the feelings like a stream of warm light moving down your arm, to your hand, to the client, filling and surrounding them. If you are not physically touching, you can touch with your heart by visualizing the feelings of love and/or appreciation as a stream of light moving from your heart to the client, surrounding them.

Love is the Key

Though I have all faith so that I could remove mountains, and have not love in my heart, I am nothing. There are three things that will remain forever—faith, hope, and love—and the greatest of these is love.

—The Bible, I Corinthians, 13

The heat is the doorway, and love is the key. When we feel love, we create a very particular vibrational frequency. That frequency opens the heart. When two hearts are open and connected, healing happens. This section suggests ideas about what love is, the physical/emotional benefits of loving, and how we can intentionally love those we hardly know, or may not like.

WHAT IS LOVE?

The word "love" brings different feelings and memories for us all. Love is a word like touch or God; it deserves some definition. In the English language, we have one word for snow. The Eskimos have 36 words that mean snow because it is so important in their daily life. The Sanskrit language of India has 96 words that mean love. We have one. Plato said that love is the pursuit of the whole. Paracelsus (1493–1541) said that the main reason for healing is love. Could loving our clients, families, and friends be a way to help create wholeness and healing?

From ancient poetry to the Star Wars saga to current scientific research, we continue to hear of the power of love to connect and to heal. Volumes have been written trying to define and understand love because it is such a powerful driving force. In the Dhamapada from around 500 B.C., the Buddha says, "In this world hate never yet dispelled hate. Only love dispels hate. This is the law, ancient and inexhaustible." (Byrom, 1993). The poems of Rumi from around 1240 A.D. speak of the depths of love. "Love is the way messengers from the mystery tell us things." (Barks, 1993).

We all want and need love. It seems to be colored differently depending on who we love, and the situation we are in. Nona B. told us this story. "I was born in West Texas in farm country shortly before harvest-time. Both Mother and Daddy had to be in the fields, so for the first months of my life I was put in a box strapped to the tractor. I imagine that every now and then a big, loving hand would reach in to touch me. To this day, when I hear very powerful motors, I feel a special sensation of familiarity, connection, and love."

But what's at the core of love? Is there something common to all love? When we discard all the unique flourishes of the situation, we find a moment of shared connection, heart to heart.

In reading about and trying to understand love; appreciation, compassion, and care often come up and are worth exploring. Sometimes these words are used interchangeably, but there are some important differences.

Compassion and Appreciation

Compassion is feeling sorry that someone is experiencing discomfort. Webster's dictionary defines compassion as: "an awareness of, and sympathy with, someone else's distress, coupled with a desire to alleviate it; a benevolent consideration for, and understanding of, the feelings of another."

Nursing is one of the most inherently compassionate of professions. Most people called to nursing have a soft spot in their hearts for people in need, and want to help. Anyone who is called to give massage to another has the desire to help brighten their day. People with stress, sore shoulders, or illness deserve compassion, and their need creates an urge to extend ourselves in service.

We can usually feel compassion for those who are suffering in one way or another. However, we have all had clients, family, or acquaintances that we wonder at times if we can even like, much less love. What do you do then? Appreciation is the first step. You can find one thing to appreciate about almost anyone. This could even be the color of their hair or eyes, or the fact that they are a fellow human being in an uncomfortable situation. **Appreciation** means to value, admire, or treasure something. We have found that simply appreciating something about our clients and friends helps us open our hearts to them. This both improves the quality of the massage we give and makes other interactions more valuable for all involved. If the client is asking for help, if nothing else, we can appreciate someone's willingness to ask. Those of us who have been seriously ill know that in such a vulnerable position, the asking for help is a plea for love and connection. No matter who the person is, that willingness to reach out is worthy of our appreciation. If he is not asking, we can appreciate that he is a fellow human being in need.

Before and during a massage, appreciating the receiver will help you focus on her as a unique human being with needs and a story to tell. You might hear the fascinating story of how she came to feel the way she does. The telling of, and listening to, this story can be a breakthrough for both you and the receiver. Even the crankiest curmudgeon was once a little boy or a little girl who scooted along the floor with eyes of innocence wide open to the discovery of a brand new world. They, like us, were conditioned to live in this very big world by the sound of human voices. Though they did not understand the words, the tempos and tones made a lasting impression on their sweet, absorbent minds. People are often bitter and demanding because they are in a very stressful condition in their lives. They feel completely out of control. Crankiness may have been the way those young minds learned to respond to a stressful world a long time ago, scooting around on the floor.

Whether or not they share their childhood stories with us, we can find something about them to value. We might wonder, what if they were happy, how would their voice sound then? What would their smile look like? You can give a great massage to the most unhappy person, even while he is complaining, if you find something about him to value. Ask him what he thinks he needs and listen to his answer. Then you may better appreciate the joy that cries out to be released. A pair of hands and a willing heart can encourage that release.

Loving and Caring

Some define love as unconditional positive regard, without judgment; or thinking of others with thoughts that are life giving or growth promoting. There is love as sexual desire, and there is loving someone just because they are another human being, recognizing that we are both sharing this unique adventure of being human.

For the purpose of this book **love** is not referring to sex or sexual feelings. It is defined as feeling warmth, nurturing, and respect. Loving another is intentionally opening a two-way heart connection with them for the purpose of helping them remember wholeness, and feel appreciated and accepted.

Erich Fromm's *Art of Loving* (1956) was, and still is, one of the most comprehensive and instructive works on what love is and how to practice it. He says that love is an attitude, an orientation to the world as a whole. Fromm suggests that love includes the basic elements of giving, responsibility, respect, care, and knowledge. To practice love requires discipline, concentration, patience, and a great desire to master the ability. The person must be sensitive to himself, being aware of bodily processes, thoughts, and emotions. To practice love, one must develop humility and the ability to see the person as they are. There must be a faith in the other person's potential. To have faith, one must have the courage to take a risk to accept pain and disappointment. Love is active, alert, and aware.

Should nurses love their patients? What was your first thought? During a class in nursing school I began asking other nurses, social workers, clergy, and spouses of nurses this question. There was never a neutral response. There was either a resounding, "No!" or a definite "Yes, of course!" Whenever there is such emotion in opposite directions, it is an issue well worth pursuing. One nurse said, "No!" at first. By the end of our discussion, she had decided that, yes, maybe it was possible, and desirable, for nurses to love their patients. We discovered that her initial hesitancy was related to her definition of love. It immediately brought up love associated with sex, which was definitely inappropriate, and that you can only love a person you know very well. Love was hard to define. Another concern about loving was that it was not professional to get too close to a client, or the institution where she worked might not approve.

I asked the nurse above to talk about times she felt love for her clients. A very strong theme that emerged was that love is a force that connects people. Love is a two-way relationship benefiting both giver and receiver. For this nurse, loving included touch, energy-based healing, and connecting to God through prayer. Love was accepting someone without judgment, being understanding and comforting. She believed the nurse's feelings for the client affected his healing process. She initially believed that she either loved a client or didn't. By the end, she could see how, with conscious intention, she could choose to love a client she had previously not really liked.

I began searching the nursing literature, and as of 2002, there are about 1,035 articles on love and 10,000 on caring. Maybe the nursing profession hesitates to address love because of the different ways people define it. As early as 1983, Carter wrote, "Rehumanizing the nursing role: A question of love." Reed (1992) mentioned giving and receiving love as a core component of feeling connected. In discussing her 10 years of research and practice addressing the psychosocial and spiritual aspects of living with HIV, Hall (1997) talked about loving self, others, and life as another way of viewing spirit and spirituality. She says, "We have had scant professional preparation for this kind of caring and use of self."

What is the difference between loving and caring? Webster's dictionary (9th ed.) defines **caring** as: "interest or concern, liking, fondness, to give care." Yet it is also defined as "feeling trouble or anxiety, disquieted state of mind involving uncertainty, apprehension, and responsibility." Loving is defined as "to hold dear, cherish, to thrive in, nurture, unselfish benevolent concern for the good of another." Perhaps there is an important difference between caring and loving. Dr. Carol Montgomery, R.N. (1991) in her study of the nurse caregiving relationship, looked at the nature of caring communication, and what it is for the caregiver. She asked whether care leads to burnout or satisfaction. Nurses whose care turned to worry and anguish for clients felt burned out, and they couldn't care anymore. True care (compassion, appreciation, connection, love) enabled the nurses to manage and maintain excellence and satisfaction with their work. Maybe when nursing students are taught to care for clients, the loving, heart aspects are not emphasized. Perhaps that is why when clients were asked to describe nurse caring behaviors, they mentioned knowing how to give shots, managing equipment, and being cheerful (Wolf, 1986).

There seem to be many different ways to define caring in nursing. In the Caring Behavior Inventory (Wolf, 1986), love was not among the top 10 caring behaviors as identified by nurses. Jean Watson (1985, 1988) has perhaps done more than any other nurse theorist to make caring and heartfelt connection a part of nursing. She discusses caring-healing as a nursing process, and that caring is the core of nursing. Pepin (1992) discusses two aspects of caring—love and labor, affective and instrumental. Nurses described love as their primary motivation in being a nurse. Some define caring as trust, being present, sharing feelings, and comforting (Swanson, 1996). Margaret Newman (1996) suggests that "nursing is the study of caring in the human health experience. A body of knowledge that does not include caring and human health experience is not nursing knowledge." According to Morse, Solberg, Neander, Bottorff, and Johnson (1996) there is not consensus in nursing regarding the definitions of caring, the components of care, or the process of caring. In reviewing 35 nursing authors' definitions of caring, they range from the legal, technical, and political aspects of caring to touch and being present in an emotional and spiritual interaction. Fitzgerald and van Hooft (2001) suggest that love is different from caring in that love takes nurses beyond what caring indicates into a dimension of committment and dedication that is beyond duty.

Watson and Smith (2002) propose a new Unified Caring Science merging aspects of Watson's transpersonal caring theory and Martha Rogers' Science of Unitary Human Beings. Transpersonal being defined as a human to human connection where both persons are influenced, going beyond the personal ego, having a spiritual dimension, connecting with deeper self, others, and the universe (Watson, 1999). She suggested that in a transpersonal caring relationship a spiritual union occurs between the phenomenal fields of the two people allowing them to become part of a deeper, larger pattern of life. This sounds very much like love as defined in the nursing and popular literature. This new Unified Caring Science suggests a place for love and HRT in nursing.

The attempt to define caring in nursing has been going on for 20 years. There seems to be reluctance to address loving as suggested by the lack of its mention in the nursing literature. Maybe this is why many nurses have confusion about what caring actually involves and how to have a caring relationship with clients. Perhaps a focus on loving is the next step in the evolution of caring science in nursing.

People care about their neighbors. Nurses care about and take care of people who are ill. It is possible to do both of these activities without really connecting with the person. Perhaps loving is being willing to connect with another, sharing heart to heart, with an attitude of nonjudgmental acceptance.

If you have been fortunate enough to feel love, you know what it is, whether it is with a spouse, friend, significant other, God, siblings, parent, child, four-legged, or winged. Love is a connection of hearts that feels safe, comfortable, soft, warm, and/or healing. You always want more (see Figure 12-2). Words are often confusing. Whatever word is used, it is here that healing happens.

Love as a Healing Force

For some people, caring does not include loving. For some, loving is part of caring only in certain circumstances. For some, caring is loving. What would happen if caring always included loving? Does love have the power to heal? From the

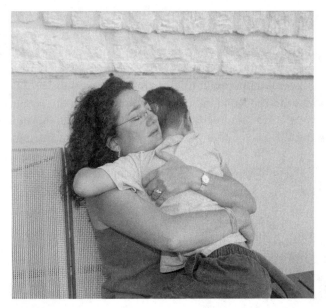

Figure 12-2

studies in HCA, feeling love seems to affect our own body in positive ways. Can love between two people create healing, or wholeness?

I am not aware of any other factor in medicine—not diet, not smoking, not exercise, not stress, not genetics, not drugs, not surgery—that has a greater impact on our quality of life, incidence of illness, and premature death from all causes, than love and intimacy.

—Dean Ornish, M.D. *Love and Survival*

In 2001, the Fetzer Institute offered $1 million in funding for research on altruistic love and compassionate love. The goal was to understand how this type of love can be learned and practiced, and what its benefits are. Ornish (1998) discusses many research studies suggesting that love is necessary for our physical, as well as emotional, survival. Of 119 men and 40 women, those who felt the most loved and supported had significantly less blockage in the arteries of their hearts. This effect was independent of risk factors such as diet, cholesterol, exercise, smoking, and family history (Seeman and Syme, 1987).

Medalie and Goldbourt (1976) found that in a study of 10,000 men, those who said their wives showed their love had half as much chest pain, even with high blood pressure and stress, than men who felt their wives did not show their love. In a study of 8,500 men, those who believed their wife loved them had 1/3 as many duodenal ulcers over the five-year study as men who did not believe their wife loved them (Medalie, et al., 1992).

In a study at Harvard in the 1950s, 126 healthy male students were randomly chosen and filled out a questionnaire asking them to describe their relationship with their mother and father (parental caring). Thirty-five years later, their medical and psychological histories were examined. Of those who rated both parents low in caring in college, 87% developed diseases in midlife, such as coronary artery disease, high blood pressure, duodenal ulcer, and alcoholism. *Perceived parental caring in college* predicted health status *35 years later.* Only 25% of those who rated both parents as caring had developed diseases (Russek and Schwartz, 1997).

The perception of love itself . . . may turn out to be a core biopsychosocial–spiritual buffer, reducing the negative impact of stressors and pathogens and promoting immune function and healing.

—Russek and Schwartz

The Meninger Clinic demonstrated that people who are in love suffer fewer colds, have a greater number of white blood cells to actively fight infections, less lactic acid in the blood, and higher endorphin levels. Having the ability to love and care about others seems to result in lower levels of the stress hormone, norepinephrine, and a higher ratio of helper/suppressor T-cells. Feeling happy with your marriage has a greater effect on levels of immune function and psychological well-being than job satisfaction or relationships with friends (Siegel, 1986).

Friedmann and Thomas (1995) studied people who had survived one year after an acute heart attack. They found that having a pet at home was a strong predictor of survival, independent of the severity of the heart disease and other psychosocial factors. Dog owners were six times less likely to die than those who didn't own a dog. In a study of women, having a dog lowered blood pressure better than the presence of a good friend (Allen, Blascovich, and Kelsey, 1991). Why might this be? Most dogs give unconditional love, something most of us are still aspiring to (Figure 12-3).

Can Our Thoughts and Feelings Affect Others at a Distance?

In LT we intentionally send our feelings of love and appreciation to another. People say, "I send my love." Have you ever wondered how it is possible to "send love"? How can a feeling affect another from a distance? LT involves new areas of research—distant intentionality and distant healing. These findings suggest that whether the nurse is touching the client, or is a few feet, or several rooms away, the nurse can affect the physical and emotional state of the client with her TF.

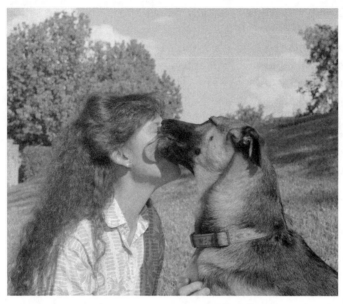

Figure 12-3

DISTANT INTENTIONALITY

The day science begins to study nonphysical phenomena, it will make more progress one decade than in all the previous centuries of its existence.

—Nikola Tesla, invent

Perhaps that decade is near. Distant intentionality and distant healing we the topics of conversation on Good Morning America in August, 2001. If y have never heard of these areas, the following studies will amaze you and perha change your view of how the world works.

Distant intentionality is divided into the effects on "non-living" and livi systems. Distant intentionality with living systems (DILS) is divided further in the intent to *just have an effect* on another at a distance and distant healing (DF DH is a conscious, intentional mental act attempting to *benefit* another's physic or emotional well-being at a distance (Sicher, et al., 1998). Distant heali involves energy-based therapies—like Therapeutic Touch, Reiki, HeartTouc Healing Touch, prayer—and other forms of spiritual and energy healing. Studi involving prayer were discussed in Chapter 11.

To suggest the extent of the research on distant intentionality, a bri overview of studies with non-living systems, and then non-human living systen will follow. These studies emphasize the importance of being aware of what v think and feel in all areas of life, especially when we are caring for others. Robert Jahn and Brenda Dunne, at the Princeton University Engineering Anomalies Research Laboratory, have the largest database ever collected studying the ability of people to affect machines. A person sits in front of a machine called a random event generator that randomly displays either positive (+) or negative (-) symbols on a screen at the rate of 1,000 per second. This random activity is said to be similar to the behavior of subatomic particles, of which everything is made. The operator uses his thoughts to try to influence the machine to display more positives or negatives. Ninety-one individual operators (2,520,000 trials) and 15 pairs of operators (256,000 trials) tried to influence the machines. **Both couples and individuals influenced the machine away from randomness and toward a pattern!** Combining the data from all trials, the operators were able to significantly influence the machines in a positive direction, $p < .01$, and negative direction, $p < .01$, at will (Jahn and Dunne, 1987; Dossey, 1993).

Peoch (1995) tested the ability of chicks to influence a machine. A light was attached to a randomly moving robot in a dark room. Chicks prefer to be in the light. Out of 80 groups of 15 chicks each, in 71% of the cases, the robot spent much of its time near the chicks. When the chicks were not there, the robot moved in random directions. The results were statistically significant, $p < .01$. It seems that even chicks can use their intention to influence machines.

If you have any doubt about distant intentionality or distant healing, read *Healing Research (vol. 1)* by Daniel Benor, M.D. (1992), which is a compilation of documented research studies demonstrating the effects of mental intent on individual cells, yeast, bacteria, plants, animals, and humans. In all of these studies, people try to either increase or decrease the functioning of an organism, at a distance, with their thoughts. He reviews at least 131 published, laboratory, controlled trials with 56 being statistically significant at $p < .01$ (meaning the results could have occurred by chance less than 1 time in 100), and another 21 studies at $p < .02–.05$. If the behavior of cells and bacteria can be affected by our thoughts to such a significant degree, think of the impact this could have on healthcare if nurses and physicians employed these methods and taught them to clients. Think how mothers and fathers could help their children when they are ill.

The following are just a few examples from Benor's book. The activity of the **enzyme,** MAO, associated with transmission of nerve signals in the body, mood states, and regulating neurotransmitters, was intentionally increased or decreased, $p < .0001$, with only 5 minutes of influence.

Looking at **cells in a laboratory** situation, a healer held his hands over a flask of red blood cells in a salt solution for 5 minutes. He was able to decrease hemolysis (destruction) of the cells caused by the salt solution. These studies were also done with the influencer in the next room directing his energy to the red blood cells. There was a significant reduction of hemolysis in both locations, p <.00096. Growth of cancer cells being incubated in a lab was inhibited by an influencer who was not in the lab but only received a photo of the bottles containing the cell cultures, p <.002.

Rein (1995) found that focused human intentionality can produce significant changes in the conformation (winding or unwinding of the DNA helix) of **human DNA** in a test tube. This suggests that we may be able to affect DNA with our thoughts.

Studying **organisms,** influencers were able to decrease the growth of cultures of fungus by concentrating on them for 15 minutes/day from up to 15 miles away, p <.00006. A group of 60 participants with no previous knowledge of having healing ability was able to inhibit the growth of E.Coli bacteria, p <.02 and promote it, p <.05, at will.

Dr. Marilyn Schlitz and Dr. William Braud have extensively studied the phenomenon of long distance intentionality. In a meta-analysis discussing 30 published experiments covering 20 years of work, Schlitz and Braud (1997) discuss distant intentionality in **humans.** Givers (influencers) affected the physical and mental states of receivers (influencees) in distant rooms of a building. The receivers and givers were connected to electrodes to measure the activity of the autonomic nervous system by measuring Galvanic skin response. The givers tried to either calm or stimulate the distant receivers, who were unaware when the attempt was being made. The giver imagined the intended state in himself using imagery or any other self-regulation technique, and then imagined that the receiver was having the same effect. In 19 studies, with 317 receivers and 105 givers, the giver could not see the one being influenced, but did have some feedback of how they were being affected. There was a significant and desired change during the periods of distant intentionality as compared with the periods of randomly interspersed control periods (no directing of thought). The experiment-wise success rate was 37%, compared to 5% which was expected due to chance alone. Schlitz and LaBerge (1999) found that when the giver viewed the receiver on a television set, he could significantly calm or activate the receiver's heart rate and respiration with the techniques used above.

Combining all 30 experiments, experiment-wise success rate was 47%, compared to 5% which was expected due to chance alone. These effects have been replicated in other studies. Sometimes the receivers reported the exact mental image that the giver was thinking, suggesting some form of mental connection. In a self-control experiment, givers tried to calm themselves using relaxing imagery. The effect of imagery on self was as effective as it was on the distant receiver, with image periods significantly different from control periods, p =.014. These studies of Schlitz and Braud (1997) suggest the importance and potential effectiveness of HCA (creating an internal state) and LT (sending a feeling to affect another).

Dr. Braud says that, *"Focusing attention upon any object establishes a two-way communication channel with that object—a channel that can be used to gain knowledge about that object or to influence it."* This is a very profound statement! Braud suggests five steps that enhanced the results in his studies of long-distance intentionality: (1) becoming relaxed first, (2) attention training—focusing on one object when the thoughts wander, like we discussed in the Relaxation Response, (3) Imagery, (4) Intentionality—intending a certain outcome, or intentionally attuning ourselves with the order of the universe and allowing the Mystery to unfold, and (5) Strong positive emotion directed toward your intention (Dossey, 1993).

Wiseman, et al., (1995) tested whether a person could detect if they were being stared at from a distance, using electrodermal activity (skin resistance) as a measurement of autonomic nervous system activity. They did not find significant results, however Schlitz and LaBerge (1994), conducting a very similar study did find significant results. Wiseman and Schlitz decided to try to find out why they got different results. In a study of distant intentionality, Wiseman and Schlitz (1997) investigated the effects that the researchers' beliefs might have on the results of an experiment, even though they may not be intentionally trying to effect the outcomes. Wiseman is a skeptic of distant intentionality, and Schlitz is a proponent. Both experimenters used the same methods, location, equipment, and subject pool, with 32 subjects acting as the receivers. The sender performed 16, 30-second trials of staring and directing their attention to the receiver, and 16 of looking and directing attention away. The receiver was in one room with the sender in another, viewing the receiver on a one-way closed circuit television. Wiseman's receivers showed no difference in test and control. Schlitz' receivers showed a significant difference.

The researchers suggested that perhaps their beliefs unintentionally created the results they desired through a distant effect. *Their individual intentions and expectations were the only factors that were different* in the two experiments. This study has extreme implications for the results of any research. It also suggests the effect that even unintentional beliefs have not only on our own physiology, but that of others.

According to Schlitz (1998), the findings from her studies suggest:

1. The ability to affect another at a distance is widely distributed in the population.

2. It is not an energy exchange because its effect does not lessen with distance.

3. The receiver has the ability to shield the intentions subconsciously and not be affected by them even when they do not know when the intentional thought is coming.

4. The effects don't always occur, but if the subject needs the effect, it is more likely to occur.

5. The effects on the receiver compare with the state generated by the giver.

A previous connection and/or emotional link seems to increase distant effects. Recall the experiments by Jahn and Dunne where people could influence machines with their thoughts. The most successful couples were those who were deeply attached to each other emotionally. The more successful individuals said they felt bonded to their machines, feeling a sense of oneness with them. If two people feel connected to each other and have the same intent, they have a greater effect on random events.

DISTANT HEALING

Now let's look at studies of distant healing (DH) where there is a definite intention to help or benefit another. In a double-blind, clinical study, 53 male patients who had undergone hernia surgery were randomly assigned to either a group receiving pre-recorded taped suggestions for quicker recovery, a group receiving DH, or a control group. The DH group showed a significant improvement, $p < .05$, compared with controls and the group hearing the suggestion tape. These differences were seen on 9 of 24 variables associated with improved recovery, including wound appearance, and subjective factors, such as less pain and more confidence in their treatment (Bentwich and Kreitler, 1994).

In a randomized, double-blind study of 40 people with advanced AIDS, distant healing was given to the experimental group 1 hour/day, 6 days/week for 10 weeks. They were assessed at 10 weeks, 4 months, and 6 months. The control group received standard medical care. Subjects were pair matched for age, CD4 count and number of AIDS defining illnesses, and randomly assigned to control or experimental groups. The healers were located all over the United States, and the subjects and healers never met. The healers were told to use whatever form of DH they used in their practices, which included Christian, Jewish, Buddhist, Native American, and graduates of schools of bioenergetic healing. At six months the treatment group, compared to the control group, had acquired fewer AIDS related diseases ($p < .05$), had lower illness severity ($p < .05$), required fewer visits to physicians ($p = .01$), had fewer hospitalizations, and fewer days of hospitalization ($p < .05$). There were no significant differences in CD4 count. Their moods were also improved (Profile of Mood States), $p < .05$ (Sicher, et al., 1998).

Published in the *Annals of Internal Medicine*, Astin, Harkness, and Ernst (2000) investigated 23 studies of distant healing, involving 2,774 human clients with controls, random assignment, peer-reviewed journals, and clinical investigation. These studies included noncontact Therapeutic Touch (11), prayer (5), and mental and spiritual healing (7). Thirteen (57%) yielded statistically significant treatment effects, nine showed no effect compared with controls, and one showed a negative effect. The effects varied widely, including a speedy recovery and decreased pain, anxiety, and wound size.

If our thoughts are powerful enough to have a healing effect, we must address the possibility for them to have a harmful effect (Dossey, 1997). Research indicates that intentions can harm bacteria and viruses. Once again we are seeing the importance of becoming aware of what we are thinking, and intentionally choosing our TF. Have you ever thought something like, "I hope you pay for what you've done"? I've heard people giving massage say, "This muscle is really tight. I don't see how you ever turn your head." Have you ever heard a parent tell a child, with great emotion, "You can't do anything right"? Have you ever heard a nurse or doctor, while walking out of a client's room, say, "This doesn't look good. I don't know if he'll make it"? Whether intentional or not, thoughts, especially with emotion, have power.

Luckily, we must have developed the ability to shield ourselves from the negative thoughts of others, or we would never have survived. Dora Kunz, one of the founders of TT, has been able to see energy fields since she was a child. She says that we have spirals that look like small tornadoes at the edges of our energy field that keep harmful vibrations from entering our field. When we are not well, physically or emotionally, these spirals open wider to allow in energy for healing. We must be aware that we are more vulnerable at these times to outside energy (Kunz, 1991). Recall that Schlitz and Braud found that the receivers could block the thoughts of the givers. They reported that even if the receivers didn't know when they were being thought about, they weren't affected if they didn't want to be.

There are many ways to protect ourselves in situations when we feel vulnerable. I once worked with a woman who was having a very difficult time dealing with her ex-husband. She said that whenever she even talked to her ex-husband on the telephone, she felt drained and helpless. I suggested that before she called him, to imagine herself inside of an oval of white light. White light seems to reflect other vibrations. She called me, amazed that she had a long conversation with him that would have previously exhausted her, and she felt perfectly fine.

There are prayers of protection, as in the 23rd Psalm, "the Lord is my Shepherd," or the Lord's Prayer, "Deliver us from evil." Some use the prayer of St. Francis of Assisi, "Lord, make me an instrument of thy peace." An Irish prayer asks that God hold you in the palm of his hand. In many prayers we have heard since childhood, there are lines with something like, "God protect us whi we are gone, one from another."

This section makes it clear that what we think and feel is very powerft Allowing our thoughts to run rampant may be as foolish as getting into a car ar stepping on the gas without holding on to the steering wheel. It is good to reali that our TF are powerful enough to bring harm to ourselves and others, so th we can become responsible for what we think and feel. It is equally important remember that we can use the power of our thoughts to connect, to protect, ar to heal.

HOW IS DISTANT INTENTIONALITY POSSIBLE?

Recall that nonlocal connection is a phenomenon in physics describing hc subatomic particles can affect each other, no matter how far apart they are. The connections are instantaneous, traveling faster than light, do not seem to use ar known signals of communication between particles, and cannot be predict (Aspect, Dalibard, and Roger, 1982). Nobel physicist Brian Josephson believ that the world is full of nonlocal influences, not only in the subatomic world, b that they underlie the events of everyday life. Replicated research suggests th two people separated by distance exhibit nonlocal connection between ther Subjects were far from each other in metal-lined boxes to block any electroma netic influences. Their EEGs (brainwave recordings) were compared. When tl subjects were just sitting quietly, there was no correlation between the patterns their brainwaves. When they connected to each other by feeling empathy or em tional closeness, their brainwave patterns began to closely resemble each oth There was no type of energy that we know of passing between them because tl effect did not diminish with distance. These researchers suggest that nonloc connections exist between human beings as they do between subatomic particl (Grinberg-Zylberbaum, et al., 1994). We know that a synchronization, or e trainment, of brainwaves can occur between professors and students, psychothe apists and clients, and two people having a good conversation (Goldman, 199; Thus, it is very likely that the TF of the nurse not only affect her own well-bein but that of her clients.

Physicist Amit Goswami has proposed a Science Within Consciousness th ory, in which consciousness is recognized as a fundamental, causal factor in tl universe, not confined to the brain, the body, or the present time. Robert Jah dean of engineering at Princeton University, has proposed a model of the mind which consciousness acts freely through space and time to create actual change the physical world (Dossey, 1997).

Learning to Intentionally Love

Love your neighbor as you love yourself.

—Jesus, Matthew 22:39

Love each other as God. Don't throw anyone out of your heart. Love people and feed them. If you cannot love each other, you cannot achieve your goal.

—Neem Karoli Baba

We have looked at some fascinating research that suggests that we can, in fact, intentionally affect others at a distance with our TF to encourage healing. We know that feeling love—within, and between people—benefits physical and emotional health. As I listened to the people I asked about nurses loving their clients, I realized that many people believe you have to know someone well, be attracted to them, or like them in order to love them. However, the words of the great teachers above are suggesting that it is possible, and desirable, to love anyone. How do we do that? How can we intentionally love someone we don't know, or don't like, or are angry with?

How do we learn about loving? We can study the words of teachers like Jesus, Neem Karoli Baba, and Buddha who were able to love all kinds of people. We can learn about love from being with loving people and observing them. I had the privilege to get to know a nurse from Thailand who is a Buddhist. I have learned much from her about self-awareness, gentleness, and love. She said that in Thailand the nursing students are all taught to love each client as if she or he was their grandma or grandpa. They even call them by those names. Wouldn't it be wonderful to be one of their clients?

Suffering enters all of our lives to a greater or lesser degree from time to time. Have you ever wondered: why do we suffer? One reason may be that we can learn about loving from encountering suffering. Suffering opens the heart. Think about it. When people are happy, we might briefly hug them and congratulate them. There may be a short burst of heart connection. We usually do not dwell for long periods discussing happiness. When we suffer, we often call on others, and the Divine. When someone is suffering, we hold them for a long time while they cry. We tend to touch them more frequently and for longer periods of time. We talk and listen, sharing similar stories, for as long as it takes to soothe the soul. Sometimes when a person's suffering is great, we may find that we want to shut ourselves off from them. We want to avoid feeling their pain for fear of losing ourselves in that pain. We sometimes insulate ourselves with an emotional distance. In order to be of help to people in circumstances such as these, we must find our own inner center, or place of strength and calm. Some people talk with others who would understand the situation. Others meditate, pray, or write about their feelings in journals, songs, or poetry. From this inner place of calm, we find the strength and courage to reach out.

We learn about love from this reaching out, or serving others. In serving another, we learn to be humble, and the heart learns to open. Rubbing the feet of another, as in massage, is a most humble service. Neem Karoli Baba says, "If you want to know God, serve people. To become enlightened, feed people. To become one with Christ, serve the poor, and remember God."

How Can We Intentionally Love Another?

1. Acceptance—Accept them as a fellow human being, see the child that they are inside
2. Compassion—Care that they are suffering
3. Appreciation—Find one thing to appreciate about them
4. Love—Relive a loving experience from your life and send that feeling to their heart, surrounding them with it
5. Connect—Be willing to open a two-way connection, giving to and receiving from

---

Bottom Line of Loving-Touch

In this step of HRT, we create a resonance with another by loving them. We use our TF to create a connection intended to benefit their health and well-being. Research in the new area of distant intentionality suggests that we can affect bacteria, cells, and people with our TF, from a distance. This effect can be one of relaxation or stimulation, depending on what we are thinking and feeling. When we use mental imagery to create a feeling state within ourselves, we can send those feelings to another and create that same state in their body and mind. We see from the research studies that when we feel love for another, mental and physical health improves, both for the receiver and giver. Feelings of caring and connection create stronger distant effects. Therefore, as nurses it is crucial that we become aware of what we think and feel. We can improve the health of our clients, and ourselves, as well as create meaningful connections by sending feelings of appreciation and love to our clients.

CONNECTING WITH HIGHER POWER

The most fundamental longing of the human heart is for union with the Divine.

—Janet Quinn, Ph.D., R.N.

In HRT, we first create a resonance within our own bodies, then we create a resonance between ourselves and another. In this final step, we create a resonance between ourselves and a Higher Power. Connecting with Higher Power (CHP) builds on Chapter 11 (energy and spirituality).

CHP has one step: through prayer, meditation, or whatever way is comfortable to you, connect with your view of a Higher Power, as a Source of Love and/or Wholeness. (Higher Power is defined in Chapter 11). If you want to connect with Higher Power, and do not have a personal method, see Chapter 11 or the meditation for moving into the heart in Appendix C.

In Chapter 11 we discussed Higher Power in detail. We reviewed research studies on prayer and spirituality, indicating that both are beneficial for health. Whether we go to church, have faith in God, believe we will be healed, or pray at home: religious/spiritual activities help the body and mind heal (Matthews and Larson, 1995). Recall that according to the Princeton Religious Research Center, 90% of the people in the United States believe that God loves them. In *Time* magazine, 82% of Americans said they believe in the healing power of prayer, 77% believe that God can intervene to cure those with a serious illness, and 73% believe that praying for another can help cure their illness (Larson, 1998). These statistics reveal that a large percentage of Americans believe that their thoughts can help to create a change in their own—or another's—body and mind, even at a distance, when they connect with God. Studies reveal that clients want their spiritual needs addressed and view them as instrumental for their healing (Matthews and Saunders, 1997).

The National Conference on Nursing Diagnosis has included spiritual distress as a category. Yet, with all the discussion and research on spirituality in nursing, many nurses still feel uncomfortable with the spiritual aspect of nursing care due to lack of clarity about what spirituality even is, inadequate education about spirituality, anxiety about discussing spirituality, and a belief that spirituality is incompatible with the scientific, professional model of nursing (Emblen and Pesut, 2001). These authors have outlined five categories for a nursing assessment of spiritual needs and interventions to address those needs.

In a study of 224 nurses, Sellers and Haag (1998) found that nurses said that if nursing is to achieve its goal of promoting health, clients must be viewed holistically, including the spiritual dimension. They believe nursing education regarding spirituality is lacking and the number of spiritual nursing interventions is insufficient, with a third of the respondents saying they felt inadequate in providing spiritual care to clients. Of those who responded, half cited the scarcity of nursing research studies examining spirituality. A second major theme was the need for the nurse's own spirituality to be developed and nurtured to provide effective spiritual care. The third theme was that spiritual care should be

expanded in all healthcare, especially the hospital setting. We hope the massa
techniques, the HRT intervention, and all of the accompanying information
this book will help to meet these needs.

Love, Higher Power, and Healing

*Whenever you find yourself dejected, bring your mind back to the splendor of t
heart, filled with love, and listen to the divine sound, So'ham.*

—Swami Chidvilasananda, *The Magic of the Hea*

People bring the Absolute into healing in different ways. Healing is abo
remembering wholeness. God is said to be everywhere and knowing all thing
the Whole. Intentionally connecting with Higher Power seems to bring abo
wholeness, or healing. We find that when we connect with Higher Power in o
massages, both the receiver and ourselves are filled with a stillness, calm, and
return to coherence.

HEALING TECHNIQUES OF CHRISTIAN SCIENCE

Virginia Harris spoke at the Spirituality and Healing in Medicine conferen
in Houston, Texas, in 1998. She has a practice of healing in the Christian Scien
tradition and described how healing happens from her view. First there
thought, and then matter develops from thought. Because thought produces t
body in the first place, the relief from pain, and the healing of any conditio
comes through a change of thought which naturally and scientifically results ir
change in the body. Her role is to help the healee realize that God is all-powerf
loving, and ever-present. Second, she helps people realize that they are inheren
healthy, whole, spiritual beings. Third, God and people are connected. Our rel
tionship with God is permanent, unbreakable, and untouched by injury or pai
She believes these three aspects apply to her and the healee. She prays for the
and with them, as they pray, remembering these principles. When someone ful
knows and believes these principles, healing of the body happens. Although the
is much more training involved in becoming a Christian Science practition
anyone can begin to use these steps to enhance the healing of self and others.

HOLOENERGETIC HEALING

Leonard Laskow is a physician who has practiced medicine for over 25 yea
He began to realize that often healing occurred that had nothing to do wi
medical treatment. In his book, *Healing with Love*, he describes Holoenerge
Healing, his technique for using love to bring about wholeness. He defines lo
as an awareness and recognition that we are a part of everything, that each of

is a part of a vast, universal order. Recall that Universal Order is one name for Higher Power.

Glen Rein, in a study at the Quantum Biology Research Laboratory in Palo Alto, California, looked at the effects of Holoenergetic Healing with Dr. Laskow on tumor cells in petri dishes. Dr. Laskow first got into a balanced, coherent state, feeling connected to and one with the cells (resonance). He then had the mental intention that the cells return to the natural order and harmony of the normal cell line. The tumor cell growth was significantly inhibited by 39%. They also found that if Laskow held a container of water in his hands while practicing the holo-energetic techniques, just using that water on the cells would cause cell inhibition. Water makes up a large part of living things, and seems to be very receptive to TF. Perhaps blessing our food before we eat does truly contribute to health.

LAWRENCE LESHAN

For over 30 years, Lawrence LeShan has been a research psychologist who has published in the areas of parapsychology, cancer as a turning point, and understanding the holistic revolution in medicine. In his book, *The Medium, the Mystic and the Physicist*, he describes his search for how healing happens. He interviewed people known for having the ability to help people heal at a distance with their thoughts. When the healer was in a state of feeling complete oneness with the universe, this was in some way transmitted to the healee. The healee no longer felt "cut off." He felt completely enfolded in the cosmos, with his individuality enhanced. Under these conditions, physical healing can happen. The healer's willingness to unite with, and hold the knowingness of unity for, the healee, seemed to allow the healing mechanism of the healee's body's to act at its greatest potential, and bring about healing.

LeShan began to practice his version of these techniques to see if they could be taught to, and learned by, anyone. He would talk with the healee for just enough time so that they were relaxed around each other. He told the healee to sit comfortably and let her mind do whatever came naturally. He closed his eyes and imagined the healee as being an individual inside her body, and at the same time, as existing as one with the universe, as energy or spirit existing to the farthest reaches of the cosmos, not limited by space or time. He focused on this image until he knew it was true. He then focused on himself until he knew that he coexisted with the healee in the same manner. At that point the healing was complete. Sometimes he would use imagery to help him, such as two trees on a hill, separate, but connected by their root systems underground. These root systems affected the ground, the rocks, the entire earth, and eventually he knew that there was nothing not affected by them, or one with them. This process took 10–15 minutes. Sometimes there were physical changes in the healee, sometimes psychological changes, sometimes there was a telepathic connection, and sometime nothing happened. Higher Power in this case was a Universe, a Cosmos not lim ited by time or space.

LeShan (1974) found that the distant healers he interviewed had two thing in common. There was a love or deep, intense caring for the person, and a view ing of the healee and themselves as one. They were united in a universe in which unity is possible. The healers went into a meditative state where they viewe themselves and the healee as one entity. There was no attempt to do anything the healee, but to meet him, be one with him. In this oneness the healer wa focused on the healee, feeling love for him. This is the essential factor. One heale Agnes Stanford, said, "Only love can generate the healing fire." Ambrose an Olga Worrall said, "We must care. We must care for others deeply and urgentl wholly and immediately; our minds, our spirits must reach out to them." For brief period of time there must be nothing else in the consciousness except on ness with the universe or God, so there is no thought, or nothing else in the fiel of knowing to prevent the healing results from occurring.

Become conscious for a single moment that Life and intelligence are . . . neither i nor of, matter, and the body will cease to utter its complaints.

—Mary Baker Edd

Healing with love is not only to use with others. We can use these techniques t bring about wholeness in ourselves. We can connect with our own cells, and fe love, thus returning their vibrations to an orderly pattern. We can enter into personal and private space with God without the help of another. Being wit God there is no doubt that we are whole and loved, completely, always, and fo ever. We are invited to remember who we are, which makes our adventures in th world much more meaningful, and fun. As we remember our connection wit

A Message from God

"My arms are always around you, I am always holding you. When your thoughts take you away to the world of form, you forget. Let go of your thoughts for only a moment, focus on the stars within, and you will feel me, see me. Know that I am always here with you. Have you ever been listening to someone, and then you thought of something else? You were in another world. They were still talking even though you cannot remember what they said. It is you who think you are separate because your thoughts take you away and create a reality for you. I never leave."

—Marsha Walker

God, it is easier to remember to love the people we encounter in daily life, even the client who angrily yells about his dinner, the child who refuses to do what you ask for the third time, the driver who rushes into the car length you left on the freeway, and the spouse who is irritated after a long day. Remembering God helps us remember love.

This message was received during a meditation involving intentional heart focus.

Bottom Line of Connecting with Higher Power

In this third step of HRT, connect with the Divine in whatever way you are comfortable. Research suggests that connection with Higher Power has many benefits to physical health and mental and emotional well-being. Spiritual connection creates hope and meaning in life for many people. Many distant healing techniques include a connection with Natural Order, the Infinite, Universal Cosmos, or God. Remembering Wholeness, we hold the opportunity for healing.

WHERE TWO OR MORE ARE GATHERED

Now that we have explored the three steps of HeartTouch, let's look at how they all work together. On this path of discovery, the breath guides us to the heart as a doorway. We have love as a key to open the door. As we enter, where does this doorway lead? Recall from our discussion of Freeze Frame that intentional heart focus—feeling love and appreciation—creates a condition where both the sympathetic and parasympathetic input to the heart are balanced. Recall from Chapter 11 that Newberg and d'Aquili found that when the sympathetic and parasympathetic nervous systems are both stimulated simultaneously, as in meditation and religious practices, the person feels the presence of God or Absolute Oneness. Perhaps then, intentionally focusing on the heart and feeling love helps us feel the presence of the Divine. Love may be the white stones shining in the night that we dropped along the path to help us remember our way Home.

Many cultures acknowledge this connection of the heart, love, and spirituality. Neem Karoli Baba, an Indian sage, says, "Cleanse the mirror of your heart and you will see God." From the Hindu tradition, God is Brahman, the ocean; the heart is Atman, a drop of water. Focus on the heart and it merges with God. Oneness with God is through love, knowledge, and service. From Siddha Yoga, "To have the vision of God, you must believe that God dwells within you, that the divine Presence is seated in your heart." From the Christian tradition, Matthew 5:8 of the Bible, "Blessed are the pure in heart, for they shall see God."

The Jewish tradition teaches that a change of heart is one of the hallmarks of the advent of loam haba, in which the "heart of stone" is changed. This inner spiritual change will transform each individual. Rabbi Kerry Baker says that in this time, "Kol Halev", the "voice of the heart", speaks to each of us of truth. The heart, not the mind, is the center of understanding. When we bring our thoughts to the heart, in its power, we are transformed.

Physicists such as John Wheeler propose the existence of many realities all operating at the same time, at different frequencies (Maudlin, 1986). This might be similar to the different frequencies of all of the radio and television stations travelling through space at the same time. We choose a station by turning the dial and selecting a frequency. The Kingdom of Heaven may be a reality of a different frequency that we can enter if we tune our radio to the right station. Perhaps to connect with God, our mind, heart, and body must be at a certain frequency, all in harmony. Recall that the heart has the ability to entrain other systems of the body to its frequency, and that feeling love as we focus on the heart, creates synchronized, coherent frequencies within the heart, as well as the body. The Bible says that God is Love, I John 4:16, and the Kingdom of God is within, Luke 17:21. If God is love, perhaps feeling love and vibrating at that frequency, takes us to the Kingdom of Heaven which is accessed through the heart space, or the energy field of the heart. Recall also that Florence Nightingale said, "Heaven is neither a place nor a time. There might be a Heaven not only here but now . . . Where shall I find God? In myself."

When you practice the three steps of HRT, you create a healing triangle. Love is the connecting feeling or frequency. First, you use love to create connection within your body. Then, sending that love to another creates a heart-to-heart connection, and their bodymind resonates with yours. When you feel love and also intend connection with Higher Power, you resonate with Higher Power. When you are connected to the client and to the Divine, the client and the Divine also connect and begin to resonate. The healing triangle forms. You might visualize this as a triangle of light or energy. You and the client then resonate with the frequency of God; a frequency that is Wholeness, Love, and Coherence, with the stronger vibration of the Divine synchronizing other vibrations to it. If disease is disharmony and cells acting out of the normal, orderly pattern, and God or Spirit is an orderly, harmonious pattern, when we attune to God, the body returns to its natural order. Health is the result.

The healing that Jesus, and others, facilitated may have been due to their ability to tune in to the heart, feel love, and connect with God. Their hearts entrained the hearts and minds of the other person, bringing about coherent functioning, or physical healing.

God Dwells within Us All

A friend shared this story with us.

"I guess I would start with what I call bookends of epiphanies, involving the relationship that I had with my partner. I remember him walking into the room, and the room sort of went away. My vision sort of became this lighted tunnel around his face. I couldn't hear anything, and I just remember seeing his incredibly brilliant dazzling white smile. That was the beginning of a 15-year relationship that I had with him.

"All of our relationship I knew that he was HIV positive. He was very, very ill for the last four years, and just went down and down and down. So the last two years of his life were incredibly difficult for him, but he had such spirit and such vibrancy. He loved life. He loved everything about it—music and art and anything that involved spectacle. About six months before he died, he had a stroke. It left him with facial paralysis on the right side of his face and he had difficulty closing his right eye. He couldn't smile on that side of his face.

"The other epiphenic moment for me is the other end of our relationship. Like every hospice patient, he had his hospital bed, and by this point was using a walker to get around in the house. I tried to help him to maintain his independence. He was on lots of different medications. So there we are in the evening, and we are standing in the bedroom next to this rolling cabinet with all of his supplies, and I was leaning against the bathroom door jam. I can so vividly, clearly see this. Oftentimes I just sort of stood by to be there so that if he did want help, I could help him. He was trying his very best to focus on a vial of medicine. I could tell that he was beginning to lose his vision at that point, and it was becoming more and more difficult for him to clearly measure off things in a syringe. He didn't want to overmedicate himself. So I said to him, 'Why don't you let me help you with that?' Time froze for an instant. He looked at me with this incredibly innocent, sweet smile. He handed me the vile and said, 'I just don't know why you love me so much.' I realized that in that moment, I was looking at the face of God.

"When you get past being able to see just the physical, he had lost 60 pounds, and there he was with all of his physical disabilities, his thin, frail frame and having to stand there with a walker. . . . You could look beyond all of that, and you could see inside of him. And now I tell healthcare providers, you know, if you can look past the physical, you can find the God within each person, because that being is there, that spirit is there. It's a once in a lifetime opportunity that he gave me. That changed my life. In large part he is responsible for the man I am today, second only to my father as being the best man I've ever known."

The heart is the doorway and at any time, in any moment, we can open the door and step through. From within, we see that all of the physical world on the other side of the door is created by our TF as a place in which to learn. We walk through the door of the heart and are swept into the arms of God. We are home.

SUMMARY

For the full HRT technique, see the HeartTouch box. In the first step of HRT, Heart-Centered Awareness, focusing on the breath brings you to the present moment. Centered, you can chose your TF. Then direct your attention to the heart area. You change your heart rhythms by changing what you are thinking and feeling. When you feel love as you focus on the heart, it functions more effi-ciently. Your heart rhythms change the frequency of your other biological oscilla-tors—respiration, digestion and the brain—synchronizing the body and mind into balance and harmony. You create resonance within your body.

In Loving-Touch you send this feeling of love to another. The frequency of the emotion, or energy, of love creates a resonant state between you and the receiver. You can be physically touching the person, as in massage, or touching only with the heart. Recall that when we touch someone, or are even in close proximity to them without touching, the electrical activity of the heart of one person can cause the brainwaves of another person to have the same rhythm. If we are angry, stressed, or judgmental our heart rhythms are erratic, which creates erratic patterns in another's EEG and may affect the electrical activity in other areas of their body. With feelings of love and appreciation, we create peace and harmony in our body and mind, and that of those around us. Love is a choice. When we intend to love another, we enter the heart. Judgments depart and per-sonalities pale. Love seems to be different than appreciation or caring, perhaps a willingness not just to stand apart and affect another, but to connect with and be affected by them. In CHP, feeling love creates a resonance between ourselves, the client, and the Divine.

HeartTouch is way of being with another. It is a way of interacting whether you are giving a massage, a medication, or a bed bath. HRT enriches a conversa-tion as you pause for a moment. It offers a way to intentionally love those you may not know very well, or that you may find hard to like. Loving someone is connecting with who they are on the inside, and knowing we are one and the same. We can use HRT to intentionally love someone even when we are not with them physically, and we can also intentionally love ourselves, nurturing who we are inside.

HeartTouch

Step 1: Heart-Centered Awareness
Go within: Feel love in the heart
Establish a resonant state within. Use the breath, prayer, or a meditative focus to center, to bring your thoughts to the present moment.

1. Centering—Take a few slow, deep breaths and bring the focus of your attention to the moment, letting go of all thoughts except being present to engage in the current situation.
2. Picture a small circle of light moving from your head, down your neck to your heart area. Once at your heart area, with each breath, allow the circle to grow.
3. Remember a situation where you felt loved, or were with someone you loved. Allow yourself to be in that situation, hear the sounds, smell the smells, see the sights, and feel the feelings.

Step 2: Loving-Touch
Connect: Touch gently
Establish a resonant state between you and the receiver. Send this loving feeling to them, to their heart area.

1. Accept the person as a worthwhile human being. Notice something about them that you can appreciate and/or love.
2. Send feelings of love from your heart area to the client. If you are touching them physically, imagine the feelings like a stream of warm light moving down your arm, to your hand, to the client, filling and surrounding them. If you are not physically touching, you can touch with your heart by visualizing the feelings of love and/or appreciation as a stream of light moving from your heart to the client, surrounding them.

Step 3: Connection with a Higher Power
Be With: Hold the Space for Change
Heal: Remember Wholeness
Establish a resonant state between you and Higher Power. See that you are one with Higher Power, an ordered, harmonious Whole, God.

Through prayer, meditation, or whatever way is comfortable to you, connect with your view of a Higher Power, as a Source of Love and/or Wholeness. (Higher Power is defined in Chapter 11). Visualize a three-way connection between you, the receiver, and Higher Power. One way to visualize this is a triangle of light. Take a few moments to allow this connection to continue.

No matter what someone else has told you, know that you deserve to love and be loved because inside you, and inside each of us, is the dwelling place of the Divine. Know it with all your heart. It is the most important Truth.

Research in healing is beginning to embrace what has always been known in the heart. Love and happiness help us heal. Considering current events the world over, it is time to bring love to all aspects of our lives, with unprecedented urgency. We can take comfort in knowing that there is a collective movement, a stirring of the Heart. Love and heart connection appear more and more on television, in books, movies, and as topics for conferences. "We" are waking up and remembering.

And now, we move to the final chapter of our journey, putting what we have learned together to give a massage with heart.

PUTTING THESE IDEAS INTO PRACTICE

1. For a moment, focus your attention on your heart area. Take a few breaths, letting your awareness remain in the heart as you breathe. Now direct that awareness or energy from your heart, down your arm, to your palm.

2. Touch something—a chair, pet, friend, yourself. Pick a feeling such as curiosity, acceptance, appreciation, or love, and let that feeling move from your heart, down your arm, to your hand, and into what you are touching. See them being filled with that feeling.

3. On a different day, each time you touch any client, take a breath, be really present with them, and intentionally feel acceptance and appreciation for them, or someone else in your life that you care about.

CHAPTER 13

Giving the Massage with Heart

When you work, you are a flute through whose heart the whispering of the hours turns to music. And what is it to work with love? It is to weave the cloth with threads drawn from your heart, even as if your beloved were to wear that cloth . . .

—Kahlil Gibran

OBJECTIVES

1. Demonstrate a massage with heart, and explain why it is different from a routine of massage strokes.
2. Describe the benefits of moving slowly when giving a massage.
3. Discuss the relevance of contemplating the question, "Who are we?" to giving a massage with heart.

Every massage is different. Even if you receive a massage from the same person two days in a row, each massage will be different. Most massages feel good. They are relaxing, and you feel better than before you got it. Your muscles are softer and discomfort is lessened. When assessing a massage, we recognize important factors such as choice of strokes and the pace, pressure, and rhythm of those strokes. But, what makes a good massage great? A great massage happens as the giver: (1) becomes more and more awake in the moment and aware of her thoughts and feelings (TF), (2) does her best to meet the needs of the receiver, and (3) gives the massage with her heart engaged.

The singing of the national anthem of the United States, "The Star Spangled Banner," is traditional before most major sports events in our country. It is a song whose words every school child knows by heart and hardly ever forgets. Occasionally someone sings this familiar melody and really puts their heart into it. Everyone who hears it is moved to tears.

If you have ever seen the words to the familiar rock and roll song, "Blue Suede Shoes," you know there is nothing particularly moving about a man who will take all the abuse you can dish out, but who finds it necessary to warn you repeatedly that you are running a great risk to your own well-being if you mess with his shoes. When Elvis sang "Blue Suede Shoes" it woke up a generation because Elvis put his heart and soul into it. Teenagers could feel it, and they heeded the call, not to go out and buy blue suede shoes (though many actually did), but to let their own souls move their own bodies like Elvis did his. The feeling behind that movement caused a collective stirring of the soul.

And finally, "The Lord's Prayer" is a simple verse known by heart by practically every Christian on Earth, and recognized by many members of other religions. The words themselves are moving, especially to those who are devoted to their meaning. Its recitation can be either mechanical or stirring, depending on the *feeling*. There is nothing quite like hearing a gifted speaker whose personal experience allows her to speak these simple, sacred words from the depths of her heart.

When we put our heart and soul into our touching of another human being, we can touch their heart and soul with our own. Hope is awakened in this place of deepest connection. It becomes easier to know that life has meaning. When we feel seen, heard, and accepted at this level, we feel loved.

A GREAT MASSAGE

What Is It?

Like everything else in life, there are many different opinions on what a great massage is. Some people like firm pressure, some light. Some like a fast pace, some like it slow. Some like talking, some don't. No matter what techniques are used, during great massage you feel like the person massaging you is completely focused on you and the massage they are doing. They are present for you. You feel they are sensitive to your individual needs and are trying to create an experience in which you can get what you want out of the massage.

Now we move into where opinions differ. We believe that after a great massage, you know you are changed. Your body feels heavy in that all the muscles are relaxed. Yet, at the same time, it's easier to move, and you almost feel as if you are gliding. Your arms hang in ways they don't usually hang, swinging freely. The tightness has been wrung out of your body, and it moves more effortlessly. You see the world in a different way. The colors are brighter, and you notice more detail. You feel a closer connection with people and everything you see. You feel peaceful and loving. It is hard to write a check, much less drive. You must sit for a while because you are moving very slowly, and you have a bit of trouble getting the thought train moving again. All the tension and stressful feelings are gone. When you look in the mirror, you are glowing. It is as if the windows have been cleaned, and you no longer look out through a fog. Your priorities are crystal clear, you are in a much better mood, and your heart is full of love.

How do you give a massage like this? Some people just do it naturally. However, most of us have to learn how. What you have learned in this book is what we feel enables you to give a massage that helps someone feel this way. When you take the techniques in Part II and add the information in Part III, you get a great massage, a massage with heart.

Giving a Great Massage

We are now going to put it all together, *briefly* describing a great massage scenario. You asked your client or family member if they would like a massage, and they agreed. Make the environment as relaxing as possible, warm the lotion, and wash your hands in warm water. Tell them to be sure to let you know if the pressure of your strokes is too much.

Recall the importance of what you think and feel while massaging the receiver. Attitude is seen in the bounce in your step. Facial expressions such as a frown or a smile convey the attitude with which we move through our day. The TF we have create the attitude we show to the world as the tone of our words, the way we view events in life, the look in our eyes, and the way we touch. Recall that endorphins, the chemicals that create feelings of happiness, are released when the corners of the mouth turn up. Smiling at yourself in a mirror makes you laugh whether you were previously happy or not.

Presence is an internal state that affects how our hands touch. Clients notice when a nurse has a healing presence. This includes being willing to give someone our undivided attention for the time we are with them. We really listen to what they have to say, accepting their opinions and feelings as real for them at that time. We recognize that they are a valuable person worthy of our time. When you are fully present in a massage, it is as if your eyes are in your fingertips, ready to notice anything their body tells you.

Here are some other simple techniques to keep your attention on the receiver.

1. Body awareness. While giving a massage, become aware of your own body. Are your shoulders relaxed? Focus on the rhythmic repetitions of the strokes.

2. Breath. In addition to simply becoming aware of your breath, breathe intentionally, without force, to focus your attention. Whenever you

become aware of holding your breath or shallow breathing, simply let your body draw in a nice deep breath. Use your breath to return your awareness always back to the receiver.

3. Listen to your hands. This focusing technique will also heighten your awareness of subtle cues picked up from the receiver's body by your hands. It will help you feel when to let your hands modify their pressure or tempo to accommodate that body's unique condition. You will begin to feel what they need. Let your hands speak to them and say, "Right now this is all I have to do. You are a good and very important person, and you deserve this."

4. Imagine that you are the one receiving the massage. What would you want?

Next, take a moment and practice the steps of HRT. Center, go to your heart, and spend a few seconds reliving a time you felt love. Send that love to the receiver's heart and encircle them with it. Intentionally love them as the playful child they are inside. If you like, connect with Higher Power and feel the three-way connection between you, the receiver, and the Divine. Ask for Healing Presence to fill you and the receiver for the highest good of all concerned.

Being centered and present, give your massage using whatever strokes you feel would be most beneficial to this individual, considering the amount of time you have. No matter what massage strokes you choose, go slow. Why do we continue to repeat, "Go Slow"? It coaxes the receiver's body to let go and soften. We are also more likely to touch them with the gentleness and care that we would a soft and delicate child. My father's cat, Lulu, reminded me of the effect of slowness. She occasionally graced me with her presence on my lap. On this day I realized that how long she stayed had a great deal to do with my energy. I was petting her as I was thinking about a million things. She started squirming and wanted down. Unconsciously I started moving my fingers very slowly and I noticed she immediately sat back down. This drew my awareness to what I was doing. I then began to squeeze her back muscles very slowly. She began to purr and knead my knee. Another very interesting thing occurred. She began to look at me directly in the eye as if to say, "Maybe there is someone in there after all."

What do we do when we are really connecting with someone, say a new romantic interest, comforting a hurt child, teaching a student a new concept, or explaining and performing a painful procedure on a client? We speak slowly in soft tones, look them in the eyes, and move our hands slowly. Slowness brings us to the present moment. Slowness engenders trust. We identify these as quality interactions that are meaningful. When we move fast, it is easier to be someplace else in our thoughts. Have you noticed that five minutes sitting still and holding

A Massage with Heart

1. Before you touch the person, create a healing environment internally and externally.
2. Practice HeartTouch and ask that the greatest healing happen that is in the best interest of all concerned.
3. Invite the receiver to be sure to give you feedback—too hard, too fast, etc.
4. Move slowly into the first touch. Touch him as if he is most fragile and precious.
5. Slow, fluid, gentle movement tells his body you are paying attention, and it can relax into safety and trust.
6. Move from strokes that are gentle and general, to firm and specific, and back to gentle and more general, from the beginning to the end of the massage. Old patterns of physical and emotional tension will more likely release if they are gently coaxed. The body gradually softens, allowing you to reach deeper and deeper layers of holding on, with the minimum amount of discomfort.
7. To reach deeply into the body, strength is not always necessary. Focus your body weight and your attention through your hands, or thumb if you are doing a deep stroke. Imagine your thumb or hand moving through the skin and down into the body to the area of tightness, with a warm, penetrating touch. See the tight areas melt under your touch.
8. With each stroke, intentionally send love from your heart through your hands and into his body. See that love permeating and surrounding him.
9. If you notice your thoughts straying, recenter. Replace the thoughts with ones that contribute to the well-being of the receiver and yourself.
10. If you are present in the moment, your fingers will become very sensitive, being able to detect even the slightest area of tension in the body. You will begin to hear, feel, and/or see from the body what it needs to release the tension. You will learn to modify your speed, pressure, and technique to give his body exactly what it is asking for.
11. If you notice that his body flinches, his breath becomes shallow and uneven, or you feel the muscles tense under your fingers, you know that the pressure needs to be less, and the speed slower. There are times we have felt the lightest pressure relax the tightest muscle.
12. *Remember to move slowly*, when doing your strokes, when recovering from your strokes, when walking around the person, when arranging the covers, when applying lotion, when breathing, and when talking. His body will entrain to yours.
13. Notice the rhythm of your strokes. If it is similar to a grandfather clock, tick-tock, or a cat kneading, it lulls his body and mind into relaxation and letting go.
14. Throughout the massage, reconnect with Higher Power and ask that Presence to fill you both.
15. At the end of the massage, stay for a moment, touching the feet, offering a blessing.

468   CHAPTER 13

the hand of a friend brings you closer than two hours of fast-paced interaction? The slower we go, the more we pay attention to what we're doing, and the person we are with. It is only when the attention is fully in the moment that we can go inside the heart. When we are able to be awake in the midst of the distractions of daily life, we are always with God.

Check your TF before the massage begins, and regularly during the massage. Recall that whenever we massage someone, our energy fields are interacting. The TF we have create energy patterns in our field. These patterns can create the same patterns of vibration in the field of whoever you are near, for bad or good. Thoughts wander amazingly. When you notice your thoughts straying to undesired ones, change them. As we learn to become aware of our TF we can create a mental landscape that is fun and relaxing. Imagine yourself in your favorite place that makes you feel warm, relaxed, and loved. Repeat the steps of HRT several times throughout the massage. These feelings cause your hands to touch in ways that feel more healing to the receiver. Being present and having the mental intention that you want to help the person initiates an energy flow that facilitates the healing process. For your own health and mental peace, and that of the receiver, fill your mind with thoughts that bring you joy.

The interest, sympathy, or compassion of the operator is literally felt by the subject. It is impossible to massage effectively while thinking of something else.

—Bertha Harmer and Virginia Henderson
Textbook of the Principles and Practice of Nursing, 1922

When you finish the massage, whether it is one or ten minutes long, sit or stand quietly beside the receiver, resting in the specialness of the moment. You might offer a prayer of thankfulness or a blessing.

WHO ARE WE?

Who is it that comes to give a massage? And who is it that receives one? We began looking at this question at the beginning of Part III, and we will end with it. For to practice HRT, to give a massage with the greatest healing potential, or to fully engage in any type of relationship, we must be asking the question, Who am I?

The Self

Researchers are recognizing the role of the Self in physical and psychological health and well-being. Dolbier, Soderstrom, and Steinhardt (2001) looked at what happens when people allow the Self to lead their life. When the Self is leading and all other aspects of the person function harmoniously, the individual moves through life as one coherent unit. In a group of 270 college students, Self-leadership was significantly related to increased optimism, hardiness, and coping effectiveness, and less interpersonal distrust. Self-leadership was also significantly related to better health status (greater perceived wellness, less perceived stress, and fewer symptoms of illness). In a sample of 160 corporate employees, Self-leadership was significantly related to better communication, increased work satisfaction, effective work relationships, quality management, less work stress, and greater perceived wellness.

The Self, as defined in this book, is the mosaic of all that we are. It is the spirit or soul, the body, the mind, the thoughts, the emotions, and all of our past, present, and future life experiences. The Self is the foundation from which we exist. Through the Self we experience and interact with our environment. The Self is also affected by the food we eat, the sleep we get, and the air we breathe. Our Self is affected by our relationships with family and friends, and the work we do. How often we are in Nature, our prayers, meditations, and our relationship with God, all contribute to the Self. All of these factors combine to create who we are, how we receive and give massage, and how we heal.

We have the capacity for self reflection. To be self reflective, or to look inside, we must step out of the soap opera of our thoughts and be willing to entertain new points from which to view. We must wake up.

There are many ways to connect with, or reflect upon, the inner Self. One is to use HRT to learn to dwell in the heart. Another method used by seekers of understanding is to sit quietly in a room alone while considering your own reflection in a mirror. Continue to gaze at the reflection in the mirror for at least five minutes, or as long as you're comfortable. Practice each day. This can be a very calming and most revealing experience, and it is no small feat. As you will soon see, this reflection is more than the image of the physical body. The mind and these techniques are like a boat to carry us across the lake and through the mist. At some point we must get out of the boat and leave the mind behind. We then experience being, love, and oneness.

Another approach might be to gently close your eyes and behold, first hand, the genuine article. The Self, as the Hindus might say, is immediate, infinite, all-pervasive, and all-knowing. The Self that we behold within, is the same Self that lives in all things. And when we behold it in ourselves, its radiance and splendor opens our hearts, filling us with its infinite compassion for all. Thus we realize first hand our intimate connection to, and oneness with, all that we behold. From a Judeo-Christian context, another way of expressing this might be, "I am

That I am," or "I and the Father are One." The Buddhists seek to become awake. We then see everything as it is, part of a Unified Whole. From the view of the Self, there is no separation. God, human, plant, and sun are all one. When we view things as separate, conflict and challenge begin. However, in order to play and learn in this world, we must, to some extent at least, entertain the illusion of separation.

Our True Nature: Information, Emotion, Connection

In this section we are going to contemplate who we are from several different points of view.

INFORMATION

Candace Pert (1997), neuroscientist and forefront researcher in the field of PNI, discusses who we are as consciousness from the view of information theory. According to information science, the movement and storage of information is intelligence. The peptides (the emotion molecules) flow all over the body, carrying information to all areas, directing the smooth functioning of all body parts. Pert suggests this flow of information is intelligence. She suggests that this flow of information is the mind. The mind may be the flow of information as it moves among the systems of the body, coordinating all functions, creating one whole, interconnected being. The mind has a material aspect which is the body including the brain, and a nonmaterial aspect that is the flow of the information. American Indians believe that consciousness resides throughout the body. Recall that Eastern Indian and Asian systems of psychology, yoga, and Ayurvedic medicine speak of specific energy centers, or chakras, throughout the body. The location of these chakras correspond to areas of high concentrations of peptide receptors along the spine. The chakras and peptide nodes are associated with different states of consciousness, intuition, and emotion.

Since the peptides, or information molecules, are released from and received by many areas throughout the body, the brain is not the center of information processing in the body, but is just another part of the information network. If intelligence doesn't come from the brain, where does it come from? Since information has an infinite capability to expand and increase, it is beyond time and space. It does not belong only to the material world that we record with our senses. Information theory seems to suggest that the mind, the consciousness, which consists of information, exists first, prior to the physical realm. It belongs to its own realm that we experience as emotion, the mind, the spirit—an "info-realm." Some call this the field of intelligence, some call it God (Pert, 1997).

EMOTION

In *Molecules of Emotion,* p. 312, Pert discusses this "big psychosomatic network in the sky," in the following way.

We are part of a psychosomatic network run by intelligence that has no bounds and is shared among all of us in a bigger network. We are all individual nodal points, each an access point into a larger intelligence. This shared connection gives us a profound sense of spirituality, making us feel connected and whole. When we think otherwise, we suffer the stress of separation from our source. What is it that flows between us all? The emotions! They are the connectors, flowing between individuals, moving us as love, sorrow, and compassion. Like information, the emotions travel between the two realms of mind and body, as peptides and their receptors in the physical realm, and as feelings in the nonmaterial realm.

As there are nodes of peptide concentration in the body affected by our feelings, we may be nodes of consciousness affected by the feelings of the larger network, or Intelligence, or the Divine.

Recall that the receptors on the walls of each cell move in wave-like patterns, receiving and transmitting vibrational frequencies. Pert suggests that the vibrations of the receptors on our cell walls can cause the receptors on the cells of another person to vibrate in response to them. This is called "extracorporeal peptide reaching." This is like the resonance we discussed in the energy chapter and in HRT. One source of vibration can synchronize another source to vibrate at the same frequency. This emotional resonance allows us to feel what others feel. Subtle energy is a fifth force in physics, identified to help explain the power of love (Pert, 1997).

Since emotions are energy waves in motion, and we are all connected by a universal energy field, it seems that our feelings may be able to travel through this field via the principle of nonlocality to communicate with, and affect others no matter how far away they are. Recall in the experiments of Grinberg-Zylberbaum, et al. (1994) on distant intentionality, EEG patterns of two people separated by distance began to resemble each other when the two people felt emotional closeness. An important point, however, is that the brains were not automatically connected. They only showed the same pattern when an emotional connection was felt between the two people. Here we see emotions as possible carriers of information between humans in a nonlocal or instantaneous manner. Emotions seem to be able to travel between individuals, connecting our hearts together, whether we are near or far.

CONNECTION

We are not only connected to other people, but apparently to all things in the universe. Information flows through the exchange of electrons in the atoms of cells. All things are made of atoms. If the flowing of information is intelligence, are cars, rocks, water, stars, computers, and refrigerators intelligent? Can information, intelligence, or consciousness connect us with all things in the universe? Recall the experiments by Jahn and Dunne where people could influence machines with their thoughts. This might be an example of emotional resonance. The most successful couples were those who were deeply attached emotionally to each other. Individuals who said that they felt bonded to their machines, feeling a sense of oneness with them, were also most successful. The results suggest that feeling love or connection enhances our ability to affect the random activity of machines.

Also recall that the opiate peptides, the endorphins, have been found in *all living things*, enabling all to experience happiness or bliss. If emotions connect, then we are connected to all who have these peptides, through feelings of happiness and love. Maybe touch is such a universal communicator because it creates emotion. Emotions may be the synchronizers of the vibrational frequencies so that everything can connect. You might say, "Rocks and machines don't have emotions." We've just seen that feelings of connection somehow affect machines. Not long ago people didn't know that emotions affect the immune system. Now we know they do.

Perhaps in the Great Design, everything was given the capacity to communicate with everything else. When we meditate, receive massage, or listen to music that is 60 beats per minute, our brainwaves move into the alpha frequency from 7–13 Hz. This is very close to that of the electromagnetic field (ionosphere) around the Earth at 7.83 Hz. (Goldman, 1992). In a special on ABC's Nightline in August of 2001, they discussed the ionosphere. It is constantly charged by the sun. There are continual electrical dances going on between 40 mile high, red and blue "sprites" and "elves" (names scientists have given these energy phenomenon). Lightning hits the Earth continually, charging it. Scientists don't yet know the significance of all of this electricity. Without the ionosphere activity, the electromagnetic energy of the Earth would drain off in 20 minutes. What would happen to life on Earth? No one yet knows. We are beings of electric, magnetic energy. All chemical reactions in the body happen as a result of electric and magnetic exchanges. We, and all on Earth, may need this energy to survive just as we need food. The ionosphere may be one way we can communicate with others, the Earth, and the Cosmos.

In the spring of 2000, we saw a PBS special on microbes. Microbes live in the dirt, on plants, in all bodies of water, on animals, on our skin, and within our bodies. In the forest, microbes are connected in a web-like structure that we don't see. They are responsible for the health of the forest, shifting nutrients to areas that need it. Scientists created a biosphere with the right amounts of water, light, and plant diversity, but plants and animals began to die. They realized they had not included microbes. Microbes may be responsible for the health of our entire planet, including ourselves, in ways we are only beginning to imagine.

Microbes all have a light detector allowing them to communicate with each other. The same photons of light that they use to communicate are exchanged in our cells in every chemical reaction. These same photons of light flood the Earth from the sun and all other stars. Remember from the physics section, as the elements combine in chemical interactions in the body, photons are given off. As photons move, they spin in harmonic progressions, in tones, like notes in a scale, like the planets in their orbits. Jean Charon, a nuclear physicist and musicologist, says that photons communicate with electrons and each other through the vibrations created by this spinning motion. Since photons move through space as light, he believes that the movement and spinning of photons (light particles) may be the way thoughts are communicated from one person to another (Berendt, 1991).

What if light is a way to connect with the stars? We know that we use only a very small portion of our brains. Now that science has mapped the entire genome, they say there are many "junk" genes. What if these genes and unused parts of the brain are intended to allow us to intentionally tune in to these pathways of connection within the universe and its inhabitants? What if emotions are the keys for opening up communication?

Dr. Hiroshi Motoyama (1981) detected photons emitting from the energy field around the heart area (heart chakra) of an experienced meditator when she intentionally projected loving energy. Physicist, Fred Alan Wolf (1986) suggests that love can affect photons. Photons are involved in all electromagnetic exchanges in humans, water, plants, and rocks. Loving thoughts then, may affect the rain forests, the elephants, and water in the rain and tides. Loving prayers may truly create change in the hearts of our fellow humans on the other side of the globe.

How are we to build a new humanity? Reverence for life. Existence depends more on reverence for life than the law and the prophets. Reverence for life comprises the whole ethic of love in its deepest and highest sense. It is the source of constant renewal for the individual and for mankind.

—Albert Schweitzer, *Reverence for Life*

My friend told me a story of two goldfish. One became ill and was staying very close to the bottom of the bowl. Days passed, and it seemed to be improving. One day my friend noticed the other fish swimming under his friend, pushing him to the top so he could eat. Penguins survive in winters that are 50 degrees below zero because they huddle in large numbers. When the outside members become too cold they are shuttled to the center where they are warmed by their fellows, and others take their place on the outside. When geese fly in a V, each bird creates an uplift for the bird following it. The flock has a 71% greater flying range than if each bird flew alone. When one goose gets sick and must go to the ground, two geese stay behind until it can fly again (Noyes, 1992). If this kind of caring and community exists in such a variety of individuals, as we love our fellows, we can create a global community in which we reach potentials we are only now beginning to imagine.

Photons of light flood the Earth from the sun and stars, photons of light move in all things, and love affects photons. All living beings contain peptides with vibrating receptors influenced by love. If God is Love, 1 John 4:16, and God is Light, 1 John 1:5, perhaps light and love are the pathways through which God reaches us, and we can reach back.

PUTTING THESE IDEAS INTO PRACTICE

1. Each week this month, give at least two people a massage with heart.
2. Set your kitchen timer for 10 minutes and create a place where you will not be disturbed. Take 10 slow, easy breaths and playfully contemplate who you are and why you are here.

SUMMARY: FINAL THOUGHTS

It is only with the heart that one can see rightly. What is essential is invisible to the eye.
—Antoine de Saint-Exupery, *The Little Prince*

Touch is one very powerful way that we convey these feelings that move in the heart. When we massage, we learn the power of this universal language of touch. We have the extreme honor to be trusted to touch the body of another at a time when it is most vulnerable. Massage brings relaxation, stillness, and peace. It helps us take a vacation from the mind, and thoughts of hurry and worry. Often all we need is a little break to help us view life from a new perspective.

Massage can be used to activate the heart. Heart connection defines a relationship. The more we open our hearts to another, the deeper the connection we feel. The giving and receiving of massage rekindles the spark of the love that has the power to heal us all.

Giving massage can also be an aid along the path of spiritual awakening. It contains many traditional practices used to increase awareness of Spirit. Focusing on the breath, the repetition of the strokes, and slow movement bring you to the moment. Observing thoughts and feelings passing through the mind, you realize that you can choose to focus on them or not, respond to them or not. Massage is an opportunity to experience connection, with Self, another, and the Divine. Focusing on the heart energy opens the door to the inner realms that always exist. God dwells in these inner realms. We begin to suspect that the outer world of things is a projection of the inner world, as the movie on a screen is the projection of the camera and film. Massage is a vehicle to release us from emotional, mental, and physical tension so that we can begin to explore what this reality truly is.

Massage is a gift. There is no way you can really know the magic of massage unless you give it to someone. And you can't fully appreciate its value unless you receive one. Massage teaches us that healing is a circle. When nothing else works, massage helps words come a little easier and hearts find a way to reach each other. You and those you massage will be changed in the giving and receiving.

Before a massage, faces are often pale, with frowns and furrowed brows. The mind is moving fast with details and deadlines. Muscles are constricted, and the spirit is often stuffed into a neat little cage. When the massage is finished, cheeks are rosy, eyes are soft, and the face is smiling. The body loosens and moves with more ease, and the mind is on vacation with words coming very slowly. The spirit is flying free.

Massage magically transforms us into the person we are in our hearts. In those moments, it is clear that the world would be a much better place if everyone received a massage.

Our time on this planet may be but a blink of an eye in our entire existence. Recall that energy and matter are continually changing from one to the other, from the subatomic level, to the activity of eating food and getting energy from it. All is connected by a universal field of energy with particles of matter arising from the field and disappearing back into it. This field may be a field of consciousness with individual patterns of consciousness arising and returning. We are these individual patterns of consciousness, arising and returning.

As we focus more and more on the outer world, we become enmeshed in thought, feeling, and things, forgetting who we really are. We view the world through the mind, whose job it is to separate, compare, and analyze. We mistakenly believe we are separate. We have the opportunity, through the heart, to move beyond the limits of the body and the teachings of separateness. We can travel to a different time and place, the kingdom within. The more we look from the heart, the more we see connection and love. The view from the mind and heart are both necessary perspectives to live in this world. The mind brings thoughts to conscious awareness so that we can choose what we think. We can also use the thoughts of the mind to take us to the heart. The more we are awake, the more we can easily shift from one view to the other whenever we desire.

Instead of a body with consciousness, we are consciousness that has created a body. To play, to interact with others in this world, we have created slightly denser aspects of ourselves, our energy fields; and slightly denser still, our physical bodies. We, as consciousness, permeate and move between all aspects of who we are, influencing and coordinating. As consciousness, we can use the emotions to influence the symphony of the inner workings of our own body and that of others. We can also use the energy of the emotions to influence the receptors on the cell walls, and photons in atoms, of others at a distance, sharing feeling, and the adventure.

Who are we? Information, emotion, light, and connection. Magnificent, multi-faceted beings of energy. We are each unique, and at the same time, One. Beyond that, it is a question you can contemplate in the comfort of your own heart. You might continue this inquiry by pondering the question, "Where are you between two thoughts?" Raja Rao, a Buddhist philosophy professor, asked me that question 28 years ago, at the beginning of my journey. I had no idea what he was talking about. That question led me to this point in the adventure, and will lead me on.

Why are we here? We are here to wake up and be conscious. We are here to learn, to serve, to love, and to have fun. Massage with heart helps us do them all.

What will the world be like as more and more of us focus our conscious attention in the present moment? What if we choose to love even those we don't know well? What will happen when we truly experience that we are—at the same time—individual, and one with others? And what will the world be like when we walk each step with the Divine, knowing that we are one with God? The Bible says, "Ask, and it shall be given you, seek, and ye shall find, knock, and it shall be opened unto you." Luke 11:9.

Life is an adventure. Touch is the highway, Massage, our vehicle. Love is the fuel, and Spirit, our destination. What happens between thoughts is like what happens between friends. This is where we find the Heart of the Matter.

Well, friend, here we are, at the end of this part of our journey together. We have so enjoyed our time with you. Perhaps one day we will meet face to face. We hope what you have found here enriches your life and that of your clients, friends, and family.

A BLESSING

Being in the presence of someone who has just received a massage and has been transported from a state of stress to one of relaxation and openness often evokes in us a wonderful, warm, and often humbling feeling. There is almost always a short moment when we can entertain a word or two in thankfulness for this person and for this moment when something good and worthwhile has been deeply embraced.

And so, here in the final quiet moments of our time together, may we entertain a word in this presence for you.

We are here, warm beings, filled with the light of life,
And we give our thanks for this moment.
May what we have been blessed to do here today
Soak into the fabric of our lives
And into the fabric of life itself.
May it remind us that we are the love in our hearts,
Nothing more, and nothing less.
We give our thanks for this beautiful, wonderful day.
And we are thankful for the heart and the compassion
That is in our hands.
May we each touch others as we hope to be touched,
By love.

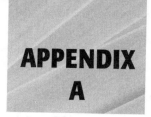

Resources and Suggestions for Additional Learning

Marsha and Jonathan Walker are available to teach workshops on:
- Healing Massage for Nurses and Families
- Reflexology for Health and Well-being
- Therapeutic Touch and Energy-based Therapies
- The Effects of Thoughts and Feelings on Stress and Health
- Heart Touch: Love, Spirituality, and Healing
- Creating Your Quality World: Using Stress as an Ally

Contact us at:
P.O. Box 3151
Austin, TX 78764-3151
walkerj@io.com

RESOURCES PRESENTED IN CHAPTER 2

1. Touch Research Institute. Further information about TRI's numerous research studies is available on their web site: http://www.corpmassage.com/html/touch_research_institute.html
2. Hospital-Based Massage Network in Fort Collins, Colorado at (970) 407–9232, or www.HBMN.com.
3. National Association of Nurse Massage Therapists, call 1-800-262-4017, visit http://members.aol.com/nanmt1 or email simpson@nebi.com.
4. Research College of Nursing in Kansas City, Missouri, Karin Roberts, robertsrcn@aol.com

Massage Courses Especially for Nurses

Contact the Mackey Health Institute in West Palm Beach, Florida (561-832-1900, bonnie@mackeyhealth.com, www.mackeyhealth.com) for more information on their courses.

As of 1997, Southampton Hospital in Long Island, New York, offered a lymphadema massage program, and the Royal College of Nursing in London and the New Center College for Wholistic Education and Research in Syosset, New York, offered general massage programs (Mower, 1997).

The American Holistic Nurses Association (AHNA) endorses a program on AMMA which is a combination of therapeutic massage and oriental health practices. Amma is taught at the New York College School of Wholistic Nursing, and occasional workshops are given in other states. A nurse can become a Certified Nurse Amma Therapist and is also eligible to be certified in oriental bodywork. AHNA also has a list of courses they have approved for CE credits on their web page which includes some on massage. Call at 1-800-278-AHNA, or http://www.ahna.org or contact the American Holistic Nurses Certification Corporation (AHNCC) in Austin, Texas, toll free at 1–877-284–0998, or e-mail at AHNCC@flash.net.

BSN Programs Based on Holistic Nursing Theory and Practice

As of June, 2001, according to the AHNCC, the following BSN programs have a curriculum based on holistic nursing theory and practice:

- College of St Catherine, St Paul, MN (651-690-6000)
- Mankato State University, Mankato MN (507-389-6022)
- Quinnipiac College, Hamden, CT
- New Jersey City University (201-200-3157)
- Georgia College and State University (706-864-1930)
- University of Akron, OH (330-972-6698)
- Mercy College, Des Moines, IA (515-643-6622)
- University of Florida, Gainesville, FL (352-846-1624)
- University of Indianapolis (317-788-3336)

The following BSN programs are endorsed by AHNCC, therefore graduates are able to sit immediately for the Holistic Nursing Certification Exam once they have received their license. They do not have to complete the year of Holistic Nursing practice, 48 contact hours, or qualitative portion of the examination process usually required to become a Certified Holistic Nurse.

- Humboldt State University, Eureka, California; Dr. Wendy Woodward
- Metro State University, St Paul, MN; Dr. Marilyn Loen (612-772-7711)
- Xavier University, Cincinnatti, Ohio; Dr. Susan Schmidt; (513-745-3814)
- Western Michigan University, Kalamazoo, Michigan; Dr. Marie Gates (616-387-2638)
- University of Colorado at Colorado Springs; Dr. Lea Gaydos (719-262-4418)

RESOURCES PRESENTED IN CHAPTER 11

Here is the contact information mentioned in the chapter.

1. Nurse Healers–Professional Associates International, Inc.
   3760 South Highland Dr., Suite #429
   Salt Lake City, Utah 84106
   801-273-3399

2. Colorado Center for Healing Touch
   12477 W. Cedar Drive, Suite 206
   Lakewood, CO 80228
   303-989-0581

3. Herbert Benson, M.D.
   The Mind/Body Medical Institute
   110 Francis Street, Suite 1A
   Boston, MA 02215
   617-632-9530

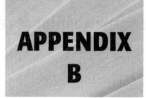

APPENDIX B

Expanded View of Physics and Energy

The following is the expanded version of physics mentioned in Chapter 11, including who we are as energy beings, and how we continually interact through our energy fields as supported by the principles of physics. We highly recommend Fritjof Capra's book (1983), *The Tao of Physics,* if you want more depth than what is offered here on how physics explores the nature of our world as energy. This book helped us realize that the world is not as it appears, in a way that we could understand.

REMEMBERING WHAT AN ATOM IS

For those of us who haven't thought about chemistry and physics for a long time, if ever, let's go back to the beginning for a moment. Everything in this universe, that we know of, is made of molecules. Molecules are made of atoms connected together. For example, our bodies are mostly water. A molecule of water is made of two hydrogen atoms and one oxygen atom, H_2O. Atoms are made of sub-atomic particles. Subatomic particles are protons (+ positive charge), neutrons, electrons (- negative charge) and photons. Every atom has a center, or nucleus, made of neutrons and protons. Electrons spin around the nucleus in predictable orbits. Photons are the subatomic particles of light. Every atom has either a positive or negative charge. These charges attract the atoms to each other to form molecules, like two magnets attract each other.

THE DISCOVERY OF ENERGY FIELDS AND ATOMS

First, the energy field. By the late 1800s, Michael Faraday and Clark Maxwell brought modern science to a turning point by discovering that when you move a magnet near a coil of copper wire, an electric current is produced—the birth of the electromagnetic (energy) field. Recall that atoms are positively or negatively charged. Each charge, positive or negative, creates a disturbance in the space around it (a field). If any other charge is nearby, it feels a force exerted on it by the field of the first charge. A field, then, can produce a force which can be felt by another charge (Capra, 1983). Each of us is made of positive and negative charges all moving, producing a field. This energy field extends throughout and away from the body. Our cells and organs perform their daily functions by the exchange of atoms with positive and negative charges. These charges produce electromagnetic fields. Field interaction within the body is a vital part of healthy functioning. When we are close to each other, each person's field exerts a force that affects the other person's field.

A law in physics called the Law of Resonance helps to explain how one moving, vibrating field of energy can affect another. This law can be applied to understand how energetic healing techniques have an effect on the bodymind and spirit. The Law of Resonance tells us that anything that moves produces vibrations, or waves of energy. All vibrations produce repeated patterns, or rhythms. These patterns look like waves that move up and down in different rhythms, or speeds (frequencies). We see these waves when we throw a pebble into a pond. Resonance means that when two objects have similar wave frequencies, and are close together, they entrain to each other. Entrainment means that their waves synchronize and have the same pattern. They have the same frequency (how many times the wave rises and falls in a certain period of time), and both together are more powerful than either alone. When a very strong rhythm is near a weaker rhythm, it can change the weaker one to the stronger wave pattern.

When clocks with pendulums are in the same room, they all tend to adjust themselves to the same rhythm. Resonance also explains how the thoughts and feelings (being waves of energy) of one person can affect the thoughts and feelings of others. Have you noticed that being around someone who is depressed can bring you down? Have you noticed that if someone is very excited, and you cannot appreciate that feeling, you become irritated? You are not "in synch." You are on "different wavelengths."

On the other hand, have you noticed that being around playful, energetic children awakens that spark of carefree abandon in us? Have you noticed that when you are listening to an inspired speaker, you become inspired? Do you remember having a conversation with someone and you are discussing exciting things that you both understand, you both begin to feel thrilled? New, creative insights occur that neither would have thought of before. We say we are "in harmony."

By 1900, it was thought that the theories of how the world worked had been discovered, and the mysteries of the universe were solved. Much to everyone's surprise, Max Planck discovered that light did not move as a continual wave, but came pulsing along in energy packets, which he called quanta. Today these quanta of light are called photons (Maudlin, 1986).

In 1905, Albert Einstein, 26 years old, had just graduated as a physicist, and was working as a patent clerk. He emerged from out of nowhere and published three papers which shook the foundation of physics, and changed the perception of our world. His first paper described how light (energy waves) had the ability to knock electrons (matter) out of metal. How was this possible? How could something not "physical" move something that was physical? There had to be a material entity to do this "knocking"; therefore, he demonstrated that light must have a dual nature. It sometimes behaves as a particle (matter), and sometimes like a wave (energy). The concrete mind may be saying "What?!" If you would, allow your mind to entertain the possibility that two opposite ideas can both be true, at the same time. Have you ever felt like you hate someone you know that you love? Because we are "matter," this suggests the possibility that we also may have a dual nature—energy and matter—both equally true at the same time.

Einstein's second paper theorized the existence of atoms. Jean Perrin carried out these experiments and demonstrated conclusively for the first time, that they did exist. In 1911, Rutherford discovered that atoms consisted of vast regions of space in which electrons (- charge) moved around a nucleus (+ charge), bound to it by electric forces. To visualize these relationships, picture an orange. If this orange was enlarged to the size of the Earth, its atoms would be enlarged to the size of cherries. To see the nucleus of the cherry-sized atoms, we expand the atom to the size of St. Peter's Cathedral in Rome. The nucleus of this atom is a grain of salt on the floor. The electrons whirling around it would be like specks of dust as far away as the ceiling of the cathedral (Capra, 1983). There is alot of space in that atom because an atom is only a nucleus with electrons whirling around. We, and all things, are made of atoms. We are all mostly space with tiny energy particles whirling around at great speeds, constantly interacting. So why do we appear to be solid?

Einstein's third paper introduced his theory of special relativity. From the theory of special relativity comes the equation you often see, $E=mc^2$. This means that energy (E) is the same as mass (matter) (m) when the mass approaches the speed of light (c) (Einstein, 1961; Lanczos, 1965). He showed that space (height, width, and length) and time are not separate entities. Both are intimately connected and form a fourth dimension, space-time. Time brings in the element of movement. To get a better idea of dimensions, in two dimensions (length and width), two discs may appear to be separate; but in three dimensions (adding height), they are parts of a circular "doughnut." In three dimensions, individuals appear to be separate. When you add the fourth dimension of time or movement, we now do not see separate individuals, but a continuous interacting field, whether looking at subatomic particles or two teams playing a game of hockey.

Space-time means that matter is always moving. Even within a table, the electrons are moving around the nucleus of every atom. A stone is full of activity. All material objects are made of atoms and subatomic particles which continually spin and vibrate. Einstein's unification of space and time suggests that matter only has the appearance of being solid. Subatomic particles have a space aspect and a time aspect. Their space aspect makes them appear as objects with a certain mass, their time aspect as constantly moving patterns of energy. These dynamic patterns of energy form the atoms of cells of matter (Capra, 1983). Being made of subatomic particles, we also have a space aspect which makes us appear as solid objects and a time aspect making us a dynamic pattern of energy, constantly changing and transforming.

The solid appearance of matter is due to the fact that a subatomic particle reacts to confinement by moving. The smaller the space of confinement, the faster it moves. The faster it moves, the more solid it appears. The velocity of electrons in an atom is 600 miles/second. The subatomic particles in the nucleus (proton and neutron) being squeezed into an extremely small space, can reach velocities of 40,000 miles/second. When a fan is turned off, we see the individual blades. We can stick a hand between the blades. When the fan is moving, the blades look like a solid disc and will repel an object thrust into the fan. In the same way, subatomic particles spin in all objects, including the human body, causing them to appear solid, and repel objects. Since all is made of subatomic particles, perhaps reality is not as concrete as it appears.

THE WORLD OF THE SUBATOMIC PARTICLE

The laws of atomic physics were formulated in the 1920s by a group of physicists working together, including Werner Heisenberg, Niels Bohr, and Erwin Schrodinger. In their exploration of the atom, these men uncovered the strange and unexpected world of subatomic particles, the building blocks of atoms. Their behaviors affect the manner in which all atoms interact. Quantum physics is the study of the behavior of, and relationships between, subatomic particles. Recall these are electrons, protons, neutrons, and photons. At first glance, the activities of subatomic particles appear to be very different from the activities of objects that we see every day. However, when we compare the characteristics of subatomic particles and people, we are strangely similar. We can't forget that all matter, including the human, is made of nothing but subatomic particles and space. Can a thing truly be so different from that of which it is made?

Continual, Dynamic Equilibrium and Transformation

Subatomic particles are continually moving, interacting, and transforming, yet there is a definite order to this change and movement that creates an appearance of stability and equilibrium. Most electrons spin like a top as they move around the nucleus, like the Earth turns on its axis as it orbits the sun (Capra, 1983). The electrons spinning around the nucleus create patterns. Atoms with a certain number of electrons and certain types of nuclei have definite patterns of energy. These stable patterns allow us to recognize them, like an atom of oxygen, or the face of a person, for example.

Because energy continuously changes to mass and mass to energy at very high speeds ($E=mc^2$), subatomic particles undergo constant transformation. We cannot think of anything being always matter or always energy. They are continuously changing back and forth, moment after moment. Subatomic particles, then, are also patterns of energy, or energy packets. Because of this, when subatomic particles interact, they exchange particles which also manifest as a ceaseless flow of energy.

When they interact, these patterns of energy rearrange themselves, sometimes forming new particles. Since energy is continually redistributed when new patterns are formed, energy is never destroyed. Since matter and energy are equal, matter is never completely destroyed. Plants use the energy from the sun to grow new cells. We eat the plants and create energy to run, think, and sing. The energy from our hands affects the vibrating receptors on cell walls (PNI). This affects all of the cells, as they create new chemicals (matter). It is somewhat like the journey of life. We are energy, then we become matter, then we transform once again into energy.

Breathing, digestion, and all processes in the body occur by chemical reactions. Chemical reactions occur when molecules of one substance interact with another. Each molecule is made of atoms with electrons circling the nucleus. This movement creates a field around the nucleus. Atoms connect to each other when the fields merge and electrons are exchanged. Photons of light are released and absorbed with this electron movement. Clouds of photons, or light, are created around each spinning electron. With all chemical reactions of the body, we give off and absorb energy in the form of light. Photons, being particles of light, can travel long distances. In this way, we are beings of light, and we send light into the world. We are also affected by light and color.

This constant movement of the subatomic particles also produces vibration, which produces sound. The continual transformation of each of us produces light and sound. Because we are constantly vibrating, we affect and are affected by, other vibrating bodies. Perhaps this is one way in which color, music, feeling, energy from the hands as in energy-based therapies, and other forms of vibration affect all chemical processes in the body. We continue to see that at the level of our subatomic particles to our peptides and emotions, continual movement, balance and transformation is our nature, and what creates health.

The Observer Affects the Observed

Physicists Niels Bohr and Werner Heisenberg developed the most accepted interpretation of quantum theory (describes subatomic particles) at this time, the Copenhagen interpretation. This divides the observed and the observer, and suggests that observation creates reality. A principle law of quantum theory is Heisenberg's uncertainty principle (Heisenberg, 1958; Capra, 1983), which shows how the observer changes the subatomic particle by what characteristic of that particle she chooses to measure. Recall that energy moves in a wave pattern. Depending upon the perspective of the observer, or what she chooses to measure, the subatomic particle may either appear to be energy or matter. For example, since a subatomic particle is an energy packet constantly moving somewhere within its wave pattern, if we want to measure the exact position of the subatomic particle, we must confine the wave to a smaller region. The subatomic particle reacts to this confinement by increasing its speed, so by measuring its position, its movement is altered. We have changed the subatomic particle by what we chose to focus on. If we measure the natural movement of the subatomic particle, its position cannot be determined precisely because it is constantly moving somewhere within its wave pattern. If we want to watch a baseball game, we cannot make the batter slow down so we can study his swing. If we did we would change the game.

Some people, such as the mathematician John von Neumann and physicist John Wheeler, propose that the dynamic (moving, interacting) attributes of the world are not objectively real, but depend on the mind of the observer. If the perspective, or method of measurement changes, the characteristics of the subatomic particle, and so what we view as reality, changes (Wheeler, 1973). The choices we make, in each moment, turn us in a direction. We choose a reality out of many possible alternatives. There is no one, objective reality that is the same for everyone. It is created and altered each moment by the one who is doing the choosing in that moment. We discussed this in light of PNI, and now we see it again from the view of physics. No doubt, what we choose, and expect to happen, creates the details of the world we experience each day, in many ways. We make decisions that create our futures based on what we believe reality to be today.

Here enters the theory of at least two, and possibly many, simultaneous realities. Physicists, Hugh Everett, Bryce DeWitt, and John Wheeler proposed the many worlds interpretation. The idea that a particle may be at many possible points (because it is constantly moving), until it is observed at one is extended to many different possible worlds (or universes). When an observation is made, a single world is chosen (Maudlin, 1986). Today we live in a world that is permeated by waves—radio, television, microwave, and cell phones. We choose a wave by turning a dial, or pushing a button. We tune into the wave we want. What if there are many possible realities at once and we tune into the one we want with our intention? We may be living in a kind of infinite dimensional space with every possibility occurring at once. Most of us only experience one possibility at a time, however. By consciously, or unconsciously, choosing a particular point of view, or action, we pick a reality or fork in the path.

There is No Separation, There is Only Connection

In 1943, Werner Heisenberg proposed the S-matrix theory to describe subatomic particles and their interactions. S-matrix theory shifts the emphasis from objects (particles) to events (interactions). Recall that $E=mc^2$ says that matter moving at very high speeds is equal to energy. Subatomic particles are always moving at very high speeds. When particles interact, they exchange particles. If particles and energy are the same at high speeds, then an interaction is energy exchanging energy. In other words, instead of two particles interacting, what we really have is an interaction, or energy interacting. These interactions build up a network of constantly interacting energy. Also, because energy equals matter at high speeds, if two particles are interacting and enough energy is added to an interaction, new particles are created (because energy=matter). Could it be possible that energy based healing modalities could interact with the energy of the body in ways yet to be discovered that affects the creation of new particles within the body? We know that if two people put enough energy into a problem, new solutions emerge.

The "bootstrap" hypothesis of Geoffrey Chew evolved out of the S-matrix principle. All things are made to exactly fit together as a whole, and all things follow this inherent pattern. There is nothing imposed from without. Each particle helps to generate other particles, which in turn generate it. The basic structure of the physical world is determined ultimately by the way each of us looks at it. Change and transformation are the primary aspects of nature, rather than the structures generated by these changes (Chew, 1968). There is no beginning and no end to the world.

Niels Bohr (1961) states that isolated material particles are abstractions, their properties being definable and observable only through their interaction with other systems. Particles are not isolated, but are interconnected patterns in a cosmic web. The nature of these patterns is to continually change and interact. Not only do the characters in the subatomic particle world appear to be inseparable, but those in the everyday world are as well. In the words of Fred Hoyle (1955),

> Present day developments in cosmology are coming to suggest rather insistently that everyday conditions could not persist but for the distant parts of the Universe, that all our ideas of space and geometry would become entirely invalid if the distant parts of the Universe were taken away. Our everyday experience even down to the smallest details seems to be so closely integrated to the grand scale features of the Universe that it is well-nigh impossible to contemplate the two being separated.

In 1964, John Bell proposed the interconnectedness theory which suggested that all things in the universe are connected in ways yet to be fully understood. This theory suggested that all individuals share a type of connected consciousness. His theory had to do with local and non-local connections between subatomic particles (Herbert, 1985). Local connections are the kinds of connections that we are familiar with between events that are separated in space. Local connections involve some kind of signal, such as a sound. The signals cannot travel faster than the speed of light. Bell proposed that non-local connections existed between subatomic particles that were instantaneous, traveling faster than light, did not seem to use any known signals, and could not be predicted.

Recall that electrons are subatomic particles that spin around the nucleus of all atoms. Electrons spin about their axis like a top spins, in either a clockwise or counter clockwise direction. Two electrons spinning together side by side can be made to spin so that their combined spin is 0, meaning one is spinning clockwise and the other counterclockwise. Bell's theory, illustrating non-local connections, proposed this experiment. Two electrons that have established a 0 spin are made to travel in opposite directions to be measured at two distant detectors. Depending on the method of measurement chosen at one detector, the electron will be made to spin clockwise or counterclockwise. One electron arrives at its detector, and is made to spin clockwise. At the instant that direction is chosen, determining the spin, the faraway electron instantaneously spins the opposite direction so that their total measured spin is still 0. How did the faraway electron "know" which way to spin?

Erwin Schrodinger proposed phase entanglement (Herbert, 1985). It was thought to be fictitious in reality until Bell's theory. Phase entanglement suggested that when the wave patterns of two subatomic particles interact, they permanently carry an aspect of the other with them. When one acts in a certain way, the other "knows" it immediately and is affected, even at great distances. If this is what is occurring in Bell's theorem, all systems that have once interacted in the past, are linked (Herbert, 1985).

In 1982, Alain Aspect conducted actual experiments measuring two photons, proving that, in fact, Bell's theorem is correct (Aspect, Dalibard, and Roger, 1982). According to Bell, the world is full of non-local influences, not only in the subatomic world, but that they underlie the events of everyday life. Research suggests that when two people have established a connection, their brains (EEG) exhibit this nonlocal phenomenon (Grinberg-Zylberbaum, et al., 1994).

So, it appears that there is no separation, on a subatomic level and in the world of daily events and interactions.

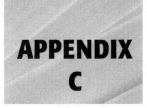

APPENDIX
C

Parting Thoughts

A MEDITATION: MOVING INTO THE HEART

This meditation is how I (Marsha) began to better know God. While practicing the Relaxation Response one day I was very relaxed and felt like I was floating. For some reason I said "God?" and I heard "Yes." From there, it has been an adventure.

When I learned the Freeze Frame (FF) technique, I added that to my meditation. Then, one afternoon in a meeting, we were led in a guided meditation where we were instructed to go to a safe place. The combination of the Relaxation Response, FF, and going to a safe place, moves me through the door of the heart. There I feel what love is like, love that is free of all judgment and conditions. You can try the meditation the way I describe it, or you can go to your own safe place. If this interests you, you may find, waiting in your own heart, the open arms of God, and the love you've always dreamed of.

In each of my meditations I have different experiences. In all of them I feel the close presence of the infinite, all loving, ever-present, God. I share this meditation with you because practicing it regularly at home makes it easier to recall the feeling while I'm giving a massage, driving down the street, or in an uncomfortable interaction with a person. I can bring the love I feel in my meditation to the client I am massaging, or to myself when I am in need.

1. Focus on the Present

   a. Create a space where you will not be disturbed, lay down, and close your eyes.

   b. Put all your irritations and worries into a helium balloon and tie it to a chair outside the room you are in. You may need to tie it outside the house.

2. Come to the Heart

   a. Focus on the top of your head and see a small light there.

    b. Watch the light as it travels slowly down your face, neck, and comes to rest in the area in and around the heart.

    c. Notice your inhale and exhale. Allow the speed and depth to be your own natural rhythm.

    d. With each inhale, watch the light grow, making an ever-larger sphere in the heart area.

3. Notice the Breath

    a. Begin to count your breaths, focusing on nothing but the next number.

    b. If your thoughts wander, return your focus to the breath, and to counting.

4. Feel Love

After 5–20 consecutive breaths, remember someone you really love, someone who really loves you, or a place you love. Let yourself be with that person or in that place. See, hear, smell, touch the interaction. Do that with two or three different scenarios, if you can.

5. Travel to a Safe Place

    a. See before you an elevator. (Mine is emerald green with gold etchings.) The door opens and you step inside. Watch as the numbers increase, counting the levels from 1 to 11 (or whatever number you like).

    b. Ding! The door opens. You walk out into a place where you feel completely safe. (I am standing on a platform in the middle of space.) The elevator disappears. What do you notice? What do you feel?

6. Expand and Explore

    a. Move into the space. (I jump into the air. I do not fall, but am supported as if on a cloud.)

    b. Experience it fully. (My body begins to evaporate, beginning with the feet and hands, and finally my entire body is gone. I am conscious energy.)

7. Connect with Love and Spirit

    a. Just be and notice. Do not consciously make anything happen. Allow yourself to be moved by the experience. (Sometimes I call for God, and hear "Yes?" Sometimes God is there waiting. Sometimes I become a spiral of energy in a unified field.) Ask questions you are pondering, and listen for the answer.

b. "Ask, and it shall be given you. Seek and ye shall find. Knock and it shall be opened unto you."

In several meditations there was a spiraling funnel of energy connecting my heart to the heart of God. It is a pathway upon which we move through the layers of vibrational frequency from the 3-D everyday experience, through the feelings, the thoughts, and into the realm of timelessness, infinity, and Spirit. Focusing on the breath and feeling love in the heart creates the necessary vibrational frequency to move through the veil between the physical and spiritual realm.

The Self can be viewed as a spiral with one end in the physical dimension and one in the spiritual dimension. As we grow and move around the spiral, we get the opportunity to experience the same situations in new ways. The coils are tightly wound when inhabiting and interacting with the physical body. The coils loosen and become more expansive, with larger circles as they interact with other beings. As the Self interacts with the energy fields of a person, the coils are wider still. As we come into oneness with God, or the Uni-verse, the spiraling movements are infinitely large. Although the movement and appearance of the coils differ in all facets of the spiral, the essence or beingness of the spiral is exactly the same when it is in the bone of the body as when it is resting in the arms of God. Massage is a holy act because it can help the aspect of our Self that touches God to awaken and rejuvenate the aspect that is so deeply rooted in the physical world that it forgets. The Self knows what we are here to learn, and guides us, sometimes with signs that we walk into and bonk our heads on, and sometimes, gently, with whispers in our ear.

SPIRITUAL HEALING: A PERSONAL EXPERIENCE

I went in for a routine mammogram. In a few days I received the dreaded call that all did not look well. The doctor wanted a repeat done because there seemed to be an unidentifiable mass in the right breast. My heart started pounding, and my life flashed before my eyes. I found myself thinking about chemotherapy or surgery. Suddenly I noticed what I was thinking, and all that I have learned about healing began to slowly permeate my brain. I began to problem solve. I decided that instead of locking in the "mass" by diagnosing it, I would take a week and do everything I could to heal my breast.

I took herbs. I expressed feelings I had been holding inside. I asked friends to pray for me. I called a friend and asked if she could give me an energy treatment every day for seven days. That night I asked Jonathan if he would also give me energy treatments. I went to my friend's home every afternoon, and we began by connecting with God through prayer. She then spent 15–20 minutes doing energy work, laying on of hands, massage, singing, and toning. At night, Jonathan did laying on of hands and energy-based therapies.

My breast got warmer and had unusual sensations. On the seventh day my friend was working on me, and I asked God to help me. I felt as if His hand reached into the area. Suddenly it seemed like a volcano of heat poured from my breast. My friend said she had felt a rush of hot energy as well. That night Jonathan said he felt no disturbance in the energy field around my breast as he had each night before.

The next day my breast was cool. I went for the repeat mammogram. After the x-ray, the technician returned and said she had to do it again because she had not gotten the right position. She returned again and said the machine must have malfunctioned, and they would have to do it again. I asked why. She said there was nothing where the mass had been. I told her what I had been doing, and that I did not want another x-ray. They did a sonogram, and again found nothing.

Whatever the mass was, I know that the love and prayers of Jonathan and my friends, my intention to do all I could, and the healing presence of God changed the disharmony in my breast to a vibration of health.

References

Abbott, J., and Abbott, P. (1995). Psychological and cardiovascular predictors of anaesthesia induction, operative and post-operative complications in minor gynaecological surgery. *British Journal of Clinical Psychology, 34,* 613–623.

Achterberg, J. (1985). *Imagery in healing.* Boston: Shambhala Publications.

Ader, R., and Cohen, N. (1981). Conditioned immunopharmacologic effects. In R. Ader (Ed.), *Psychoneuroimmunology.* New York: Academic Press.

Adler, J. (1999). How stress attacks you and what works to bust it. *Newsweek,* June 14, 56–63.

Aguilera, D. C. (1967). Relationship between physical contact and verbal interaction between nurses and patients. *Journal of Psychiatric Nursing, 5(1),* 5–21.

Allen, K., Blascovich, J., and Kelsey, R. (1991). Presence of human friends and pet dogs as moderators of autonomic responses to stress in women. *Journal of Personality and Social Psychology, 61,* 582–89.

Anderson, G. (1995). Touch and the kangaroo care method. In T. Field, (Ed.), *Touch in early development.* Mahwah, New Jersey: Lawrence Erlbaum Associates.

Antai-Otong, D. (2001). Creative stress-management techniques for self-renewal. *Dermatology Nursing, 13(1),* 31–32, 35–39.

Archer, T., and Leier, C. (1992). Placebo treatment in congestive heart failure. *Cardiology, 81,* 125–33.

Armstrong, K. (1993). *A history of God: The 4,000-year quest of Judaism, Christianity, and Islam.* New York: Knopf.

Armour, J., and Ardell, J. (Eds.). (1994). *Neurocardiology.* New York: Oxford University Press.

Aspect, A., Dalibard, J., and Roger, G. (1982). Experimental Test of Bell's Inequalities Using Time-Varying Analyzers. *Physics Review Letters, 49,* 1804.

Astin, J., Harkness, E., and Ernst, E. (2000). The efficacy of "distant healing": A systematic review of randomized trials. *Annals of Internal Medicine, 132,* 903–910.

Babbitt, E. (1967). *The principles of light and color.* Secausus, New Jersey: Citadel Press.

Bakker, A. (2000). Effort-reward imbalance and burnout among nurses. *Journal of Advanced Nursing, 31(4),* 884–891.

Barber, T. (1978). Chapter 10. In J. L. Foshage and P. Olsen (Eds.), *Healing implications for psychotherapy.* New York: Human Science Press.

Barefoot, J., and Schroll, M. (1996). Symptoms of depression, acute myocardial infarction, and total mortality in a community sample. *Circulation, 93,* 1976–1980.

Barnard, K., and Brazelton, T. (Eds.). (1990). *Touch: The foundation of experience.* Connecticut: International Universities Press, Inc.

Barrios-Choplin, B., McCraty, R., and Cryer, B. (1997). A new approach to reducing stress and improving physical and emotional well-being at work. *Stress Medicine, 13,* 193–201.

Beck, M. (1994). *Theory and practice of therapeutic massage.* New York: Milady Publishing Company.

Becker, R., and Selden, G. (1985). *The Body Electric: Electromagnetism and the foundation of life.* New York: William Morrow.

Bell, A. (1964). Massage and the physiotherapist. *Physiotherapy, 50,* 406–408.

Benor, D. J. (1992). *Healing research, vol.1.* Deddington, England: Helix Editions Ltd.

Benson, H. (1996). *Timeless healing.* New York: Simon and Schuster.

Benson, H., and Friedman, R. (1996). Harnessing the power of the placebo effect and renaming it 'remembered wellness.' *Annual Review of Medicine, 47,* 193–99.

Bentwich, Z., and Kreitler, S. (1994). *Psychological determinants of recovery from hernia operations.* Paper presented at the Dead Sea Conference, Tiberias, Israel.

Berendt, J. (1991). *The world is sound.* Rochester, Vermont: Destiny Books.

Berkman, L., and Syme, S. (1979). Social networks, host resistance, and mortality: a nine-year follow-up study of Alameda County residents. *American Journal of Epidemiology, 109,* 186–204.

Bliss, J., McSherry, E., and Fassett J. (1995). Chaplain intervention reduces costs in major DRGs: An experimental study. In H. Hefferman, E. McSherry, and R. Fitzgerald, (Eds.), *Proceedings NIH Clinical Center Conference on Spirituality and Health Care Outcomes.* March 21.

Blalock, E., Harbour-McMenamin, D., and Smith, E. (1985). Peptide hormones shaped by the neuroendocrine and immunologic systems. *The Journal of Immunology, 135(2),* 858–861.

Blumenthal, J. (1997). Stress management and exercise training in cardiac patients with myocardial ischemia: Effects on prognosis and evaluation of mechanisms. *Archives of Internal Medicine, 157,* 2213–2223.

Bosma, H., Hemingway, H., Brunner, E., and Stansfeld, S. (1997). Contribution of job control and other risk factors to social variations in coronary heart disease incidence. *The Lancet, 350,* 235–239.

Brennan, B. (1988). *Hands of light*. New York: Bantam Books.

Brigham, D., and Toal, P. (1990). The use of imagery in a multimodal psychoneuroim-munology program for cancer and other chronic diseases, in *Mental imagery*, edited by R. Kunzendorf. New York: Plenum Press.

Bruyere, R. (1994). *Wheels of light*. New York: Simon and Schuster.

Buchanan, G., Gardenswartz, C., and Seligman, M. (1999, December). Physical health following a cognitive-behavioral intervention. *Prevention and Treatment, 2(10)*, [np.]. Retrieved August 14, 2002, http://journals.apa.org/prevention/volume2/pre0020011a.html..

Burr, H. (1972). *The fields of life*. New York: Ballantine Books.

Burroughs, S. (1976). *Healing for the age of enlightenment*. Kailua, Hawaii: Stanley Burroughs.

Byers, D. (1983). *Better health with foot reflexology*. Florida: Ingham Publishing.

Byrd, R. (1988). Positive therapeutic effects of intercessory prayer in a coronary care unit population. *Southern Medical Journal, 81(7)*, 826–29.

Cady, S., and Jones, G. (1997). Massage therapy as a workplace intervention for reduction of stress. *Perceptual & Motor Skills. 84(1)*, 157–58.

Caine, J. (1991). The effects of music on the selected stress behaviors, weight, caloric and formula intake, and length of hospital stay of premature and low birthweight neonates in a newborn intensive care unit. *Journal of Music Therapy, 28(4)*, 180–92.

Calabria, M., and Macrae, J. (1994). *Suggestions for thought by Florence Nightingale*. Philadelphia: University of Pennsylvania Press.

Capra, F. (1983). *The tao of physics*. Boston: New Science Library.

Carpenito, L. (Ed.). (1995). *Nursing diagnosis: application to clinical practice*. 6th edition, Philadephia: Lippincott, pp. 355–358.

Carson, V., and Green, H. (1992). Spiritual well-being: a predictor of hardiness in patients with acquired immunodeficiency syndrome. *Journal of Professional Nursing, 8(4)*, 209–20.

Carson, V. (1989). *Spiritual dimensions of nursing practice*. Philadelphia, PA: WB Saunders.

Carter, S. (1983). Rehumanizing the nursing role: a question of love. *Topics in Clinical Nursing*, 11–17.

Caudill, M., Schnable, R., Zuttermeister, P., Benson, H., and Friedman, R. (1991). Decreased clinic use by chronic pain patients: Response to behavioral medicine intervention. *The Journal of Clinical Pain, 7(4)*, 305–310.

Charkin, D., Eisenberg, D., Sherman, K., Barlow, W., Kaptchuk, T., Street, J., and Deyo, R. (2001). Randomized trial comparing traditional Chinese acupuncture, therapeutic massage, and self care education for chronic low back pain. *Archives of Internal Medicine, 161(8)*, 1081–88.

Childre, D. L. (1996). *Cut-Thru*. Boulder Creek, California: Planetary Publications.

Childre, D. (1994). *Freeze frame*. Boulder Creek, California: Planetary Publications.

Childre, D., and Martin, H. (1999). *The HeartMath solution.* San Francisco: Harper-Collins Publishers.

Chopra, D. (1993). *Ageless Body, timeless mind.* New York: Harmony Books.

Cohen, S., Doyle, W., Skoner, D., Rabin, B., and Gwaltney, J. (1997). Social ties and susceptibility to the common cold. *Journal of the American Medical Association, 277(24),* 1940–44.

Collinge, W. (1996). Massage therapy and bodywork: Healing through touch. *The American Holistic Health Associations complete guide to alternative medicine,* Warner Books.

Cousins, N. (1989). *Head first.* NewYork: E.P. Dutton.

d'Aquili, E., and Newberg, A. (1998). The neuropsychological basis of religions, or why God won't go away. *Zygon-The Journal of Religion and Science, 33(2),* 187–201.

David-Neel, A. (1936). *Tibetan journey.* London: John Lane.

Davis, M., Matthews, K., and McGrath, C. (2000). Hostile attitudes predict elevated vascular resistance during interpersonal stress in men and women. *Psychosomatic Medicine, 62,* 17–25.

Davis, M., Eshelman, E., and McKay, M. (1995). *The relaxation and stress reduction workbook.* Oakland, California: New Harbinger Publications.

Day, M. (1947). *Basic science in nursing arts.* St. Louis: C.V. Mosby Co.

de Groot, K., Boeke, S., van den Berge, H., Duivenvoorden, H., Bonke, B., and Passchier, J. (1997). The influence of psychological variables on postoperative anxiety and physical complaints in patients undergoing lumbar surgery. *Pain, 69,* 19–25.

DeDomenico, G., and Wood, E. (1997). *Beard's massage, 4th edition.* Philadelphia: W.B. Saunders.

Diamond, M. (1990). Evidence for Tactile Stimulation Improving CNS Function. In K. Barnard and T. Brazelton, (Eds.), *Touch: The foundation of experience.* Connecticut: International Universities Press, Inc.

Doczi, G. (1994). *The power of limits.* Boston, Massachusetts: Shambhala Publications.

Dolbier, C., Cocke, R., Leiferman, J., Steinhardt, M., Schapiro, S., Nehete, P., Perlman, J., and Sastry, J. (2001). Differences in functional immune responses of high vs. low hardy healthy individuals. *Journal of Behavioral Medicine, 24(3),* 219–229.

Dolbier, C., Soderstrom, M., and Steinhardt, M. (2001). The relationships between self-leadership and enhanced psychological, health, and work outcomes. *Journal of Psychology, 135(5),* 469–485.

Dossey, B., Keegan, L., and Guzzetta, C. (2000). *Holistic nursing: a handbook for practice.* Gaithersburg, Maryland: Aspen.

Dossey, L. (1993). *Healing words.* San Francisco: HarperCollins Publishers.

Dossey, L. (1997). *Be careful what you pray for . . .* San Francisco: HarperCollins Publishers.

Drinker, C., and Yoffey, J. (1941). *Lymphatics, lymph and lymphoid tissue: their physiological and clinical significance.* Cambridge: Harvard University Press.

Dunn, K., and Horgas, A. (2000). The prevalence of prayer as a spiritual self-care modality in elders. *Journal of Holistic Nursing, 18(4)*, 337–352.

Easter, A. (2000). Construct analysis of four modes of being present. *Journal of Holistic Nursing, 18(4)*, 362–378.

Eisenberg, D., Davis, R., Ettner, S., Appel, S., Wilkey, S., Van Rompay, M., and Kessler, R. (1998). Unconventional medicine in the United States. *New England Journal of Medicine, 328(4)*, 246–252.

Emblen, J., and Pesut, B. (2001). Strengthening transcendent meaning: A model for the spiritual nursing care of patients experiencing suffering. *Journal of Holistic Nursing, 19(1)*, 42–57.

Erickson, H., Tomlin, E., and Swain, M. (1988). *Modeling and role modeling.* Englewood Cliffs, NJ: Prentice-Hall, Inc.

Estabrooks, C. A., and Morse, J.M. (1992). Toward a theory of touch: the touching process and acquiring a touching style. *Journal of Advanced Nursing 17*, 448–456.

Fakouri, C., and Jones, P. (1987). Relaxation Rx: Slow Stroke Back Rub. *Journal of Gerontological Nursing, 13(2)*, 32–35.

Fanslow, C. (1990). Touch and the Elderly. In K. Barnard and T. Brazelton, (Eds.), *Touch: The foundation of experience.* Connecticut: International Universities Press, Inc.

Fawzy, F. I., Fawzy, N., Hyun, C., Elashoff, R., Guthrie, D., Fahey, J., and Morton, D. (1993). Malignant melanoma: Effects of an early structured psychiatric intervention, coping, and affective state on recurrence and survival 6 years later. *Archives of General Psychiatry, 50:* 681–689.

Ferrell-Torry, A., and Glick, O. (1993). The use of therapeutic massage as a nursing intervention to modify anxiety and the perception of cancer pain. *Cancer Nursing, 16(2)*, 93–101.

Field, T. (1998). Massage therapy effects. *American Psychologist, 53(12)*, 1270–1281.

Field, T. (1995). Infant Massage Therapy. In T. Field, (Ed.), *Touch in early development.* Mahwah, New Jersey: Lawrence Erlbaum Associates.

Field, T., Grizzle, N., Scafidi, F., Abrams, S., and Richardson, S. (1996). Massage therapy for infants of depressed mothers. *Infant Behavior and Development, 19*, 109–114.

Field, T., Scafidi, F., and Schanberg, S. (1987). Massage of preterm newborns to improve growth and development. *Pediatric Nursing, 13*, 385–387.

Field, T., Hernandez-Reif, M., Seligman, S., Krasnegor, J., Sunshine, W., Rivas-Chacon, R., Schanberg, S., and Kuhn, C. (1997). Juvenile rheumatoid arthritis: benefits from massage therapy. *Journal of Pediatric Psychology 22(5)*, 607–17.

Field, T., Hernandez-Reif, M., Shaw, K., LaGreca, A., Schanberg, S., and Kuhn, C. (1997). Glucose, levels decreased after giving massage therapy to children with Diabetes Mellitus. *Diabetes Spectrum, 10*, 23–25.

Field, T., Hernandez-Reif, M., Quintino, O., Wheeden, C., Schanberg, S., and Kuhn, C. (1997). Elder retired volunteers benefit from giving massage therapy to infants. *Journal of Applied Gerontology, 17*, 229–239.

Field, T., Ironson, G., Scafidi, F., Nawrocki, T., Goncalves, A., Burman, I., Pickens, J., Fox, N., Schanberg, S., and Kuhn, C. (1996). Massage therapy reduces anxiety and enhances EEG pattern of alertness and math computations. *International Journal of Neuroscience. 86(3–4)*, 197–205.

Field, T., Lasko, D., Mundy, P., Henteleff, T., Talpins, S., and Dowling, M. (1997). Autistic children's attentiveness and responsivity improved after touch therapy. *Journal of Autism and Development Disorders, 27,* 329–334.

Field, T., Morrow, C., Valdeon, C., Larson, S., Kuhn, C., and Schanberg, S. (1992). Massage reduced anxiety in child and adolescent psychiatric patients. *Journal of the American Academy of Child and Adolescent Psychiatry, 31(1),* 125–31.

Field, T., Quintino, O., and Hernandez-Reif, M. (1998). Adolescents with attention deficit hyperactivity disorder benefit from massage therapy. *Adolescence, 33,* 103–108.

Field, T., Scafidi, F., and Schanberg, S. (1987). Massage of preterm newborns to improve growth and development. *Pediatric Nursing, 13,* 385–387.

Field, T., Schanberg, S., Kuhn, C., Fierro, K., Henteleff, T., Mueller, C., Yando, R., Shaw, S., and Burman, I. (1998). Builimic adolescents benefit from massage therapy. *Adolescence, 33(131),* 555–63.

Field, T., Schanberg, S., Scafidi, F., Bauer, C., Vega-Lahr, N., Gracia, R., Nystrom, J., and Kuhn. (1986). Tactile/kinesthetic stimulation effects on preterm neonates. *Pediatrics, 77,* 654–658.

Field, T., Sunshine, W., Hernandez-Reif, M., Quintino, O., Schanberg, S., Kuhn, C., and Burman, I. (1997). Chronic fatigue syndrome: Massage therapy effects on depression and somatic symptoms in chronic fatigue. *Journal of Chronic Fatigue Syndrome, 3,* 43–51.

Fitzgerald, L., and van Hooft, S. (2001). A Socratic dialogue on the question 'what is love in nursing?' *Nursing Ethics, 7(6),* 481–490.

Forrest, S. (1999). Creativity on the edge of chaos. *Seminars for Nurse Managers, 7(3),* 136–40.

Fraser, J., and Kerr, J. (1993). Psychophysiological effect of back massage on elderly institutionalized patients. *Journal of Advanced Nursing, 18,* 283–245.

Frasure-Smith, N., Lesperance, F., and Talajic, M. (1993). Depression following myocardial infarction: impact on 6 month survival. *Journal of American Medical Association, 270*(15): 1819–1861.

Fredriksson, L. (1999). Modes of relating in a caring conversation: A research synthesis on presence, touch and listening. *Journal of Advanced Nursing, 30(5),* 1167–1176.

Friedman, E., and Thomas, S. (1995). Pet ownership, social support, and one-year survival after acute myocardial infarction in the Cardiac Arrhythmia Suppression Trial. *American Journal of Cardiology, 76(17),* 1213–1217.

Friedman, R., Sobel, D., Myer, P., Caudill, M., and Benson, H. (1995). Behavioral medicine, clinical health psychology, and cost offset. *Health Psychology, 14,* 509–518.

Fritz, S. (1995). *Fundamentals of therapeutic massage.* St. Louis: Mosby-Year Books, Inc.

Fromm, E. (1956). *The Art of Loving.* New York: Harper and Brothers Publishers.

Furman, C. (1996). *Effectiveness of music therapy procedures: Documentation of research and clinical practice* (2nd ed.). Silver Spring, Maryland: National Association for Music Therapy.

Gahery, Y., and Vigier, D. (1974). Inhibitory effects in the cuneate nucleus produced by vago-aortic afferent fibers. *Brain Research, 75,* 241–46.

Gerard, R. (1985). *Differential effects of colored lights on psychophysiological functions.* Unpublished doctoral dissertation, University of California, Los Angeles.

Gerber, R. (1988). *Vibrational medicine.* Santa Fe, NM: Bear and Co.

Ghadiali, D. (1933). *Spectro-Chrome metry encyclopedia.* Malaga, New Jersey: Spectro-Chrome Institute.

Gherman, E. (1981). *Stress and the bottomline.* New York: American Management Associations.

Giedt, J. (1997). Guided imagery: A psychoneuroimmunological intervention in holistic nursing practice. *Journal of Holistic Nursing, 15(2),* 112–127.

Giese, L. (2000). Complementary health care practices. *Gastroenterology Nursing, 23(4),* 192–193.

Glasser, W. (1994). *Control theory manager.* New York: HarperCollins Publishers, Inc.

Gleick, J. (1987). *Chaos: Making a new science.* New York: Viking Penguin, Inc.

Godkin, J. (2001). Healing presence. *Journal of Holistic Nursing, 19(1),* 5–22.

Goldberg, B. (1998). Connection: an exploration of spirituality in nursing care. *Journal of Advanced Nursing, 27(4),* 836–42.

Goldberg Group. (1993). *Alternative medicine.* Washington: Future Medicine Publishing.

Goldman, J. (1992). Sonic Entrainment. In R. Spintge and R. Groh, (Eds.), *MusicMedicine* (pp. 194–209). St. Louis, MO: MMB Music, Inc.

Goleman, D., and Gurin, J. (Eds.). *Mind body medicine.* New York: Consumer Reports Book.

Goodman, M. (1996). Hostility predicts restenosis after percutaneous transluminal coronary angioplasty. *Mayo Clinic Proceedings, 71,* 729–734.

Gottfried, A. (1990). Touch as an organizer of development and learning. In K. Barnard and T. Brazelton, (Eds.), *Touch: The foundation of experience.* Connecticut: International Universities Press, Inc.

Grealish, L., Lomasney, A., and Whiteman, B. (2000). Foot massage: A nursing intervention to modify the distressing symptoms of pain and nausea in patients hospitalized with cancer. *Cancer Nursing, 23(3),* 237.

Green, E.. and Green, A. (1977). *Beyond biofeedback.* New York: Delacorte Press.

Grinberg-Zylberbaum, J., Delaflor, M., Attie, L., and Goswami, A. (1994). The Einstein-Podolsky-Rosen Paradox in the Brain: The Transferred Potential. *Physics Essays 7, 4,* 422–28.

Groer, M., Mozingo, J., Droppleman, P., Davis, M., Jolly, M., Boynton, M., Davis, K., and Kay, S. (1994). Measures of salivary secretory immunoglobulin A and state anxiety after a nursing back rub. *Applied Nursing Research, 7(1),* 2–6.

Grossarth-Maticek, R., Eysenck, H., Vetter, H. (1988). Personality type, smoking habit, and their interaction as predictors of cancer and coronary heart disease. *Personality and Individual Differences, 9(2),* 479–495.

Grossbart, T. (1993). The skin: matters of the flesh. In D. Goleman and J. Gurin, (Eds.), *MindBody medicine.* New York: Consumer Reports Books.

Gullette, E., Blumenthal, J., Babyak, M., Jiang, W., Waugh, R., Frid, D., O'Connor, C., Morris, J., and Krantz, D. (1997). Effects of mental stress on myocardial ischemia during daily life. *Journal of the American Medical Association, 277,* 1521–1526.

Gump, B., and Matthews, K. (2000). Are vacations good for your health? The 9-year mortality experience after the multiple risk factor intervention trial. *Psychosomatic Medicine, 62,* 608–612.

Hall, B. (1997). Spirituality in terminal illness. *Journal of Holistic Nursing, 15(1),* 82–96.

Hall, B. (1994). Ways of maintaining hope in HIV disease. *Research in Nursing and Health, 17,* 283–293.

Hall, H., Minnes, L., and Olness, K. (1993). The psychophysiology of voluntary immunomodulation. *International Journal of Neuroscience, 69:* 221–234.

Hammett, F. (1922). Studies of the thyroid apparatus: V. *Endocrinology, 6,* 221–229.

Harlow, H. F. (1958). The nature of love. *The American Psychologist, 13,* 673–685.

Harmer, B. (1924). *Text-book of the principles and practice of nursing.* New York: Macmillan Co.

Harmer and Henderson. (1939). *The principles and practice of nursing.* New York: Macmillan Co.

Harris, W., Gowda, M., Kolb, J., Strychacz, C., Vacek, J., Jones, P., Forker, A., O'Keefe, J., and McCallister, B. (1999). A randomized, controlled trial of the effects of remote, intercessory prayer on outcomes in patients admitted to the coronary care unit. *Archives of Internal Medicine, 159,* 2273–2278.

Herbert, T., and Cohen, S. (1993). Stress and immunity in humans: A meta-analytic review. *Psychosomatic Medicine, 55(4),* 364–379.

Hernandez-Reif, M., Field, T., Hart, S., Theakston, H., Schanberg, S., Kuhn, C., Burman, I. (1999). Pregnant women benefit from massage therapy. *Journal of Psychosomatic Obstetrics and Gynecology,* 20(1), 31–38.

Hernandez-Reif, M., Field, T., Krasnegor, J., Theakton, H., and Burman, I. (2001). Chronic lower back pain is reduced and range of motion improved with massage therapy. *International Journal of Neuroscience, 106(3–4)*, 131–45.

Herron, R., Hillis, S., and Mandarino, J. (1996). The impact of the Transcendental Meditation program on government payments to physicians in Quebec. *American Journal of Health Promotion, 10,* 208–216.

His Holiness the Dalai Lama. (1995). *The Dalai Lama's book of wisdom.* London: HarperCollins Publishers.

Hobza, P., and Zahradnik, R. (1988). *Intermolecular complexes.* New York: Elsevier-Science Publishing Co., Inc.

Hollinger, L. M., and Buschmann, M. B. (1993). Factors influencing the perception of touch by elderly nursing home residents and their health caregivers. *International Journal of Nursing Studies, 30 (15):*445–461.

Hotz, R. (1997, October 29). Response to religion may lie in brain makeup, study says. *The Austin American Statesman*, A1, A11.

House, J., Landis, K., and Umberson, D. (1988). Social relationships and health. *Science, 241,* 540–545.

Hover-Kramer, D., Mentgen, J., and Scandrett-Hibdon. (1996). *Healing touch.* New York: Delmar Learning.

Hoyle, F. (1955). *Frontiers of astronomy.* New York: Harper.

Hunt, V. (1995). *Infinite mind, the science of human vibrations.* Malibu, CA: Malibu Publishing Company.

Iribarren, C., Sidney, S., Bild, D., Liu, K., Markovitz, J., Roseman J., and Matthews K. (2000). Assocation of hostility with coronary artery calcification in young adults: The CARDI study. *Journal of the American Medical Association, 283,* 2546–2551.

Ironson, G., Field, T., Scafidi, F., Kumar, M., Patarca, R., Price, A., Gonclaves, A., Hashimoto, M., Kumar, A., Burman, I., Tetenman, C., and Fletcher, M. (1996). Massage therapy is associated with enhancement of the immune system's cytotoxic capacity. *International Journal of Neuroscience, 84,* 205–218.

Jahn, R., and Dunne, B. (1987). *Margins of reality.* San Diego: Harcourt Brace and Co.

Janssen, P., de Jonge, J., and Bakker, A. (1999). Specific determinants of intrinsic work motivation, burnout and turnover intentions: A study among nurses. *Journal of Advanced Nursing, 29(6),* 1360–1369.

Jensen, P. (1998). Touching lives in Romania. *Professional Bodyworkers Journal,* Spring.

Jivanjee, P. (1994). Enhancing the well-being of family caregivers of patients with Alzheimer's disease. *Journal of Gerontological Social Work, 23(1/2),* 31–48.

Jones, S. (1994). *The right touch.* Cresskill, New Jersey: Hampton Press, Inc.

Joseph, R. (1999). The neurology of traumatic "dissociative" amnesia: commentary and literature review. *Child Abuse Neglect, 23(8),* 715–27.

Justice, B. (1988). *Who gets sick?* Los Angeles: Jeremy P. Tarcher, Inc.

Kaard, B., and Tostinbo, O. (1989). Increase of plasma beta endorphins in a connective tissue massage. *General Pharmacology, 20(4),* 487–89.

Kabat-Zinn, J. (1993). Mindfulness meditation: Health benefits of an ancient Buddhist practice. In D. Goleman and J. Gurin (Eds.). *Mindbody medicine.* New York: Consumer Reports Books.

Kabat-Zinn, J., Wheeler, E., Light, T., Skillings, A., Scharf, M., Cropley, T., Hosmer, D., and Bernhard, J. (1998). Influence of a mindfulness meditation-based stress reduction intervention on rate of skin clearing in patients with moderate to severe psoriasis undergoing phototherapy (UVA) and photochemotherapy (PUVA). *Psychosomatic Medicine, 60(5),* 625–632.

Karagulla, S., and Kunz, D. (1989). *The chakras and the human energy fields.* Wheaton, IL: Theosophical Publishing House.

Karasek, R. (1979). Job demands, job decision latitude, and mental strain: implications for job redesign. *Administrative Science Quarterly, 24,* 285–308.

Kaufman, M. (1964). Autonomic responses as related to nursing comfort measures. *Nursing Research, 13,* 45–55.

Kaye, J., Morton, J., Bowcutt, M., and Maupin, D. (2000). Stress, depression, and psychoneuroimmunology. *Journal of Neuroscience Nursing, 32(2),* 93–100.

Keegan, L. (1995). Touch: connecting with the healing power. In B. Dossey, L. Keegan, C. Guzzetta, and L. Kolkmeier, *Holistic nursing: A handbook for practice.* Gaithersburg, Maryland: Aspen Publishers.

Kelley, I. (1936). *Text-Book of nursing technique.* Philadelphia: W.B. Saunders Co.

Kennedy, P., and Grey, N. (1997). Stress: I can't take anymore. *Nursing Times, 93(29),* 26–32.

Keyes, L. (1973). *Toning, the creative power of the voice.* Marina del Rey, CA: De Vorss and Co.

Kiecolt-Glaser, J., and Glaser, R. (1997). Marital conflict in older adults: endocrinological and immunological correlates. *Psychosomatic Medicine, 59(4),* 339–49.

Kiecolt-Glaser, J., Dura, J., Speicher, C., Trask, O., and Glaser, R. (1991). Spousal caregivers of dementia victims: Longitudinal changes in immunity and health. *Psychosomatic Medicine, 53,* 345–362.

Kiecolt-Glaser, J., and Glaser, R. (1995). Psychoneuroimmunology and health consequences: Data and shared mechanisms. *Psychosomatic Medicine, 57(3),* 269–274.

Kiecolt-Glaser, J., Glaser, R., Williger, D., Stout, J., Messick, G., Sheppard, S., Ricker, D., Romisher, S., Briner, W., Bonnell, G., Donnerberg, R. (1985). Psychosocial enhancement of immunocompetence in a geriatric population. *Health Psychology, 4,* 25–41.

Kiecolt-Glaser, J., Malarkey, W., Chee, M., Newton, T., Cacioppo, J., Mao, H., and Glaser, R. (1993). Negative behavior during marital conflict is associated with immunological down-regulation. *Psychosomatic Medicine, 55(5),* 395–409.

Kiecolt-Glaser, J., Marucha, P., Malarkey, W., Mercado, A., and Glaser, R. (1995). Slowing of wound healing by psychological stress. *Lancet, 346(8984),* 1194–96.

Kiecolt-Glaser, J., Page, G., Marucha, P., MacCallum, R., and Glaser, R. (1998). Psychological influences on surgical recovery: Perspectives from psychoneuroimmunology. *American Psychologist, 53(11),* 1209–1218.

Kime, Z. (1980). *Sunlight.* Penryn, California: World Health Publications.

King, M., Pettigrew, A., and Reed, F. (2000). Complementary, alternative, integrative; have nurses kept pace with their clients? *Dermatology Nursing,12(1),* 41–44, 47–50.

Klein, A. (1989). *The healing power of humor.* Los Angeles: Jeremy P. Tarcher.

Knaster, M. (1998). Tiffany Field provides proof positive, scientifically. *Massage Therapy Journal, 37(1).*

Koenig, H. (1998). *The effects of religion on health: What science has to say.* Paper presented at the Spirituality and Healing in Medicine Conference, Houston, TX.

Koenig, H., and Larson, D. (1997). Use of hospital services, church attendance, and religious affiliation. Presented at Spirituality and Healing in Medicine Conference, Houston, 1998.

Koenig, H., Cohen, H., George, L., Hays, J., and Blazer, D. (1997). Attendance at religious services, interleukin-6, and other biological indicators of immune function in older adults. *International Journal of Psychiatry in Medicine, 27(3),* 233–50.

Krakov, S. (1942). Color vision and autonomic nervous system. *Journal of the Optical Society of America, June.*

Krebs, K. (2001). The spiritual aspect of caring—An integral part of health and healing. *Nursing Administration, 25(3),* 55–60.

Krieger, D. (1979). *The therapeutic touch.* New York: Prentice Hall.

Kunz, D. (1991). *The personal aura.* Wheaton, IL: Quest Books.

Lacey, J., and Lacey, B. (1970). Some autonomic–central nervous system interrelationships. In P. Black (Ed.), *Physiological correlates of emotion.* New York: Academic Press.

Landsbergis, P. (1988). Occupational stress among healthcare workers. *Journal of Organizational Behavior, 9,* 217–239.

Larson, D. (1998). *Spirituality and medical outcomes.* Paper presented at the Spirituality and Healing in Medicine Conference, Houston, TX.

Laskow, L. (1992). *Healing with love.* San Francisco: HarperCollins Publishers.

Lazarus, R., and Folkman, S. (1984). *Stress, appraisal, and coping.* New York: Springer.

LeShan, L. (1974). *The medium, the mystic, and the physicist.* New York: The Penguin Group.

LeShan, L. (1994). *Cancer as a turning point.* New York: Plume Books.

Levin, J., Larson, D., and Puchalski, C. (1997). Religion and spirituality in medicine: research and education. *Journal of the American Medical Association, 278(9),* 792–93.

Lewis, P. (1996). A review of prayer within the role of the holistic nurse. *Journal of Holisitic Nursing, 14(4),* 308–316.

Libster, M. (2001). *Demonstrating care.* New York: Delmar Thomson Learning.

Lieberman, J. (1991). *Light, medicine of the future.* Santa Fe, NM: Bear and Company.

Lingerman, H. (1983). *The healing energies of music.* Wheaton, Illinois: Theosophical Publishing House.

Lynch, J. (1998). *The broken heart: The medical consequences of loneliness.* Baltimore: Bancroft Press.

Madrid, M., and Winstead-Fry, P. (2001). Nursing research on the health patterning modalities of Therapeutic Touch and imagery. *Nursing Science Quarterly, 14(3),* 187–194.

Malarkey, W., Kiecolt-Glaser, J., Pearl, D., and Glaser, R. (1994). Hostile behavior during marital conflict alters pituitary and adrenal hormones. *Psychosomatic Medicine, 56(1),* 41–51.

Markowitsch, H. (1999). Functional neuroimaging correlates of functional amnesia. *Memory, 7(5–6),* 561–83.

Marmot, M., Bosma, H., Hemingway, H., Brunner E., and Stansfeld, S. (1997). Contribution of job control and other risk factors to social variations in coronary heart disease incidence. *The Lancet, 350,* 235–239.

Maslach, C., and Leiter, M. (1997). *The truth about burnout.* San Fransisco: Jossey-Bass Publishers.

Mason, J. (1999). Massage; the nursing touch. *American Journal of Nursing, 99(4),* 44.

Mast, D., Meyers, J., and Urbanski, A. (1987). Relaxation techniques: a self-learning module for nurses, Unit I and II. *Cancer Nursing, 10(3, 4),* 141–147, 217, 223.

Matthews, D., and Larson, D. (1995). *The faith factor: An annotated bibliography of clinical research on spiritual subjects: Vol. III.* Rockville, MD: National Institute for Health Care Research.

Matthews, D., and Saunders, D. (1997). *The faith factor: An annotated bibliography of clinical research on spiritual subjects: Vol. IV.* Rockville, MD: National Institute for Health Care Research.

Maudlin, J. (1986). *Particles in nature.* Blue Ridge Summit, PA: TAB Books, Inc.

McCorkle, R. (1974). Effects of touch on seriously ill patients. *Nursing Research, 23(2),* 125–132.

McCormack, G. L. (1990). Neurophysiology of sensorimotor approaches to treatment. In L. Pedretti, (Ed.), *Occupational therapy practice skill for physical dysfunction.* St. Louis, Missouri: C.V. Mosby, Co.

McCraty, R., Atkinson, M., Tiller, W., Rein, G., and Watkins, A. (1995). The effects of emotions on short-term power spectrum analysis of heart rate variability. *American Journal of Cardiology, 76:* 1089–1093.

McCraty, R., Atkinson, M., and Tomasino, D. (1998). The electricity of touch: detection and measurement of cardiac energy exchange between people. In K. Pribam, (Ed.),

Brain and values: Is a biological science of values possible? (pp. 359–379). Mahwah, NJ: Lawrence Erlbaum Associates.

McCraty, R., Atkinson, M., Tiller, W. A., Rein, G., and Watkins, A. D. (1995). The effects of emotions on short term power spectrum analysis of heart rate variability. *American Journal of Cardiology, 76 (14),*1089–1093.

McDonald, S. (1982). Effect of visible light waves on arthritis pain: A controlled study. *International Journal of Biosocial Research, 3(2),* 49–54.

McEwen, B. (1990). Hormones and the nervous system. *Advances, 7:1*: 50–54.

Mead, M. (1935). *Sex and temperament in three primitive societies.* New York: William Morrow.

Meaney, M., Aitken, D., Bhatnagar, M., Bodnoff, S., Mitchell, J., and Sarrieau, A. (1990). Neonatal handling and the development of the adrenocortical response to stress. In N. Gunzenhauser, T. Brazelton, and T. Field (Eds.), *Advances in touch.* Skillman, New Jersey: Johnson and Johnson.

Medalie, J., and Goldbourt, U. (1976). Angina pectoris among 10,000 men. II. Psychosocial and other risk factors as evidenced by a multivariate analysis of a five year incidence study. *American Journal of Medicine, 60(6),* 910–21.

Medalie, J., Stange, K., Zyzanski, S., and Goldbourt, U. (1992). The importance of biopsychosocial factors in the development of duodenal ulcer in a cohort of middle-aged men. *American Journal of Epidemiology, 136(10),* 1280–87.

Meek, S. (1993). Effects of slow stroke back massage on relaxation in hospice clients. *Image: Journal of Nursing Scholarship, 25(1),* 17–21.

Melland, H., and Clayburgh, T. (2000). Complementary therapies: introduction into a nursing curriculum. *Nurse Educator, 25(5),* 247–250.

Meltzoff, A. (1995). Understanding the intentions of others: re-enactment of intended acts by 18-month-old children. *Developmental Psychology, 31(5),* 838–850.

Melzak, R., and Wall, P. (1965). Pain mechanisms: A new theory. *Science, 150,* 971–978.

Merriam-Webster's Collegiate Dictionary (9th ed.). (1987). Springfield, MA: Merriam-Webster.

Merritt, S. (1990). *Mind, music, and imagery.* New York: Plume Publications.

Mitzel-Wilkinson, A. (2000). Massage therapy as a nursing practice. *Holistic Nursing Practice, 14(2),* 48–56.

Montagu, A. (1986). *Touching: The human significance of the skin.* New York: Harper and Row.

Montgomery, C. (1991). The care-giving relationship: Paradoxical and transcendent aspects. *Journal of Transpersonal Psychology, 23(2),* 91–103.

Morse, J., Solberg, S., Neander, W., Bottorff, J., and Johnson, J. (1996). Concepts of caring and caring as a concept. In J. Kenney (Ed.), *Philosophical and theoretical perspectives.* Boston: Jones and Bartlett Publishers.

Motoyama, H. (1981). A biophysical elucidation of the meridian and Ki-energy. *International Association For Religion and Parapsychology, 7,* 1.

Mower, M. (1997). Massage returns to nursing. *Massage Magazine, September/October,* 47–55.

Muruta, T., Colligan, R., Malinchoc, M., and Offord, K. (2000). Optimists vs. pessimists: Survival rate among medical patients. *Mayo Clinic Proceedings, 75,* 140–43.

Nerem, R., Levesque, M., Cornhill, J. (1980). Social environment as a factor in diet-induced atherosclerosis. *Science, 208(4451):* 1475–76.

Newman, M. (1999). *Health as expanding consciousness.* New York: National League for Nurses Press.

Newman, M., Sime, A., and Corcoran-Perry, S. (1996). The focus of the discipline of nursing. In J. Kenney (Ed.), *Philosophical and theoretical perspectives.* Boston: Jones and Bartlett Publishers.

Nightingale, F. (1957). *Notes on nursing.* Philadelphia: J.B. Lippincott Co.

Nixon, M., Teschendorff, J., Finney, J., and Karnilowicz, W. (1997). Expanding the nursing repertoire: the effect of massage on post-operative pain. *Australian Journal of Advanced Nursing, 14(3),* 21–26.

Noyes, H. (1992). *The Goose Story.* ARCS News, 7(1).

Omdahl, B., and O'Donnell, C. (1999). Emotional contagion, empathic concern and communicative responsiveness as variables affecting nurses' stress and occupational commitment. *Journal of Advanced Nursing, 29(6),* 1351–1359

Ornish, D. (1998). *Love and survival.* New York: HarperCollins.

Ornish, D., Brown, S., Scherwitz, L., Billings, J., Armstrong, W., Ports, T., McLanahan, S., Kirkeeide, R., Brand, R., and Gould, K. (1990). Can lifestyle changes reverse coronary heart disease? *Lancet, 336,* 129–33.

Ott, J. (1988). Color and light: Their effects on plants, animals, and people. *International Journal of Biosocial Research, 10,* part 4, 111–116.

Oxman, T., Freeman, D. Jr., Manheimer, E. (1995). Lack of social participation or religious strength and comfort as risk factors for death after cardiac surgery in the elderly. *Psychosomatic Medicine, 57(1):* 5–15.

Payne, R. (2001). Occupational stressors and coping as determinants of burnout in female hospice nurses. *Journal of Advanced Nursing, 33(3),* 396–405.

Peden, A., Hall, L., Rayens, M., and Beebe, L. (2000). Reducing negative thinking and depressive symptoms in college women. *Journal of Nursing Scholarship, 32(2),* 145–151.

Pelletier, K., and Peper, E. (1976). Alpha EEG feedback as a means for pain control. *Journal of Clinical and Experimental Hypnosis, 25(41),* 361–371.

Pellitier, K., Marie, A., Krasner, M., and Haskell, W. (1997). Current trends in the integration and reimbursement of complementary and alternative medicine by managed care, insurance carriers, and hospital providers. *American Journal of Health Promotion, 12(2),* 112–123.

Pennix, B., van Tilburg, T., and Kriegsman, D. (1997). Effects of social support and personal coping resources on mortality in older age: the longitudinal aging study–Amsterdam. *American Journal of Epidemiology. 146(6)*, 510–519.

Peoc'h, R. (1995). Psychokinetic action of young chicks on the path of an illuminated source. *Journal of Scientific Exploration, 9(2)*, 223–29.

Pepin, J. (1992). Family caring and caring in nursing. *Image: Journal of Nursing Scholarship, 24(2)*, 127–131.

Pert, C. (1986). The wisdom of the receptors: neuropeptides, the emotions, and bodymind. *Advances, 3(3)*, 8–16.

Pert, C. (1987). Neuropeptides: The emotions and bodymind. *Noetic Sciences Review, 2*, 13–18.

Pert, C. (1997). *Molecules of emotion.* New York: Scribner.

Pert, C., Pasternak, G., and Snyder, S. (1973). Opiate agonists and antagonists discriminated by receptor binding in brain. *Science, 182*(4119), 1359–1361.

Pert, C., Ruff, M., Weber, R., and Herkenham, M. (1985). Neuropeptides and their receptors: A psychosomatic network. *The Journal of Immunology, 135*(2), 820–826.

Prescott, J., and Wallace, D. (1976). *Developmental sociobiology and the origins of aggressive behavior.* Paper presented at the Twenty-First International Congress of Psychology, Paris.

Pressman, P., Lyons, J., Larson, D., and Strain, J. (1990). Religious belief, depression, and ambulation status in elderly women with broken hips. *American Journal of Psychiatry, 147*, 758–760.

Prigogine, I., and Stengers, I. (1984). *Order out of chaos: Man's new dialogue with nature.* New York: Bantam Books.

Prudden, B. (1980). *Pain erasure: The Bonnie Prudden way.* New York: M. Evans and Company, Inc.

Quinn, J., and Strelkauskas, A. (1993). Psychoimmunologic effects of Therapeutic Touch on practitioners and recently bereaved recipients: a pilot study. *Advances in Nursing Science, 15(4)*, 13–26.

Rama, S., Ballentine, R., and Hymes A. (1979). *Science of breath.* Honesdale, Pennsylvania: Himalayan Institute.

Reed, P. (1991). Preferences for spiritually-related nursing interventions among terminally ill and nonterminally ill hospitalized adults and well adults. *Applied Nursing Research, 4(3)*, 122–28.

Reed, P. (1992). An emerging paradigm for the investigation of spirituality in nursing. *Research in Nursing and Health, 15(5)*, 349–57.

Reed, F., Pettigrew, A., and King, M. (2000). Alternative and complementary therapies in nursing curricula. *Journal of Nursing Education, 39(3)*, 133–139.

Rees, B. (1995). Effect of relaxation with guided imagery on anxiety, depression, and self-esteem in primiparas. *Journal of Holistic Nursing, 13(3)*, 255–267.

Rein, G. (1995). The in vitro effect of bioenergy on the conformational states of human DNA in aqueous solutions. *Acupuncture Electrotherapy Research, 20(3–4)*, 173–80.

Rein, G., Atkinson, M., and McCraty, R. (1995). The physiological and psychological effects of compassion and anger. *Journal of Advancement in Medicine, 8(2)*: 87–105.

Reite, M. (1990). Touch, attachment and health: Is there a relationship? In K. Barnard and T. Brazelton, (Eds.), *Touch: The foundation of experience.* Connecticut: International Universities Press, Inc.

Roberts, K. (1999). Nursing students elect to pursue wellness. *Nurse Educator, 24(4)*, 10.

Rogers, M. E. (1970). *An introduction to the theoretical basis of nursing.* Philadephia: F. A. Davis.

Rossi, E. (1986). *The psychobiology of mind body healing.* New York: W.W. Norton and Company, Inc.

Rossi, E., and Cheek, D. (1988). *Mind-body therapy.* New York: W.W. Norton and Company.

Routasalo, P. (1999). Physical touch in nursing. *Journal of Advanced Nursing, 30(4)*, 843–850.

Rozman, D., Whitaker, R., Beckman, T., and Jones, D. (1995). A new intervention program which significantly reduces psychological symptomatology in HIV-seropositive individuals. *Psychosomatics, 36(2)*, 207.

Ruff, M., and Pert, C. (1984). Small cell carcinoma of the lung: Macrophage-specific antigens suggest hemopoieticstem cell origin. *Science, 225*, 1034–1036.

Russek, L., and Schwartz, G. (1997). Perceptions of parental caring predict health status in midlife: a 35-year follow-up of the Harvard mastery of stress study. *Psychosomatic Medicine, 59(2)*, 144–49.

Sarter, B. (1997). Philosophical sources of nursing theory. In L. Nicoll (Ed.), *Perspectives on nursing theory.* New York: Lippincott.

Scafidi, F., and Field, T. (1996). Massage therapy improves behavior in neonates born to HIV positive mothers. *Journal of Pediatric Psychology, 21*, 889–898.

Schanberg, S. (1994). Genetic basis for touch effects. In T. Field, (Ed.), *Touch in early development.* Mahwah, New Jersey: Lawrence Erlbaum Associates.

Schaufeli, W., Van Dierendonck, D., and Van Gorp, K. (1996). Burnout and reciprocity: towards a dual-level social exchange model. *Work and Stress, 10*, 225–237.

Schlitz, M. (1998, March). *Possible healing effects of intercessory prayer and distant intentionality.* Paper presented at the Spirituality and Healing in Medicine Conference, Houston, TX.

Schlitz, M., and Braud, W. (1997). Distant intentionality and healing: Assessing the evidence. *Alternative Therapies, 3(6)*, 62–73.

Schlitz, M., and LaBerge, S. (1999). Covert observation increases skin conductance in subjects unaware of when they are observed. *Journal of Parapsychology, 63(2)*, 182–84.

Schlitz, M., and LaBerge, S. (1994). Autonomic detection of remote observation: Two conceptual replications. In D. J. Bierman (Ed.) *Proceedings of Presented Papers, The Parapsychological Association 37th Annual Convention,* The Netherlands, 352–360.

Schneider, E., and Havens, L. (1915). Changes in the blood flow after muscular activity and during training. *American Journal of Physiology, 36,* 259.

Schneider, J., Smith, C., Minning, C., Whitcher, S., and Hermanson, J. (1990). Guided imagery and immune system function in normal subjects: A summary of research findings. In *Mental imagery,* edited by R. Kunzendorf. New York: Plenum Press.

Schrader, K. (1996). Stress and immunity after traumatic injury: The mind-body link. *AACN Clinical Issues, 7(3),* 351–358.

Schroeder, C., and Likkel, J. (1999). Integrative health care: The revolution is upon us. *Public Health Nursing, 16(4),* 233–234.

Scofield, M. (1990). Are we there yet? Anticipating the future of worksite health promotion. *Occupational Medicine, 5(4),* 863–75.

Scull, W. (1945). Massage-physiologic basis. *Archives of Internal Medicine, 26,* 159–167.

Seeman, T., and Syme, S. (1987). Social networks and coronary relations as predictors of disease: A comparison of the structure and function of social relations as predictors of disease. *Psychosomatic Medicine, 49(4),* 341–54.

Seligman, M. (1990). *Learned optimism.* New York: Alfred Knopf.

Sellers, S., and Haag, B. (1998). Spiritual nursing interventions. *Journal of Holistic Nursing, 16(3),* 338–354.

Selye, H. (1974). *Stress without distress.* New York: Signet.

Selye, H. (1976). *Stress in health and disease.* Boston: Butterworths.

Sicher, F., Targ, E., Moore, D., and Smith, H. (1998). A randomized double-blind study of the effect of distant healing in a population with advanced AIDS. *Western Journal of Medicine, 169,* 356–363.

Siegel, B. (1986). *Love, medicine, and miracles.* New York: Harper and Row.

Siegrist, J., Peter, R., Junge, A., Cremer, P., and Seidel, D. (1990). Low status control, high effort at work and ischemic heart disease; prospective evidence from blue-collar men. *Social Science and Medicine, 31,* 1127–1134.

Siegrist, J. (1996). Adverse health effects of high effort-low reward conditions. *Journal of Occupational Health Psychology, 1,* 27–41.

Silverman, A., Pressman, M., and Bartel, H. (1973). Self-esteem and tactile communication. *Journal of Humanistic Psychology, 13,* 73–77.

Simonton, D., Matthews-Simonton, S., and Creighton, J. (1978). *Getting well again.* Los Angeles: Tarcher-St.Martins.

Sims, S. (1986). Slow stroke back massage for cancer patients. *Nursing Times, 82,* 47, 57–50.

Sister Regina Elizabeth. (1966). Sensory stimulation techniques. *American Journal of Nursing, 66,* 281–285.

Snyder, M., Egan, E., and Burns, K. (1995). Efficacy of hand massage in decreasing agitation behaviors associated with care activities in persons with dementia. *Geriatric Nursing, 16(2)*, 60–63.

Sobel, D., and Ornstein, R. (1996). *Healthy mind, healthy body handbook.* Los Altos, California: DRx.

Song, L., Schwartz, G., and Russek, L. (1998). Heart-focused attention and heart-brain synchronization: Energetic and physiological mechanisms. *Alternative Therapies in Health and Medicine, 44(5)*, 44–62.

Spiegel, D., Bloom, J., Kraemer, H., and Gottheil, E. (1989). Effect of psychosocial treatment on survival of patients with metastatic breast cancer. *Lancet, 14(2)*, 888–91.

Spintge, R., and Droh, R. (1992). *MusicMedicine.* St. Louis, MO: MMB Music, Inc.

Steele, J. (1984). Brain research and essential oils. *Aromatherapy Quarterly, 3*, 5.

Stone, A., Neale, J., Cox, D., Napoli, A., Valdimarsdottir, H., and Kennedy-Moore, E. (1994). Daily events are associated with a secretory immune response to an oral antigen in humans. *Health Psychology, 13*, 440–446.

Sunshine, W., Field, T., Schanberg, S., Quintino, O., Kilmer, T., Fierro, K., Burman, I., Hashimoto, M., McBride, C., and Henteleff, T. (1997). Massage therapy and transcutaneous electrical stimulation effects on fibromyalgia. *Journal of Clinical Rheumatology, 2*, 18–22.

Suomi, S. (1995). Touch and the immune system in rhesus monkeys. In T. Field, (Ed.), *Touch in early development.* Mahwah, New Jersey: Lawrence Erlbaum Associates.

Swanson, K. (1996). Empirical development of a middle-range theory of caring. In J. Kenney (Ed.), *Philosophical and theoretical perspectives.* Boston: Jones and Bartlett Publishers.

Tappan, F. (1978). *Healing massage techniques.* Virginia: Reston Publishing Co., Inc.

Temple, K. (1967). The back rub. *American Journal of Nursing, 67*, 2102–2103.

Tiller, W., McCraty, R., and Atkinson, M. (1996). Cardiac coherence: A new non-invasive measure of autonomic system order. *Alternative Therapies, 2(1)*, 52–65.

Tilley, B., Alarcon, G., Heyse, S., Trentham, D., Neuner, R., Kaplan, D., Clegg, D., Leisen, J., Buckley, L., Cooper, S., Duncan, H., Pillemer, S., Tuttleman, M., and Fowler, S. (1995). Minocycline in rheumatoid arthritis: A 48 week, double-blind, placebo-controlled trial. *Annals of Internal Medicine, 122*, 81–89.

Todaro-Franceschi, V. (2001). Energy: A bridging concept for nursing science. *Nursing Science Quarterly, 14(2)*, 132–140.

Tompkins, P., and Bird, C. (1973). *The secret life of plants.* New York: Harper and Row.

Tracy, M. (1938). *Nursing: An art and a science.* St. Louis, MO: C.V. Mosby Co.

Turner, J., Deyo, R., Loesner, J., Von Korff, M., and Fordyce, W. (1994). The importance of placebo effects in pain treatment and research. *Journal of the American Medical Association, 271*, 1609–14.

Tusek, D., Church, J., Strong, S., Grass, J., and Fazio, V. (1997). Guided imagery: A significant advance in the care of patients undergoing elective colorectal surgery. *Diseases of the Colon and Rectum, 40(2)*, 172–78.

Tyler, D., Winslow, E., Clark, A., and White, K. (1990). Effects of a one-minute back rub on mixed oxygen saturation and heart rate in critically ill patients. *Heart-Lung, 19(5)*, 562–555.

Uchino, B., Cacioppo, J., Kiecolt-Glaser, J. (1996). The relationship between social support and physiological processes: A review with emphasis on underlying mechanisms and implications for health. *Psychological Bulletin, 119(3)*, 488–531.

Villaire, M. (1999). In our unit. Healing Touch therapy makes a difference in surgery unit. *Critical Care Nurse, 19(1)*, 104.

Walker, M. (1998). Spirituality in nursing: journey to the heart. Workshop presented at the University of Texas at Austin School of Nursing Continuing Education Holistic Nursing Series. Austin, Texas.

Walker, M. (1996). Presented in workshops of the Holistic Nursing Series at the University of Texas School of Nursing, 1995–1997, Austin, TX.

Walsh, M. (2000). Chaos, cosmology and evolution: The key to understanding practice. *British Journal of Perioperative Nursing, (7)*, 378, 380–82.

Watson, J. (1985). *Nursing: Human science and human care.* Norwalk, CT: Appleton-Century-Crofts.

Watson, J. (1999). *Postmodern nursing and beyond.* New York: Churchill Livingstone.

Watson, J., & Smith, M. (2002). Caring science and the science of unitary human beings: A trans-theoretical discure for nursing knowledge development. *Journal of Advanced Nursing, 37(5)*, 452–461.

Watson, M. J. (1988). New dimensions of human caring theory. *Nursing Science Quarterly, 1(4)*, 175–181.

Weber, S. (1996). The effects of relaxation exercises on anxiety levels in psychiatric inpatients. *Journal of Holistic Nursing, 14(3)*, 196–205.

Weinrich, S., and Weinrich, M. (1990). The effect of massage on pain in cancer patients. *Applied Nursing Research, 3(4)*, 140–145.

Weiss, S. (1990). Parental touching: correlates of a child's body concept and body sentiment. In K. Barnard and T. Brazelton, (Eds.), *Touch: The foundation of experience.* Connecticut: International Universities Press, Inc.

Wells-Federman, C., Stuart, E., Deckro, J., Mandle, C., Baim, M., and Medich, C. (1995). The mind-body connection: The psychophysiology of many traditional nursing interventions. *Clinical Nurse Specialist, 9(1)*, 59–66.

Wetzel, M., Eisenberg, D., Kaptchuk, T. (1998). Courses involving complementary and alternative medicine at US medical schools. *Journal of the American Medical Association, 280(9)*, 784–787.

Wheeden, A., Scafidi, F., Field, T., Ironson, G., Bandstra, E., Valdeon, C., and Schanberg, S. (1993). Massage effects on cocaine-exposed preterm neonates. *Journal of Developmental and Behavorial Pediatrics, 14,* 318–322.

Williams, J., Paton, C., Siegler, I., Eigenbrodt, M., Nieto, F., and Tyroler, H. (2000). Anger proneness predicts coronary heart disease risk. *Circulation, 101,* 2034–2039.

Williams, R. (1993). *Anger Kills.* New York: Random House.

Wilson, D. (1995). Therapeutic touch: foundations and current knowledge. *Alternative Health Practitioner, 1(1),* 55–66.

Wirth, Daniel. (1990). The effect of non-contact therapeutic touch on the healing rate of full thickness dermal wounds. *Subtle Energies,* 1(1), 1–20.

Wiseman, R., and Schlitz, M. (1997). Experimenter effects and the remote detection of staring. *Journal of Parapsychology, 61,* 197–207.

Wiseman, R., Smith, B., Freedman, D., Wasserman, T., and Hurst, C. (1995). Two further experiments concerning the remote detection of an unseen gaze. *Proceedings of the Parapsychological Association 38th Annual Convention.* Parapsychological Association, 480–490.

Witt, A. (1997). Can science prove God exists: Contact. *Tropic, August 17,* 6–12. The Herald.

Wolf, F. A. (1986). *The body quantum.* New York: Macmillan.

Wolf, Z. (1986). The caring concept and nurse identified caring behaviors. *Topics in Clinical Nursing, 8(2),* 84–93.

Woloshin, S., Schwartz, L., Tosteson, A., Chang, C., Wright, B., Plohman, J., and Fisher, E. (1997). Perceived adequacy of tangible social support and health outcomes in patients with coronary artery disease. *Journal of General Internal Medicine, 12(10),* 613–618.

Wood, E., and Becker, P. (1981). *Beard's Massage.* Philadelphia: W.B. Saunders Company.

Yates, J. (1990). *Physician's guide to therapeutic massage.* British Columbia, Canada: Massage Therapists' Association of British Columbia.

Zeller, J., and McCain, N. (1996). Psychoneuroimmunology: An emerging framework for nursing research. *Journal of Advanced Nursing, 23(4),* 657–664.

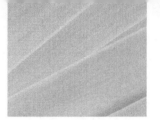

Index

In the index, an "f" following a page number indicates a figure.